I0060963

Epidemiology I

Theory, Research and Practice

Epidemiology I – Theory, Research and Practice

Publisher: iConcept Press Ltd.
Cover design: Pineapple Design Ltd.
Interior design: iConcept Press Ltd.
Typesetting and copy editing: iConcept Press Ltd. and Pineapple Design Ltd.

ISBN: 978-1-922227-82-9

This work is subjected to copyright. All rights are reserved, whether the whole or part of the materials is concerned, specifically the rights of translation, reprinting, re-use of illustrations, recitation, broadcasting, reproduction on microfilms or in other ways, and storage in data banks. Duplication of this publication or parts thereof is only permitted under the provisions of the authors, editors and/or iConcept Press Ltd.

Printed in the United States of America

Copyright © iConcept Press 2014

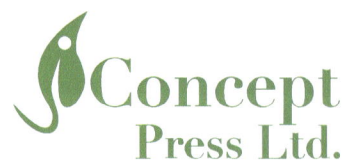

ɸConcept
Press Ltd.

www.iconceptpress.com

Contents

Preface

Epidemiology is the study (or the science of the study) of the patterns, causes, and effects of health and disease conditions in defined populations. Epidemiology has developed into a vibrant scientific discipline that brings together the social and biological sciences, incorporating everything from statistics to the philosophy of science in its aim to study and track the distribution and determinants of health events. *Epidemiology I – Theory, Research and Practice* presents the latest epidemiologic principles, concepts and research outcomes as well as the practical uses of epidemiology in public health and in clinical practice.

There are totally 14 chapters in this book. Chapter 1 proposes to assess whether caries restorative treatment can result in the selection and/or emergence of cariogenic mutans streptococci (MS) genetic strains in children with severe early childhood caries, and also characterizes the xylitol-resistance properties of select dominant and minor MS strains. Chapter 2 describes and explores a new research model of dental practce-based research network by reviewing the current dietary evidence collected from clinical epidemiology research, describing the Dental PBRN, and presenting the results from research conducted using the Dental PBRN model. Chapter 3 discusses the biological effects of solar radiation, describes the risk factors, incidence and mortality rates for skin cancer and melanoma. In addition, it also describes the necessity of sun protection knowledge especially in children and teens and gives information for the most famous sun education programs all over the world. Chapter 4 discusses basal cell carcinoma which comprises the vast majority of skin cancers. It predominantly affects fair-skinned individuals, and its incidence is rising rapidly. Etiology may be multifactorial, but sun exposure appears to play a critical role. When detected early, the prognosis is excellent. Thus appropriate diagnosis, treatment, and surveillance are of utmost importance.

Chapter 5 highlights possible detrimental effects associated with persistent exposure to antimicrobial agent-containing consumer products, particularly medicated soaps. It also provides practical and laboratory-based evidences demonstrating the some negative impacts of medicated soaps usage with special emphasis on toxicity and development of antimicrobial cross-resistance with clinically used antibiotics because of some shared target binding sites in microorganisms. Chapter 6 discusses the course of melanoma in patients post-organ transplant and in the settings of iatrogenic and lymphoproliferative disease-associated immunosuppression. It concludes with a discussion of potential new targets and therapeutic modalities for the treatment of malignant melanoma. Chapter 7 summarizes a comprehensive methodology to evaluate new technology in Radiation Oncology. With rapidly expanding technology in Medicine, decision makers are forced to make choices as to how to provide care for their population. This Chapter also introduces with examples an analytical method to aid in the decision making process. Chapter 8 discusses the neuroprotective effects of endogenous carbon monoxide (CO) and use of exogenous CO as a neuroprotective and neurotherapeutic agent. It is worth noting that exogenous administration of inhaled carbon monoxide or carbon monoxide releasing molecules impart similar neurophysiological responses as the endogenous gas.

Chapter 9 reviews an extremely rare pathology where miliary brain metastases are associated with poor prognosis. This chapter aims at providing detailed information on this condition and review the recent literature. Chapter 10 gives an up-to-date review and provides a synthesis of our collective knowledge regarding the application of computational epidemiologic modeling and risk analysis in addressing HIV/AIDS in both macro- and micro-settings. The role and importance of computational epidemiologic modeling and a new avenue of research, involving the application of risk assessment are discussed in solving public health problems. Chapter 11 discusses the relationship between HIV and maternal mortality in Africa and suggests some methods for addressing the problem. Chapter 12 analyses cellular gene expression profiles by comparing HBV producing cells to its parental HBV non-producing cells. It shows that considerable numbers of gene expression level was altered by HBV amplification.

Chapter 13 proposes current computer models for the prediction of particle deposition in the respiratory tracts of children and adults. The theoretical approach considers different shapes of inhaled particles and additionally allows the calculation of regional particle deposition fractions (extrathoracic, bronchial, alveolar) under various breathing conditions. Chapter 14 discusses epidemiology in tilapia fish. Most of the chapters in this book focuses on human beings, whereas this chapter focuses on some other species, hoping to let our readers to get borden their vision on epidemiology.

Editing and publishing a book is never an easy task. Each chapter in this book has gone through a peer review, a selection and an editing process so as to guarantee its quality. Without the supports and contributions of the authors and reviewers, this book can never be able to complete. We would like to thank all of the authors in this book and all of the reviewers who participated in the reviewing process: Nihat Akbulut, Harith Jabbar Fahad Al-Mathkhury, Samad Amini-Bavil-Olyaee, Dawit G Ayele, Carlos Bellot-Arcis, M L Casanova, Yue Chen, Eidi Christensen, Celso Cunha, Daiane Cobianchi da Costa, Ziad Daoud, Najla S Dar-Odeh, Isabelle de Zoysa, Michael D. Diamantidis, Sibel Dosler, Chandradhar Dwivedi, Jimmy Thomas Efird, Silvano Gallus, Alan Geater, Raquel Santos Gil-Gouveia, Maximilien C. Goris Gbenou, William B Grant, Jeffrey Greenspoon, Toby M. Hall, Yue Huang, Lidia Moraes Ribeiro Jordao, Richard W Joseph, Pauline Lorena Kale, Saurabh Karmakar, Saori Kashima, Yumiko Kawashita, Pratima Devi Khumanthem, Chiaki Kitamura, Noriaki Koizumi, Charalampos Konstantinidis, Rebecca Korner, K-M Lee, Erika Lencova, Jiabin Li, Wengui Li, Zhen Li, Carlos Anselmo Lima, Nicola Martinelli, Yoshiro Maru, Jaime Matta, Tim A. McAllister, Lesley McGee, John C. Meade, Rani Mol.P, Marcelo Moreno, Claude P. Muller, Fawaz Mzayek, Hiroaki Naka, Rose Nathan, Adebola Onanuga, Helena Parfenova, Viness Pillay, Ali Pouryasin, Michael A. Purdy, SM Rezayat, Eduardo Ricci-Júnior, Jan Rustemeyer, Sheeba Saini, Nathanael Salako, Erika M Santos, G. Singh, LI-XIN SUN, Varsha K Vaidya, Frank van Bel, Michele Viana, Andrea Vierkotter, Xin Wang, XING-HUAN WANG, Solomon Assefa Woreta, Q. Jackie Wu, Kentaro Yasuchika, Eman Zahran and Sten G Zelle. We hope that you, the reader, will find this book interesting and useful. Any advices please feel free and are always welcome to tell us.

iConcept Press Ltd
October 2014

Mutans Streptococci Genetic Strains in Children with Severe Early Childhood Caries: Implications for Caries Incidence and Treatment Outcome

Kenneth C. Gilbert, Alexander Sonesson, Nhu Nguyen
Academic DMD Program, School of Dentistry
Oregon Health & Science University, USA

Uyen Nguyen
Department of Integrative Biosciences, School of Dentistry
Oregon Health & Science University, USA

Alex H. Vo
Graduate Orthodontic Residency Program, School of Dentistry
Oregon Health & Science University, USA

Elizabeth A. Palmer
Department of Pediatric Dentistry, School of Dentistry
Oregon Health & Science University, USA

Tom Maier
Departments of Integrative Biosciences and Pathology and Radiology, School of Dentistry
Oregon Health & Science University, USA

Curtis A. Machida
Departments of Integrative Biosciences and Pediatric Dentistry, School of Dentistry
Oregon Health & Science University, USA

1   Introduction

1.1   Cariogenic Microorganisms and Severe Early Childhood Caries

Dental caries represents one of the most common chronic diseases affecting young children (Banas, 2004), and is a multifactorial disease involving complex interactions of genetic, dietary, environmental, behavioral, and microbial risk factors (Fejerskov, 2004). It is now accepted that dental caries is the result of changes in the plaque biofilm ecology brought about primarily by increased consumption of processed and simple carbohydrates. This leads to frequent and prolonged acidification of the plaque biofilm, resulting in selective pressures that lead to a more cariogenic oral microbiome dominated by acidophilic and aciduric microorganisms. Research over many decades strongly implicates several species of streptococci (especially mutans streptococci), lactobacilli, and actinomyces as among the most cariogenic of the well-characterized oral microbes (Kanasi *et al.*, 2010). However over the last decade, DNA-based technologies have dramatically altered the view of the oral microbiome and expanded our understanding of the microbes associated with dental health and disease (Dewhirst, *et al.*, 2010). This research has expanded the number of microorganisms associated with dental caries to include not only species of mutans streptococci, lactobacilli, and actinomyces, but also other species of non-mutans streptococci, bifidobacteria, and scardovia (Gross *et al.*, 2012, Peterson *et al.*, 2013). This has led to a refinement of the ecologic concept of caries (Marsh, 2003) to one defined by pathogenic communities (Jenkinson, 2011), similar to the current understanding of periodontal disease, another common plaque biofilm-associated pathology (Socransky & Haffajee, 2005).

Still it is widely acknowledged that *S. mutans* and *S. sobrinus* are among the most cariogenic microorganisms that reside in the oral cavity, and represent key bacteria associated with dental caries. There are distinct genotypes of *S. mutans* in saliva and dental plaque (Napimoga *et al.*, 2005; Tabchoury *et al.*, 2008), with some genotypes having preferred or dominant sites of localization in the oral environment (Napimoga *et al.*, 2005; Tabchoury *et al.*, 2008; Svensater *et al.*, 1997). The coexistence and concurrent virulence of multiple mutans streptococci (MS) genotypes in caries-active individuals may serve as important determinants for increased caries incidence, as well as treatment success or failure (Svensater *et al.*, 1997).

The development of dental caries requires consumed food substrates containing fermentable carbohydrates, susceptible tooth structures of the host, and the presence of cariogenic microorganisms (Zafar *et al.*, 2009). Cariogenic microorganisms, including MS and lactobacilli, ferment the consumed carbohydrates and produce organic acids as by-products, which in turn demineralize tooth enamel hydroxyapatite and ultimately results in carious lesions (Zafar *et al.*, 2009). Saliva is an important protective factor against caries development because it dilutes and buffers the acid produced by cariogenic microorganisms and provides calcium phosphate for remineralization. Saliva also contains IgA antibodies developed after the first exposure to the microorganisms (Cunha-Cruz *et al.*, 2013).

The 1988-94 National Health and Nutrition Examination Survey (NIANES) found that 8.4 percent of 2-year old children had at least one decayed or filled tooth and that by age 5, 40.4 percent of the children were affected (Drury *et al.*, 1999). Additionally, approximately 10.9% of children had frank caries and even higher percentages were found with enamel decalcifications or soft plaque accumulation (Yoon *et al.*, 2012). Although there is a significant need for preventive and restorative treatment, only 11.7% of children in the United States received dental treatment in 2007 due to the limited access to dental care and the behavioral difficulties in restorative procedures for young children (Yoon *et al.*, 2012).

S-ECC is defined in children ages 3-5 years old as: one or more cavitated, missing (due to caries) or smooth filled surfaces in primary maxillary anterior teeth, or dmfs (decayed, missing, filled and surface) score of >4 (age 3), >5 (age 4), or >6 (age 5) (Drury *et al.*, 1999; Evans, 2013).

1.2   Mutans Streptococci and Virulence Factors for Dental Caries

S. mutans encode several potential virulence factors including biofilm formation, adhesion, acidogenesis, and acid tolerance. These would all be important factors when determining the epidemiology of dental caries. The ability of *S. mutans* to form biofilms on saliva-covered surfaces has been correlated with increased incidence of dental caries (Banas, 2004; Lemos *et al.*, 2005; Nakano *et al.*, 2002; Shemesh *et al.*, 2007; Wen *et al.*, 2004). Biofilm formation by *S. mutans* is essential for its ability to survive and thrive in a highly competitive environment. Two pathways of biofilm formation have been identified: sucrose-dependent and sucrose-independent adherence. The sucrose-dependent pathway is the more significant mechanism in the development of dental caries (Lemos *et al.*, 2005). The major factors in the mechanism of sucrose-dependent adhesion are glucan-binding proteins (*gbp*) A, and C, and glucosyltransferase (*gtf*) B, C, and D, which promote adhesion (Lemos *et al.*, 2005; Fujita *et al.*, 2011; Bowen & Koo, 2011; Shemesh *et al.*, 2007; Nakano *et al.*, 2005). In the mouth, ingested dietary sucrose undergoes cleavage via *gtf* to glucose and fructose. Fructose is used as fuel by *S. mutans* whereas glucose is converted into dextran. These dextran chains allow for adhesion to enamel and constitute the scaffold in which *S. mutans* can colonize and form biofilm. Recently, the ComCDE operon, and the genetic regulators *luxS*, *relA*, and *ccpA*, have also been associated with biofilm formation (Lemos *et al.*, 2005; Wen *et al.*, 2004).

Adhesion of *S. mutans* is a major potential virulence factor of dental caries, and may also be involved in the development of infective endocarditis (Abranches *et al.,* 2011). In the oral cavity, surface-associated protein P1 (*spaP1*) displays adherence to both collagen and enamel components (Lemos *et al.*, 2005). *Gbp* and *gtf* also play significant roles in adhesion (Bowen *et al.*, 2011; Fujita *et al.*, 2011; Nakano *et al.*, 2005; Shemesh *et al.*, 2007). High levels of acid are major environmental stressors that affect the survivability of oral microorganisms (Banas, 2004; Guo *et al.*, 2013; Lemos *et al.*, 2005). Microorganisms that can survive at low pH would have distinct advantages in surviving in dental plaque (Wen & Burne, 2004; Matsui & Cvitkivitch, 2010; Lemos *et al.*, 2005). The ability of *S. mutans* to tolerate acidic environments and compete with other bacterial flora is well documented and is a significant virulence factor. The major concern with acidic environments is the potential to acidify the intracellular cytoplasm. Detrimental effects of this acidification include DNA and protein damage, alteration of enzyme activity, and cell membrane damage. Acid tolerance mechanisms utilized by *S. mutans* include 1) an F-ATPase proton pump used to restore cytoplasmic pH, 2) DNA repair molecules *uvrA* and AP endonucleases, 3) use of cytoplasmic enzymes with a wide pH range such as LGL and *pdhA*, and 4) addition of membrane components to maintain physiological composition such as *fabM*, *Dcp*, *Ffh*, and *Dgk* (Wen & Burne, 2004; Matsui & Cvitkivitch, 2010; Lemos *et al.*, 2005; Cotter & Hill, 2003). The unique ability of *S. mutans* to maintain proper function under harsh acidic conditions has provided selective advantages for successful colonization of the oral dentition.

Acidogenesis is another important virulence factor that helps *S. mutans* compete in the oral cavity. *S. mutans* utilizes dietary sugars to produce and secrete lactic acid as an end-product of glycolysis (Palmer *et al.*, 2012a; Banas, 2004; Dashper & Reynolds, 1996; Guo *et al.*, 2013; Harris *et al.*, 1992). As mentioned above, the acid tolerance of *S. mutans* is higher than in most bacteria; thus this microorganisms' ability to acidify the environment eliminates or diminishes competing bacteria and allows for enhanced colonization (Wen & Burne, 2004; Lemos *et al.*, 2005). More importantly, acid generation is the main cause of tooth demineralization and tooth decay (Banas, 2004; Dashper & Reynolds, 1996; Guo *et al.*, 2013; Harris *et al.*, 1992). In addition to biofilm formation, dextran and other sugar polymer chains can serve as a carbon reservoir and ultimately increase the production of lactic acid (Lemos *et al.*, 2005).

1.3   Prevention and Treatment of Dental Caries

Over the past few decades there has been considerable scientific progress that has greatly increased knowledge of the pathogenesis of dental caries. With these advances in scientific knowledge, combined with improved clinical techniques and dental materials, the clinical approach of treatment has evolved from an invasive surgical model to a minimal intervention medical model that attempts to address the cause of dental disease and not just the symptoms (Featherstone *et al.*, 2012; Mount, 2007; Zero *et al.*, 2001). These preventive treatment models involve assessing each individual's risk for caries, or caries risk assessment (American Academy of Pediatric Dentistry Council on Clinical Affairs, 2013; Featherstone, 2003; Featherstone, 2004a, Litt *et al.*, 1995; Nicolau *et al.*, 2003). Once an individual's risk has been assessed, a specific plan or "care path" can be implemented along with an adjunct customized restorative plan based on level of risk (American Academy of Pediatric Dentistry Council on Clinical Affairs, 2013; Ramos-Gomez & Ng, 2011). Multiple factors are taken into account when assigning caries risk status including socio-economic status, demographic background, attitude towards oral health, oral health habits, and systemic health and medications (American Academy of Pediatric Dentistry Council on Clinical Affairs, 2013; Featherstone, 2003, Featherstone, 2004b; Gao *et al.*, 2013; Litt *et al.*, 1995; Nicolau *et al.*, 2003). Caries risk assessment has been shown to be an effective method of significantly reducing caries risk in individuals labeled as high and moderate risk (Featherstone *et al.*, 2012).

Following the determination of caries risk status as low, moderate, or high, specific care paths can then be determined. This involves the use of minimally invasive restorative procedures based on evaluation of the extent of carious lesions as well as a customized oral hygiene regimen based on risk (Tassery *et al.*, 2013). Two key tools that can be utilized to decrease or reverse caries progression are antibacterial agents and remineralizing agents (Featherstone & Doméjean, 2012). One of the most common agents utilized in caries prevention that works as both an antibacterial agent and remineralizing agent is fluoride (ten Cate & Featherstone, 2012). Fluoride has been widely known to prevent caries since the 1930s when naturally fluoridated water was shown to decrease caries prevalence in communities (Dean *et al.*, 1938). It has since been demonstrated in numerous clinical trials that fluoride is an effective anticaries agent and is recognized as playing a central role in the decline of caries prevalence in many developed countries (Stookey, 1990; Hargreaves *et al.*, 1983). Individuals of all different caries risk statuses will benefit from fluoride use, including use in dentifrices, topical applications, and mouthrinses (Zero, 2005). In addition to fluoride treatment, individuals at all caries risk levels may also benefit from a professional prophylactic cleaning and the use of a calcium phosphate-based paste (Tassery *et al.*, 2013).

When discussing caries prevention, it is important to understand that caries is an infectious and transmissible disease. With this knowledge it is not surprising that colonization of cariogenic bacteria in the oral cavity of a child is generally the result of transmission from the child's primary caregiver (Seki *et al.*, 2006). In fact, a direct relationship can usually be found between levels of cariogenic bacteria in children and their primary caregivers (Douglass *et al.*, 2008). It is now recognized that the implementation of an effecting perinatal program to improve a mother's oral health may delay the acquisition of oral bacteria and the development of early childhood caries in their children (Ramos-Gomez, 2006). Following suit with the prevention and treatment techniques determined by caries risk assessment, it is critical that the parent/caregiver's oral health be addressed when treating children (Ramos-Gomez *et al.*, 2010). Such an assessment includes the determination of biological and lifestyle risk factors that support the development and progression of caries (Ramos-Gomez *et al.*, 2012*)*.

1.4   Use of Xylitol in Prevention of Dental Caries

The use of xylitol as a preventive measure for dental caries has been controversial. This five-carbon sugar alcohol, which has been implemented as a food sweetener, is capable of reducing plaque formation, inhibiting enamel demineralization, and suppressing growth of plaque bacteria (Marsh *et al.*, 2009). Xylitol, which can be delivered in numerous forms including lozenges, wipes, gum, and candy is widely considered to reduce caries by inhibiting the growth of MS (Marsh *et al.*, 2009). It has been shown that consumption of xylitol can lead to a decrease in MS bound to dental plaque and a reduction in plaque acidogenicity (Marsh *et al.*, 2009; Soderling, 2009). With these characteristics the use of xylitol as a preventive strategy for dental caries seems promising, however recent results from a placebo-controlled randomized trial of 691 participants suggests that the use of xylitol as an anticaries therapy for adults does not significantly reduce caries (Bader *et al.,* 2013). This is contradicted by past studies where xylitol has been shown to significantly reduce caries incidence in young children (Milgram *et al.*, 2012; Zhan *et al.,* 2012). These contrasting results suggest the possibility that children may possess distinct MS strains with differing xylitol resistant properties.

The inhibitory effects of xylitol on MS may be credited to the inhibition of key bacterial glycolytic enzymes (e.g. phosphofrucokinase). Xylitol is taken up by many strains of bacteria even if it cannot be metabolized (Waler & Rølla, 1990). This leads to the intracellular accumulation of xylitol 5-phosphate and the subsequent competition with bacterial glycolytic enzymes (e.g. phosphofructokinase), arrest of glycolysis, and impaired growth (Lee *et al.*, 2012; ten Cate & Featherstone, 2012). Long-term xylitol consumption has been shown to cause the emergence of strains of xylitol-resistant MS. However, these xylitol resistant MS strains have been found to form biofilms of reduced depths and shed more easily from plaque into saliva (Trahan *et al.*, 1992; Soderling *et al.*, 1996). These less cariogenic traits result in reduced amounts of MS bacteria in plaque and potential decrease in transmission and colonization between individuals (Soderling *et al.*, 1996; Palmer *et al.*, 2012b).

The anticariogenic traits of xylitol may be compounded when taken in a chewing gum form. Chewing gum is known to increase salivary flow rates (Rebelles *et al.*, 2010). Numerous oral health benefits can be credited to increased salivary flow. This includes more rapid oral clearance of sugars, neutralization of plaque acidic pH, and enhanced mineralization of early-carious lesions (Dodds, 2012). Due to these benefits, xylitol chewing gum may be a key tool in the prevention and treatment of dental caries.

1.5   Implications of Xylitol-Resistant Mutans Streptococci Strains in Children with Severe Early Childhood Caries

As the use of xylitol-containing products continues to gain popularity, questions emerge concerning the potential adaptation of plaque microorganisms, including MS, to xylitol and the possible selection of xylitol-resistant MS strains with increased cariogenic potential. Studies conducted in young children, as opposed to studies conducted with adults, indicate that xylitol (40% solution) may not significantly suppress *S. mutans* counts or plaque accumulation (Ramos-Gomez *et al.*, 2012). Thus, caries-active children may potentially possess distinct MS genetic strains with differential xylitol resistance properties, with some strains also exhibiting increased cariogenic potential. One objective of this 1-year follow-up study was to provide insight on the use of xylitol treatment as an effective maintenance practice for caries preventive therapy in pediatric dental patients.

In this 1-year follow-up study, we examined the profiles of MS genotypic strains from a pediatric patient cohort that had been diagnosed with severe early childhood caries [S-ECC]. In the original study, isolates were collected both prior to and following full-mouth dental rehabilitation, which included the removal and/or repair of carious lesions and application of antimicrobial rinse and fluoride varnish. In this chapter, we examine the MS genetic strains that are dominant at 1-year post-dental rehabilitation and the emergence of six new previously undetected minor MS strains. We also characterize the xylitol resistance properties of select dominant and minor strains.

2   Methods

2.1   Patient Selection and Treatment

As described in our prior reports (Palmer *et al.*, 2012a; Palmer *et al.*, 2012b), participants for this study were selected from patients seen at the OHSU Pediatric Dentistry clinic. The inclusion parameters for recruitment were young children with S-ECC, but otherwise who had good general health. Exclusion criteria included children treated with antibiotics, topical fluoride application, and/or antiseptic mouth rinses within the previous three months, or undergoing orthodontic therapies. Study participants all underwent full-mouth dental rehabilitation therapy, conducted under general anesthesia at Doernbecher Children Hospital [located within OHSU], because this permitted the completion of full-mouth caries restorative therapy during a single patient visit. These individuals were all between 3-5 years of age.

The patient demographics, including decayed, missing and filled teeth (dmft); and decayed, missing and filled surfaces (dmfs) scores have been reported previously (Palmer *et al.*, 2012b), and are summarized in Table 1. Dental rehabilitation therapy included application of 0.12% chlorhexidine gluconate to the gingiva and dentition using a sterile gauze to prepare the surgical area prior to beginning the procedure, followed by amalgam (Valiant® PH.D®), composite (Pulpdent ® Etch-Rite 38% Phosphoric Acid Etching Gel, Optibond™, Z100™ and Filtek™ Supreme), and stainless steel crown restorations (3M ES-PE, Unitek), formocresol pulpotomies (Patterson Dental), extractions, sealants (Patterson Dental), dental prophylaxis (NUPRO® prophylaxis paste [1.23% fluoride]), and sodium fluoride varnish (Cavity Shield™) application with a brush.

2.2   Plaque Sampling Procedure

For 1-year follow-up study described here, plaque samples were taken from each participant and compared to specimens collected at the three previous time points: 1) prior to the initiation of dental rehabilitation therapy, 2) within the 2-4 weeks post-rehabilitation visit, and 3) at the 6-month recall visit following dental rehabilitation.

2.3   Selection of Mutans Streptococci (MS) Isolates and Control Streptococci Strains

As described in Fazilat *et al.* (2010) and Palmer *et al.* (2012a), plaque specimens were plated on mitis salivarius agar (MSA; product number 229810, Difco, Becton, Dickinson and Company, Sparks, MD), supplemented with 1% sodium tellurite and the antibiotic bacitracin (0.2 Units/ml), to isolate MS. Colonies were grown on MSA plates for 48-72 hours (37°C, 5% CO_2), and then individual colonies were selected based on typical MS morphology. Control streptococci strains include *S. mutans* ATCC strains 25175 and 35668, *S. sobrinus* ATCC 33478, and non-MS oral streptococci strain *S. salivarius* ATCC 13419.

		G	J	K	L	M
	Sex	Female	Male	Male	Male	Male
Treatment Day	**Treatment Age[1]**	5 years	5 years	3 years	3 years	5 years
	Teeth Present[2]	A-T	A-T	A-T	A-T	A-T
	DMFT Score[3]	11	13	18	13	12
	DMFS Score[4]	25	38	61	48	41
1 Year Recall Exam	**Teeth Present[2]**	A-K, M-T	3, A-C, H-J, 14, 19, K-M, 23-26, R-T, 30	A-T	A-T	A-C, H-T
	Condition of Restorations	Satisfactory	Satisfactory	Satisfactory	Missing 1 restoration	Satisfactory
	Number of New Carious Lesions	1	2	1	2	1
	Lesion at Margin of Existing Restoration	Yes	No	No	Yes	No

[1] Treatment Age: Age of patient on day of full-mouth dental rehabilitation.

[2] Teeth Present: Teeth present on day of either full-mouth dental rehabilitation or at the 1-year recall exam. Letters denote primary teeth and numbers denote permanent teeth present following the Primary Universal Numbering System.

[3] DMFT: The sum of the primary teeth that is decayed (d), missing (m) or filled (f) due to dental caries.

[4] DMFS: The sum of the primary tooth surfaces that is decayed (d), missing (m) or filled (f) due to dental caries.

Table 1: Demographics of Patients (G, J, K, L, and M) Returning for One-Year Recall Exam. This table was shown in part in Palmer *et al.* (2012a) and Palmer *et al.* (2012b) and is reproduced here with the kind permission of the American Academy of Pediatric Dentistry and CoAction Publishing, the publisher of the *Journal of Oral Microbiology*, respectively.

2.4   Genomic DNA Isolation, Conventional Polymerase Chain Reaction [PCR] and Arbitrarily Primed PCR (AP-PCR)

Genomic DNA was extracted from overnight liquid cultures, and *S. mutans* were independently identified using conventional PCR (Palmer *et al.*, 2012a). Highly-specific primers for *S. mutans* and *S. sobrinus*, in addition to thermal cycling parameters, have been defined (Igarashi *et al.*, 2000; Chen *et al.*, 2007), and are also described in our previous reports (Palmer *et al.*, 2012a; Palmer *et al.*, 2012b). The amplification parameters for AP-PCR were similar to conventional PCR, with the exception of annealing at reduced temperatures (35°C for 30 seconds).

2.5   Xylitol-Susceptibility Assays and Statistical Curve-Fitting Analyses

MS genetic strains were grown overnight in BHI broth to ensure bacteria were in exponential growth-phase, prior to xylitol-susceptibility experiments. Cultures were then grown with various concentrations of xylitol, and growth curves were determined by measuring absorbance (A=600 nm) every hour from 0-10 hours, and finally at 24 hours. Independent cultures were treated with varying xylitol concentrations (0-5%). Xylitol concentrations were selected based on concentrations used in similar *in vitro* xylitol inhibition assays (Söderling *et al.*, 2008) and are thought to bracket the effective dose of xylitol in saliva released from oral xylitol-containing products. Curve fitting analysis using cubic and quadratic models

(Raudenbush & Bryk, 2002; Hox, 2002; Skrondal & Rabe-Hesketh, 2004) was conducted to determine the xylitol concentration (w/v) that results in 50% inhibition of growth, using the absorbance value of the 0% xylitol control at peak logarithmic phase (typically at 9-10 hours) for normalization at 100%.

3   Results

3.1   Description of Study Participants

Nine patients were originally enrolled in this pilot study; seven (Patients G, H, I, J, K, L and M) were available for their initial 2-4 week recall visits, and only five patients (Patients G, J, K, L and M) made all appointments, including their 6-month and 1-year post-dental rehabilitation visits. Table 1 shows information collected from the five patients who completed all four sample collection visits. The pediatric dentistry patients were between the ages of 3 and 5 years old on the day of dental rehabilitation and in good health (American Society of Anesthesiologists [ASA] physical status I). The patients were all diagnosed with severe-early childhood caries (S-ECC) with dmft and dmfs scores ranging from 11-18 and 25-61 respectively (Palmer *et al.*, 2012a) (see also Table 1). All patients in our study underwent full-mouth dental rehabilitation therapy under general anesthesia. They all also had antimicrobial chlorhexidine rinse, and fluoride varnish applied.

3.2   Identification of Mutans Streptococci Strains

Based on growth and colony morphology on mitis salivarius agar (MSA) and Gram stain analysis, up to 60 isolates were obtained from each plaque specimen originating from every patient at all collection periods, with each isolate confirmed as bacitracin-resistant, Gram-positive, oral streptococci. Using primers specific for *S. mutans* or *S. sobrinus* (both members of mutans streptococci, MS), and testing genomic DNA from isolates obtained from the seven patients (Patients G, H, I, J, K, L and M), we identified 37 genotypic strains of *S. mutans*, two strains [K2 and K3 strains] of *S. sobrinus*, and seven non-MS strains during the entire study (pre-rehabilitation, 2-4 week post-rehabilitation, 6-month post-rehabilitation and 1-year post-rehabilitation) (Palmer *et al.*, 2012b), including the appearance of six new MS strains found only at the 1-year collection (Figure 1 and Table 2). For the five pediatric patients who completed the entire 1-year study, we identified 30 genotypic strains of *S. mutans*, two genotypic strains [K2 and K3 strains] of *S. sobrinus*, and five non-MS strains (Table 2; also Palmer *et al.*, 2012b). Several of the new strains identified at 1-year post-dental rehabilitation were found only as single isolates, or were highly-related to other genotypes that differ by only single bands in their AP-PCR genetic profiles (Figure 1 and Table 2; e.g. compare L1c found only at the 1-year collection to dominant strain L1 and other minor MS strains L1a and L1b). Genomic DNA from several isolates were not amplified, or only weakly amplified using *S. mutans*-specific primers, and comprised seven additional genetic strains of bacitracin-resistant Gram-positive oral streptococci, which we termed non-MS strains. As described previously (Palmer *et al.*, 2012a), these seven genotypic strains were subjected to 16S ribosomal RNA gene sequencing, which identified them as three strains of *S. gordonii*, three strains of *S. anginosus*, and one strain of *Granulicatella adiacens*, previously known as *S. adjacens* (Woo *et al.*, 2003).

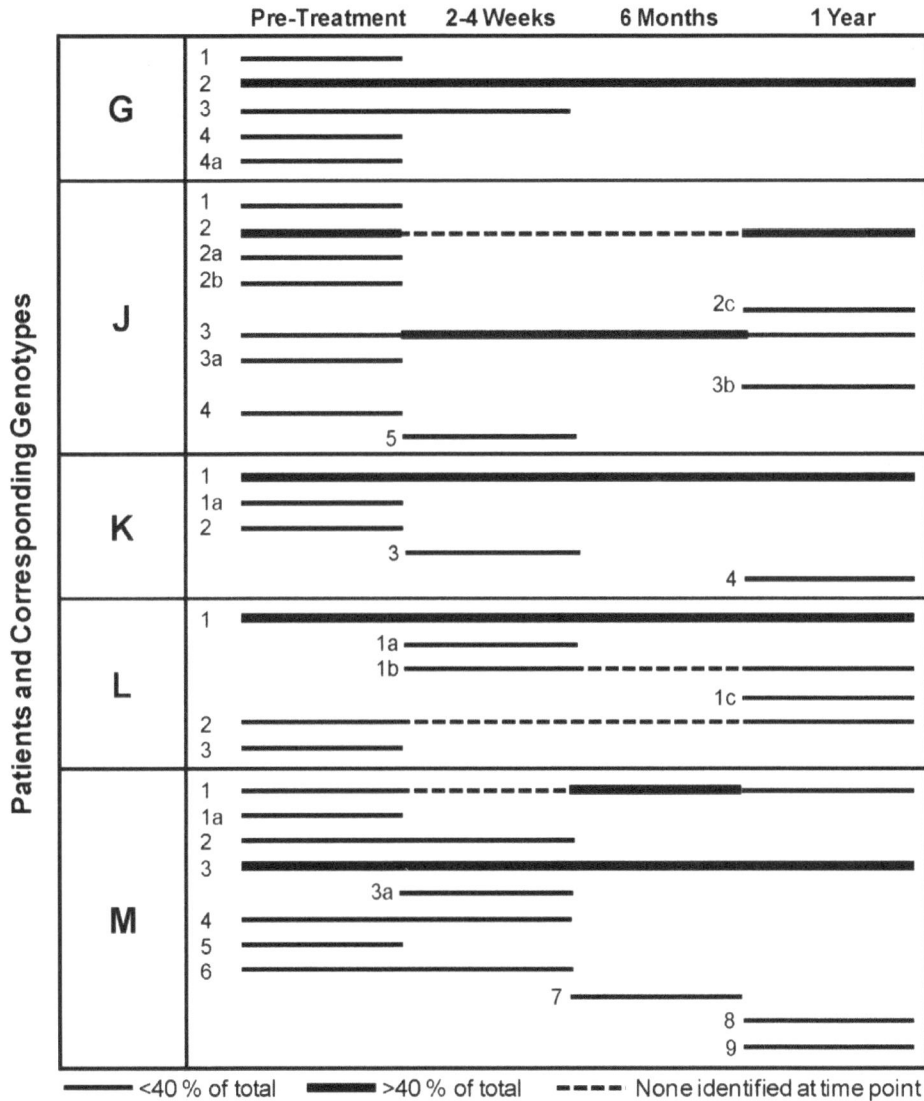

Figure 1: Genotypic strain diversity in pediatric dentistry patients at pre- and post-dental rehabilitation therapy (2-4 weeks, 6 months and 12 months). Each line represents distinct genotypes identified by AP-PCR. The dominant genotypes are marked in bold at each collection point (greater than 40% of the isolates). Dotted lines indicate the periods when genotypes were detected at one time point but were not detected at subsequent time points. Isolates were genotyped numerically within each patient (G, J, K, L and M). Only data for Patients G, J, K, L and M, who completed all recall visits, including the 12-month post-therapy visit, are included in this analysis. Portions of this figure were previously displayed in Palmer et al. (2012a) and in full in Palmer et al. (2012b) and were reproduced with the kind permission of the American Academy of Pediatric Dentistry and CoAction Publishing (the publisher of the *Journal of Oral Microbiology*), respectively.

Patient G

Patient Visit	Percentage of Genotypes S. mutans[1]				No. of Genotypes	Dominant Strain
	G1	G2	G4	G4a		
Pre-Treatment	18	56	16	3	5	G2 (56%)
Post-Treatment (4 weeks)	0	98	0	0	2	G2 (98%)
Post-Treatment (6 months)	0	100	0	0	1	G2 (100%)
Post-Treatment (1 year)	0	100	0	0	1	G2 (100%)

Patient J

Patient Visit	Percentage of Genotypes S. mutans										No. of Genotypes	Dominant Strain
	J1	J2	J2a	J2b	J2c	J3	J3a	J3b	J4	J5		
Pre-Treatment	13	56	7	2	0	16	4	0	2	0	7	J2 (56%)
Post-Treatment (2 weeks)	0	0	0	0	0	98	0	0	0	2	2	J3 (98%)
Post-Treatment (6 months)	0	0	0	0	0	100	0	0	0	0	1	J3 (100%)
Post-Treatment (1 year)	0	60	0	0	4	32	0	4	0	0	4	J2 (60%)

Patient K

Patient Visit	Percentage of Genotypes S. mutans			No. of Genotypes	Dominant Strain
	K1[2]	K1a	K4		
Pre-Treatment	90	7	0	3	K1 (90%)
Post-Treatment (2 weeks)	57	0	0	2	K1 (57%), K3 (43%)
Post-Treatment (6 months)	100	0	0	1	K1 (100%)
Post-Treatment (1 year)	98	0	2	2	K1 (98%)

Patient L

Patient Visit	Percentage of Genotypes S. mutans						No. of Genotypes	Dominant Strain
	L1	L1a	L1b	L1c	L2	L3		
Pre-Treatment	96	0	0	0	2	2	3	L1 (96%)
Post-Treatment (4 weeks)	96	2	2	0	0	0	3	L1 (96%)
Post-Treatment (6 months)	100	0	0	0	0	0	1	L1 (100%)
Post-Treatment (1 year)	89	0	6	3	2	0	4	L1 (89%)

Patient M

Patient Visit	Percentage of Genotypes S. mutans							No. of Genotypes	Dominant Strain
	M2	M3	M3a	M5	M7	M8	M9		
Pre-Treatment	14	44	0	2	0	0	0	7	M3 (44%)
Post-Treatment (4 weeks)	2	88	4	0	0	0	0	5	M3 (88%)
Post-Treatment (6 months)	0	40	0	0	12	0	0	3	M3 (40%), M1 (48%)
Post-Treatment (1 year)	0	93	0	0	0	2	2	4	M3 (93%)

[1] Genotypes confirmed as *S. mutans* by conventional PCR with *S. mutans* specific primers. Note that genotypes containing an "a", "b", or "c" suffix as in G4a or J2a and J2b differ from the its matched comparison strains (in this case: G4 and J2) with the addition of one or more AP-PCR fragments ("a" suffix implies one additional band, "b" suffix implies two additional bands and "c" suffix implies three additional bands, all when compared to the AP-PCR profile of its matched genotypic strain). Note that individual MS genotypes were determined for comparison within each patient alone, and thus, comparisons of MS genotypes were conducted at only the intra-patient level. Please note that non-MS strains were also identified and published in Palmer et al. (2012a), but not reflected in this table for space considerations, and that the genotype percentages were calculated based on the sum total of all MS and non-MS genotypes observed at each time collection point.

[2] Genotype K1 isolates obtained at the 2 week post-treatment collection did not yield robust PCR products using *S. mutans*-specific primers and conventional PCR; however, these isolates were defined in the MS group because they retained identical AP-PCR fingerprints when compared to other K1 isolates.

Note: This table was shown in part in Palmer et al. (2012a) and Palmer et al. (2012b) and is reproduced here with the kind permission of the AAPD and CoAction Publishing, the publisher of the *Journal of Oral Microbiology*, respectively.

Table 2: Identification and Percentage of MS and Oral Streptococci Genotypes at Each Visit.

3.3   Genotypic Strains Remain Dominant and New Minor Strains Appear at 1-Year Post-Rehabilitation

The numbers of genotypic strains identified from any one patient over the entire collection period ranged from 3-9, or from any one visit from 3-7 (Figure 1 and Table 2). In all five patients who completed all recall visits, including the 1-year recall, the highest number of strains was observed at the pre-treatment visit, and dominant strains representing >44% of the population examined emerged at post-rehabilitation collections. Four out of these five patients (Patients G, K, L, and M), had the same dominant genotypic strain at 6 months post-rehabilitation as at 1-year post-rehabilitation (Figure 1 and Table 2). Interestingly, in four patients (Patients J, K, L and M), the number of MS strains became more diverse at 1-year post-rehabilitation, with the emergence of new minor strains. Also, in almost all cases and collection times (with the exception of Patient J), there was only one dominant strain, each representing >56% of the strain population examined (Figure 1 and Table 2). In Patient J, genotype J2 was the dominant MS strain at pre-dental rehabilitation, disappearing (perhaps below detection) during the 2-week and 6-month collections, and then reappearing as the dominant strain at 1-year post-rehabilitation. Genotype J3 remained throughout the entire sampling period, and was the dominant MS strain during the 2-week and 6-month post-rehabilitation sampling times. The genotypic distribution patterns for the patient cohort were distinctive and unique for each patient; all comparisons of genotypes were conducted with strains collected within each individual patient, and not between patients. Inter-patient comparisons of MS strains were not conducted as part of this study.

3.4   Xylitol-Susceptibility of Dominant and Minor MS Genetic Strains

Using an *in vitro* growth assay, we determined the 50% xylitol inhibition values for select MS strains ranged between 2.48% to 33.3% xylitol, using the absorbance value of the control 0% xylitol group at peak logarithmic phase (typically at 9-10 hours) as the 100% normalization value for each strain (Figures 2 and 3). *S. mutans* ATCC strains 25175 and 35668, generally considered to be laboratory attenuated strains, had very similar 50% xylitol inhibition values of 3.35% and 3.30%, respectively (Figures 2 and 3). The majority of the MS genetic strains analyzed (15 out of 23 strains from Patients G, J, K, L and M) exhibited 50% xylitol inhibition values ranging from 2.48% - 5.58%, similar to the two *S. mutans* ATCC control strains. In patients where 1-year post-dental rehabilitation specimens were collected, dominant strains G2, J3, K1, L1, and M3 exhibited 50% xylitol inhibition values of 2.95%, 3.26%, 3.45%, 7.06% and 3.86%, respectively (Figures 2 and 3). In Patient J, dominant strain J3 at 6 months post-rehabilitation therapy was highly xylitol-resistant with a 50% xylitol inhibition value of 33.3%, but was replaced as the dominant strain at 1-year post-therapy by dominant strain J2, which displayed typical xylitol-susceptibility (Figure 2). In the five pediatric patients who completed all post-rehabilitation recall visits [Patients G, J, K, L and M], the dominant MS genotypic strain at the 1-year post-rehabilitation collection exhibited 50% xylitol inhibition values similar or close to the values retained by the *S. mutans* ATCC control strains.

4   Discussion

Dental caries is one of the most common chronic diseases found throughout the world. Dental caries results from multifactoral and complex interactions at the tooth surface between certain oral bacteria and

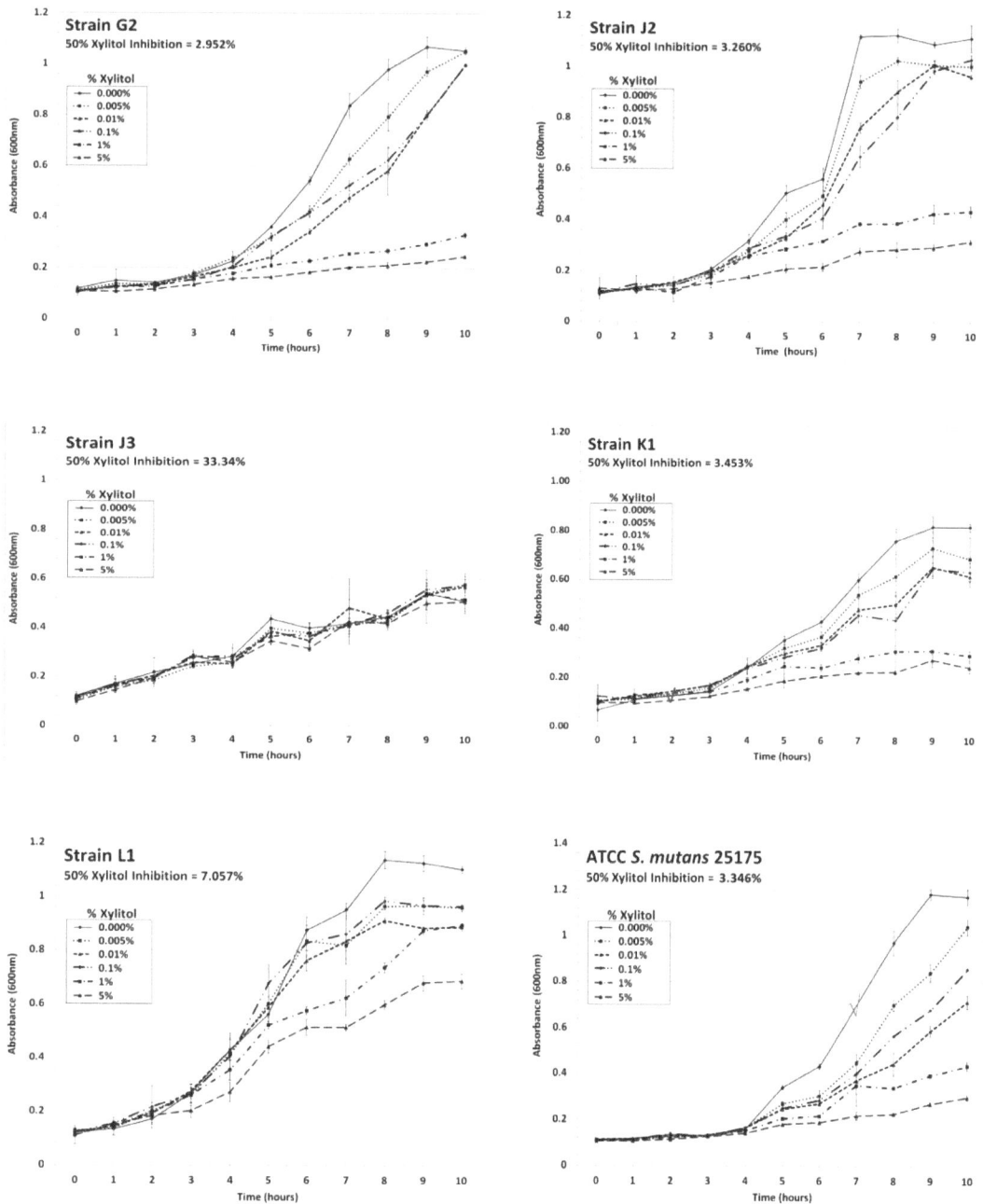

Figure 2: Xylitol susceptibility curves for dominant MS strains and *S. mutans* ATCC 25175. Dominant MS strains G2, J2, J3, K1 and L1, and *S. mutans* ATCC 25175 were propagated in BHI for 24 hours at 37°C, and subsequently diluted in fresh BHI to an absorbance (600 nm) level of 0.1 to initiate logarithmic growth in the presence or absence of xylitol (final concentrations of 0%, 0.001%, 0.01%, 0.1%, 1% and 5% xylitol). Cultures were measured spectrophotometrically every hour for 10 hours and then at 24 hours, using four replicates per time point for each xylitol concentration. Plots were constructed and then curve fitted using cubic or quadratic models (Raudenbush & Bryk, 2002; Hox, 2002; Skrondal & Rabe-Hesketh, 2004) to determine the theoretical xylitol concentrations for 50% inhibition of growth, using the peak absorbance of the 0% xylitol control as the normalization factor at 100%. This figure was previously displayed in Palmer *et al.* (2012b) and was reproduced with the kind permission of CoAction Publishing (the publisher of the *Journal of Oral Microbiology*).

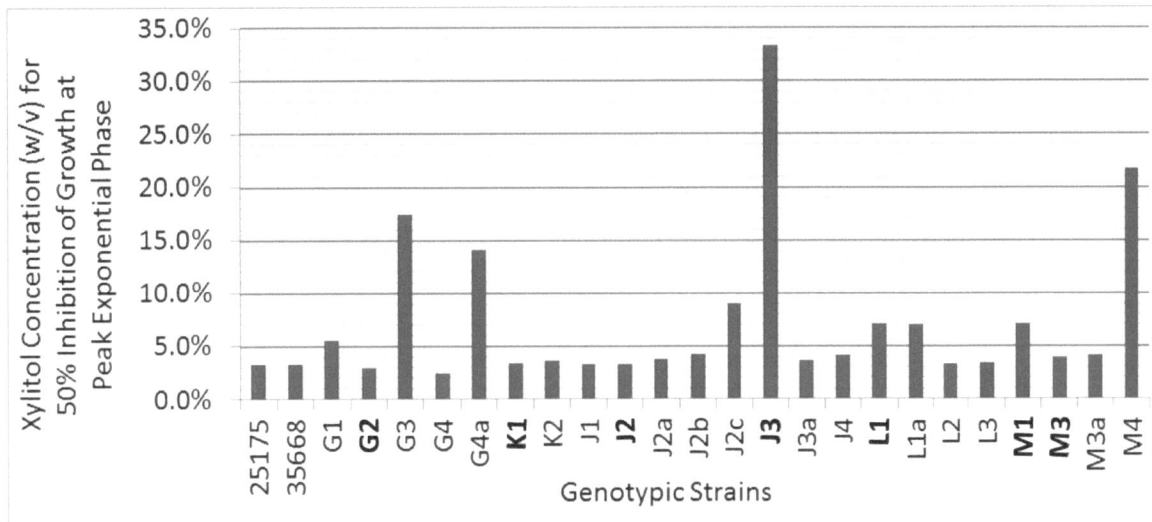

Figure 3: Bar graphs illustrating xylitol concentrations (w/v) for 50% inhibition of growth for dominant MS strains and select minor MS strains from Patients G, J, K, L and M. 50% inhibition values are also displayed for *S. mutans* ATCC 25175 and 35668. Dominant strains are in bold. Xylitol concentrations (w/v) for 50% inhibition of growth for: 1) *S. mutans* ATCC 25175 and 35668 are 3.35% and 3.30%, respectively; 2) Strains G1, G2, G3, G4, and G4a are 5.58%, 2.95%, 17.4%, 2.48% and 14.1%, respectively; 3) Strains K1 and K2 are 3.45% and 3.61%, respectively; 4) Strains J1, J2, J2a, J2b, J2c, J3, J3a, and J4 are 3.35%, 3.26%, 3.77%, 4.28%, 9.05%, 33.3%, 3.65% and 4.12%, respectively; 5) Strains L1, L1a, L2 and L3 are 7.06%, 7.00%, 3.35% and 3.43%, respectively; and 6) Strains M1, M3, M3a and M4 are 7.07%, 3.86%, 4.10% and 21.7%, respectively. M3 was the dominant strain in Patient M throughout the entire 1-year collection period. M1 was an additional co-dominant strain in Patient M at 6 months post-rehabilitation therapy and was defined as a non-MS strain (Palmer *et al*, 2012a). This figure was previously displayed in Palmer *et al*. (2012b) and was reproduced with the kind permission of CoAction Publishing (the publisher of the *Journal of Oral Microbiology*).

their products, salivary constituents, and dietary carbohydrates. Many bacteria have been implicated in caries formation, but research has shown that *S. mutans* is essential in the pathogenesis of dental caries. *S. mutans* is thought to be highly cariogenic because of multiple virulence factors including acidogenicity and acid tolerance, and its ability to generate copious biofilms made of insoluble extracellular glycans. Distinct strains of *S. mutans* produce differential levels of these virulence factors, including differing amounts of glucosyltransferase enzymes (Alaluusua *et al.*, 1996). Further, caries-active individuals have been shown to often harbor larger numbers of MS genotypes with increased capacity to synthesize water-insoluble glycans, which are essential for extracellular matrix production in dental plaque biofilms (Napimoga *et al.*, 2005). Thus, this genetic diversity among the various *S. mutans* genetic strains, with their corresponding differences in virulence gene expression must now be taken into consideration when thinking about the overall pathogenesis and epidemiology of dental caries.

We originally designed our pilot study to begin to understand this genetic diversity of *S. mutans* and how it is displayed in a small group of children with S-ECC. We also wanted to determine if any changes occurred in the genotypic population within each of these patients following full-mouth dental rehabilitation therapy. Prior to treatment these children with S-ECC harbored multiple different strains of

MS (i.e., *S. mutans* and *S. sobrinus*), whose relative numbers changed dramatically after treatment (Palmer *et al.*, 2012a). Continuing these studies, using the remaining members of the original patient cohort, we have demonstrated in our primary article (Palmer *et al.*, 2012b) and also now show the continued presence of dominant MS genotypic strains and the emergence of additional minor MS strains at 1-year post-dental rehabilitation. We also describe the *in vitro* xylitol resistance of dominant and select minor MS genotypic strains.

4.1   Genetic Analysis and Identification of MS Strains

Investigations by several research groups, including Napimoga *et al.* (2005), Lembo *et al.* (2007), and Baca *et al.* (2008) have validated the use of arbitrarily primed-PCR (AP-PCR) in discriminating MS genotypes within individuals, and have formed the basis of both our original pilot study, and the studies outlined here. We also now find that AP-PCR profiles of MS isolates obtained at 1-year post-rehabilitation therapy can be reproducibly and reliably compared to profiles of MS isolates obtained earlier in the original study. Thus, AP-PCR and the genetic profiling of MS strains allow longitudinal epidemiology studies to be conducted over the 1-year post-rehabilitation therapy period.

4.2   MS Colonization and Genotypic Diversity in Children with Severe Early Childhood Caries

Mitchell *et al.* (2009) have suggested that the composition of strains within the MS population, or the acquisition and loss of specific MS strains, is a dynamic, active process in S-ECC patients. We also observed similar MS population shifts in patients described in our study, for all time periods including 1-year post-rehabilitation. As described in our previous reports (Palmer *et al.*, 2012a; Palmer *et al.*, 2012b), the re-appearance of genotype J2 at 1-year post-rehabilitation in Patient J, as well as the appearance of new minor MS strains in four patients (Patients J, K, L and M) at 1-year post-rehabilitation, may be due to re-infection from external sources. Alternatively, genotype J2, undetected at the 2-4 week and the 6-month collections, may have been present at numbers below the threshold of our detection. In the case of Patient J, and other individuals with S-ECC, it is probable that MS genotypes were acquired either vertically from their mother or horizontally from other members of their family or extended care group. The diagnoses of ECC and S-ECC are associated with several risk factors including caregivers with high levels of MS and untreated carious lesions, frequent ingestion of sucrose-rich diets, and poor oral hygiene practices. In combination, these factors can result in MS colonization at earlier ages, with higher bacterial levels and greater number of MS genotypes than in caries-free children (Napimoga *et al.*, 2005; Napimoga *et al.*, 2004; Lembo *et al.*, 2007; Baca *et al.*, 2008; Mitchell *et al.*, 2009; Poggio *et al.*, 2009). They may also predispose these patients to easier re-colonization by MS strains after caries treatment.

As described here and in our previous report (Palmer *et al.*, 2012a), our enrolled children with S-ECC, ages 3-5 years, exhibited 3-7 MS genotypes prior to dental rehabilitation therapy, and most exhibited only 1-3 genotypes 6 months post-therapy. Single dominant genotypes, were identified in four of five pediatric patients 6-months post-rehabilitation therapy. By 1-year post-therapy however, the diversity of MS genotypes increased in four out of five patients [e.g.: Patients J, K, L and M], with the appearance of six new minor MS strains.

Our primary objective in these studies was to define changes that occur in the composition of MS genetic strains in caries-active children, after full-mouth dental rehabilitation therapy. Collectively our results are most similar to those of Pieralisi *et al.* (2010), where we observe a wide diversity of genetic MS strains in children with S-ECC prior to treatment, but we also demonstrate that dental rehabilitation therapy results in the appearance of single dominant MS strains by 6-months post-therapy. Unfortunately we were unable to determine if the reduction of MS strains and appearance of single dominant strains were due to the selective effects of the antimicrobial rinse, application of fluoride varnish, the restorative procedure itself, or a combination of these therapies. We also found that by 1-year post treatment, genetic diversity of MS strains again increased within most of the S-EEC patients studied, perhaps indicative of a return to circumstances more similar to pre-treatment within these individuals' mouths.

4.3   Full-Mouth Dental Rehabilitation Therapy and Effects on Diversity of MS Strains

In our original study (Palmer *et al.*, 2012a; Palmer *et al.*, 2012b), we examined the diversity of genotypic strains of MS and other non-MS streptococci from seven pediatric patients who had S-ECC, with an additional objective of evaluating the effects on these MS strains of the standard regimen for full-mouth dental rehabilitation therapy. In most patients, dental rehabilitation therapy reduced the diversity of oral MS from many genotypic strains to only 1-2 dominant strains by 6 months post-therapy. We presume that the treatment of the carious lesions, as well as the antimicrobial rinse and fluoride treatment reduced the total bacterial numbers of all strains immediately following dental rehabilitation, but the effectiveness of the therapy was time-limited, with dominant strains appearing by 6 months post-rehabilitation. In most of the patients examined, and as described in our previous reports (Palmer *et al.*, 2012a; Palmer *et al.*, 2012b), dental rehabilitation therapy eliminated several non-MS strains and allowed specific strains of highly acidogenic *S. mutans* bacteria to become dominant strains. Finally as shown here, new minor MS strains appeared at 1-year post-therapy, as a result of re-infection from the primary care giver or other external sources.

Our studies do not address how patient compliance with at home dental care instructions might have impacted the appearance of the MS dominant strains by 6-months, or the appearance of new minor strains by 1-year post-rehabilitation therapy. This of course is an area of research that needs to be examined further.

We understand that we have limited numbers of patients in both the pilot study (Palmer *et al.*, 2012a) and in the 1-year follow-up study (Palmer *et al.*, 2012b), but believe that this work is statistically substantiated by Cheon *et al.* (2011), who have used probabilities to determine the minimum number of MS isolates from an individual required to fully evaluate diversity of bacterial genotypes. Cheon *et al.* (2011) determined theoretically that screening seven MS isolates from any one specimen collection was sufficient for the detection of up to four MS genotypes with a success probability of 78%. In our studies we screen at least ten MS isolates per oral specimen, thus increasing the probability of identifying all MS strains present.

4.4   Xylitol-Susceptibility of MS Strains

One commonly used caries prevention modality is xylitol. Even though xylitol has been studied for decades, its use as a caries preventive tool is still controversial. Even so many pediatric dentistry organizations throughout the world, including The American Academy of Pediatric Dentistry, have officially recognized the benefits of xylitol as a caries preventative measure for use in children. Therefore, we sought to determine the *in vitro* xylitol susceptibility of the some of the MS strains, including the dominant strains, isolated from our S-ECC patients.

Our xylitol inhibition experiments indicate that most of the dominant MS strains are similar in xylitol resistance to the attenuated *S. mutans* ATCC control strains, with some strains being variably inhibited by xylitol *in vitro*. Moraes *et al.* (2011) indicate that xylitol (40% solution) may not significantly suppress *S. mutans* counts or plaque accumulation in young children, as opposed to adults, potentially implicating the existence of xylitol-resistant MS strains. Our studies support Moreas *et al.* (2011) and affirm the existence of MS strains showing variable inhibition, including strains dramatically more xylitol-resistant. The presence of these xylitol-resistant MS strains would no doubt impact the effectiveness of any xylitol preventive treatments in individuals.

Acknowledgements

Support was provided to KCG as a 2013 OCTRI Student Research Fellow, to AS as a 2013 AADR Student Research Fellow, and to NN as a 2013 Dean's Research Fellow. UN is a 2013 graduate in Biology/Organismal Biology from Portland State University. This research was supported in part by the Oregon Clinical and Translational Research Institute (OCTRI), grant numbers TL1 RR024159 and UL1 RR024140 from the National Center for Research Resources (NCRR), a component of the National Institutes of Health (NIH), and NIH Roadmap for Medical Research. Support for the original research was also obtained from the Pediatric Dentistry residency fund. EAP, TM, and CAM are faculty supported by the OHSU School of Dentistry. Portions of this manuscript, including the figures, tables and text, were displayed in part from Palmer *et al.* (2012a), with the kind permission of the American Academy of Pediatric Dentistry, and from Palmer *et al.* (2012b), with the kind permission of CoAction Publishing (the publisher of the *Journal of Oral Microbiology*). The authors also thank and acknowledge support and encouragement from Samyia Chaudhry, Nicole Paterson, Trusha Patel, Sam Nazaretyan, Ryan Fromme, Kendra Flann, Asmita Sharma, John Peterson and John Engle.

References

Abranches J., Miller J. H., Martinez A. R., Simpson-Haidaris P. J., Burne R. A., & Lemos J. A. (2011). *The collagen-binding protein Cnm is required for Streptococcus mutans adherence to and intracellular invasion of human coronary artery endothelial cells. Infection and Immunity, 79(6), 2277-2284.*

Alaluusua S., Mättö J., Grönroos L., Innilä S., Torkko H., Asikainen S., Jousimies-Somer H., & Saarela M. (1996). *Oral colonization by more than one clonal type of mutans streptococci in children with nursing bottle dental caries. Archives in Oral Biology, 41(2), 167-173.*

Amaechi B. T. , Higham S. M. , & Edgar W. M. (1999). *Caries inhibiting and remineralizing effect of xylitol in vitro. Journal of Oral Science, 41(2), 71-76.*

American Academy of Pediatric Dentistry Council on Clinical Affairs (2013). *Guidelines on caries-risk assessment and management for infants, children and adolescents. Pediatric Dentistry, 35, 118-125.*

Baca P., Castillo A. M., Baca A. P., Liebana M. J., Junco P., & Liebana L. (2008). *Genotypes of Streptococcus mutans in saliva and dental plaque. Archives of Oral Biology, 53(8), 751-754.*

Bader J. D., Vollmer W. M., Shugars D. A., Gilbert G. H., Amaechi B. T., Brown J. P., Laws R. L., Funkhouser K. A., Makhija S. K., Ritter A. V., & Leo M. C. (2013). *Results from the xylitol for adults caries trial (X-ACT). Journal of American Dental Association, 144(1), 21-30.*

Banas J. A. (2004). *Virulence properties of Streptococcus mutans. Frontiers of Bioscience, 1;9, 1267-1277.*

Bowen, W. H. & Koo H. (2011). *Biology of Streptococcus mutans-derived glucosyltransferases: Role in Extracellular Matrix Formation of Cariogenic Biofilms. Caries Research, 45(1), 69–86.*

Chen Z., Saxena D., Caufield P. W., Ge Y., & Li Y. (2007). *Development of species-specific primers for detection of Streptococcus mutans in mixed bacterial samples. FEMS Microbiology Letters, 272(2), 154-162.*

Cheon K., Moser S. A., Whiddon J., Osgood R. C., Momeni S., Ruby J. D., Cutter G. R., Allison D. B., & Childers N. K. (2011). *Genetic diversity of plaque mutans streptococci with rep-PCR. Journal of Dental Research, 90(3), 331-335.*

Cotter P. D. & Hill C. (2003). Surviving the acid test: responses of Gram-positive bacteria to low pH. *Molecular Biology Reviews, 67(3),* 429–453.

Cunha-Cruz J., Scott J. A., Rothen M., Mancl L., Lawhorn T., Brossel K., & Berg J. (2013). Salivary characteristics and dental caries: Evidence from general dental practices. *Journal of American Dental Association, 144(5),* e31-e40.

Dashper S. G. & Reynolds E. C. (1996). Lactic acid excretion by Streptococcus mutans. *Microbiology, 142(1),* 33-39.

Dean H. T., McKay F. S., & Elvove E. (1938). Mottled enamel survey of Bauxite, Ark., ten years after a change in the public water supply. *Public Health Reports, 53(39),* 1736-1748.

Dewhirst F. E., Chen T., Izard J, Paster B. J., Tanner A. C., Yu W.-H., Lakshmanan A., & Wade W. G. (2010). The Human Oral Microbiome. *Journal of Bacteriology, 192:* 5002-5017.

Dodds M. W. (2012). The oral health benefits of chewing gum. *Journal of Irish Dental Association, 58(5),* 253-261.

Douglass J. M., Li Y., & Tinanoff N. (2008). Association of mutans streptococci between caregivers and their children. *Pediatric Dentistry, 30(5),* 375-387.

Drury T. F., Horowitz A. M., Ismail A. I., Haertens M. P., Rozier R. G., & Selwitz R. H. (1999). Diagnosing and reporting early childhood caries for research purposes. A report of a workshop sponsored by the National Institute of Dental and Craniofacial Research, the Health Resources and Services Administration, and the Health Care Financing Administration. *Journal of Public Health Dentistry, 59(3),* 192-197.

Fazilat S., Sauerwein R., McLeod J., Finlayson T., Adam E., Engle J., Gagneja P., Maier T., & Machida C. A. (2010). Application of adenosine triphosphate-driven bioluminescence for quantification of plaque bacteria and assessment of oral hygiene in children. *Pediatric Dentistry, 32(3),* 195-204.

Featherstone J. D. (2003). The caries balance: Contributing factors and early detection. *Journal of California Dental Association, 31(2),* 129-33.

Featherstone J. D. (2004). The caries balance: The basis for caries management by risk assessment. *Oral Health & Preventive Dentistry, 2(Suppl 1),* 259-264.

Featherstone J. D. & Doméjean S. (2012). The role of remineralizing and anticaries agents in caries management. *Advances in Dental Research, 24(2),* 28-31.

Featherstone J. D., White J. M., Hoover C. I., Rapozo-Hilo M., Weintraub J. A., Wilson R. S., Zhan A., & Gansky S. A. (2012). A randomized clinical trial of anticaries therapies targeted according to risk assessment (Caries Management by Risk Assessment). *Caries Research, 46(2),* 118-129.

Fejerskov O. (2004). Changing paradigms in concepts on dental caries: Consequences for oral health care. *Caries Research, 38(3),* 182-191.

Fujita K., Takashima Y., Inagaki S., Nagayama K., Nomura R., Ardin A. C., Grönroos L., Alaluusua S., Ooshima T., & Matsumoto-Nakano M. (2011). Correlation of biological properties with glucan-binding protein B expression profile in Streptococcus mutans clinical isolates. *Archives of Oral Biology, 56(3),* 258–263.

Gao X., Di Wu I., Lo E. C., Chu C. H., Hsu C. Y., & Wong M. C. (2013). Validity of caries risk assessment programmes in preschool children. *Journal of Dentistry, 41(9),* 787-795.

Giertsen E., Arthur R. A., & Guggenheim B. (2010). Effects of xylitol on survival of mutans streptococci in mixed six-species in vitro biofilms modeling supragingival plaque. *Caries Research, 45(1),* 31-39.

Gross E. L., Beall C. J., Kutsch S. R., Firestone N. D., Leys E. J. & Griffen A. L. (2012). Beyond Streptococcus mutans: Dental Caries Onset Linked to Multiple Species by 16S rRNA Community Analysis. *PLoS ONE 7(10):* e47722. doi:10.1371/journal.pone.0047722

Guo L., Hu W., He X., Lux R., McLean J., & Shi W. (2013). Investigating acid production by Streptococcus mutans with a surface displayed pH-sensitive green fluorescent protein. *PLoS ONE, 8(2),* e57182.

Hallett K. B. & O'Rourke P. K. (2006). Pattern and severity of early childhood caries. *Community Dentistry and Oral Epidemiology, 34(1),* 25–35.

Hargreaves J. A., Thompson G. W., & Wagg B. J. (1983). Changes in caries prevalence of Isle of Lewis children between 1971 and 1981. *Caries Research, 17(6),* 554-559.

Harris G. S., Michalek S. M., & Curtiss R. III (1992). Cloning of a locus involved in Streptococcus mutans intracellular polysaccharide accumulation and virulence testing of an intracellular polysaccharide-deficient mutant. *Infection and Immunity, 60(8),* 3175-3185.

Hox J. (2002). Multilevel analysis: Techniques and applications. Mahwah, NJ: Lawrence Erlbaum Associates.

Igarashi T., Yamamoto A., & Goto N. (2000). PCR for detection and identification of Streptococcus sobrinus. Journal of Medical Microbiology, 49(12), 1069-1074.

Jenkinson H. F. (2011). Beyond the oral microbiome. Environmental Microbiology, Dec;13(12):3077-87.

Kanasi E., Johansson I., Lu S. C., Kressin N. R., Nunn M. E., Kent R. Jr, & Tanner A. C. (2010). Microbial risk markers for childhood caries in pediatricians' offices. Journal of Dental Research, Apr;89(4):378-83.

Lee S. H., Chi B. K., & Kim Y. J. (2012). The cariogenic characters of xylitol-resistant and xylitol-sensitive Streptococcus mutans in biofilm formation. Archives in Oral Biology, 57(6), 697-703.

Lembo F. L., Longo P. L, Ota-Tsuzuki C., Rodrigues C. R. M. D., & Mayer M. P. A. (2007). Genotypic and phenotypic analysis of Streptococcus mutans from different oral cavity sites of caries-free and caries-active children. Oral Microbiology and Immunology, 22(5), 313-319.

Lemos J,. Abranches J., & Burne R. A. (2005). Responses of cariogenic streptococci to environmental stresses. Current Issues in Molecular Biology, 7(1), 95-108.

Litt M. D., Reisine S., & Tinanoff N. (1995). Multidimensional causal model of dental caries development in low-income preschool children. Public Health Reports, 110(5), 607-617.

Madigan M. T & Martinko J. M. (2006). Brock Biology of Microorganisms 11th edition. Pearson Prentice Hall, Upper Saddle River, NJ.

Marsh P. D. (2003). Are dental diseases examples of ecological catastrophes? Microbiology, Feb;149(Pt 2):279-94.

Marsh P. D., Martin M. V., Lewis M. A., & Williams D. W. (2009). Oral Microbiology. 5th ed. Edinburgh, UK: Elsevier.

Matsui R. & Cvitkovitch D. (2010). Acid tolerance mechanisms utilized by Streptococcus mutans. Future Microbiology, 5(3), 403–417.

Milgram P., Soderling E. M., Nelson S., Chi D. L., & Nakai Y. (2012). Clinical evidence for polyol efficacy. Advances in Dental Research, 24(2), 112-116.

Mitchell S. C., Ruby J. D., Moser S., Momeni S., Smith A., Osgood R., Litaker M., & Childers N. (2009). Maternal transmission of mutans streptococci in severe-early childhood caries. Pediatric Dentistry, 31(3), 193-201.

Moraes R. S., Modesto A., dos Santos K. R. N., & Drake D. (2011). The effect of 1% chlorhexidine varnish and 40% xylitol solution on Streptococcus mutans and plaque accumulation in children. Pediatric Dentistry, 33(7), 484-490.

Mount G. J. (2007). A new paradigm for operative dentistry. Australian Dental Journal, 52(4), 264-270.

Nakano K., Matsumura M., Kawaguchi M., Fujiwara T., Sobue S., Nakagawa I., Hamada S., & Ooshima T. (2002). Attenuation of glucan-binding protein C reduces the cariogenicity of Streptococcus mutans: Analysis of strains isolated from human blood. Journal of Dental Research, 81(6), 376-379.

Nakano K., Fujita K., Nishimura K., Nomura R., & Ooshima T. (2005). Contribution of biofilm regulatory protein A of Streptococcus mutans, to systemic virulence. Microbes and Infection, 7(11-12), 1246–1255.

Napimoga M. H., Höfling J. F., Klein M. I., Kamiya R. U., & Gonçalves R. B. (2005). Transmission, diversity and virulence factors of Streptococcus mutans genotypes. Journal of Oral Science, 47(2), 59-64.

Napimoga M. H., Kamiya R. U., Rosa R. T., Rosa E. A., Hofling J. F., Mattos-Graner R. O., & Goncalves R. B. (2004). Genotypic diversity and virulence traits of Streptococcus mutans in caries-free and caries-active individuals. Journal of Medical Microbiology, 53(Pt7), 697-703.

Nguyen Q. L., Thiffeault M., & Trahan L. (1991). Adherence to hydroxyapatite, aggregation properties and hydrophobicity of xylitol-resistant S. mutans. Journal of Dental Research, 70:411.

Nicolau B., Marcenes W., Bartley M., & Sheiham A. (2003). A life course approach to assessing causes of dental caries experience: The relationship between biological, behavioural, socio-economic and psychological conditions and caries in adolescents. Caries Research, 37(5), 319-326.

Palmer E. A., Nielsen T., Peirano P., Nguyen A. T., Vo A., Nguyen A., Jackson S., Finlayson T., Sauerwein R., Marsh K., Edwards I., Wilmot B., Engle J., Peterson J., Maier T., & Machida C. A. (2012a). Children with severe early childhood caries: pilot study examining mutans streptococci genotypic strains after full-mouth caries restorative therapy. Pediatric Dentistry, 34(2), e1-e10.

Palmer E. A., Vo A., Hiles S. B., Peirano P., Chaudhry S., Trevor A., Kasimi I., Pollard J., Kyles C., Leo M., Wilmot B., Engle J., Peterson J., Maier T., & Machida C. A. (2012b). Mutans streptococci genetic strains in children with severe early childhood caries: follow-up study at one-year post-dental rehabilitation therapy. Journal of Oral Microbiology, 4 (e-pub); doi, 10.3402.

Peterson S. N., Snesrud E., Liu J., Ong A. C., Kilian M., Schork N. J. & Bretz W. (2013). The Dental Plaque Microbiome in Health and Disease. PLoS ONE 8(3): e58487. doi:10.1371/journal.pone.0058487

Pieralisi F. J., Rodriques M. R., Segura V. G., Maciel S. M., Ferreira F. B. A., Garcia J. E., & Poli-Federico R. C. (2010). Genotypic diversity of Streptococcus mutans in caries-free and caries-active preschool children. International Journal of Dentistry, e-pub.

Poggio C., Arciola C. R., Rosti F., Scribante A., Saino E., & Visai L. (2009). Adhesion of Streptococcus mutans to different restorative materials. The International Journal of Artificial Organs, 32(9), 671-677.

Ramos-Gomez F. (2006). Bacterial salivary markers' role in ECC risk assessment in infants. Journal of Dental Research, 85B, poster 0516.

Ramos-Gomez F., Crystal Y. O., Doméjean S., & Featherstone J. D. (2012). Minimal intervention dentistry: part 3. Paediatric dental care-prevention and management protocols using caries risk assessment for infants and young children. British Dental Journal, 213(10), 501-508.

Ramos-Gomez F., Crystal Y. O., Ng M., Crall J., & Featherstone J. D. (2010). Pediatric dental care: Prevention and Management Protocols based on caries risk assessment. Journal of California Dental Association, 38(10), 746-761.

Ramos-Gomez F. & Ng M. (2011). Into the future: keeping teeth caries free: pediatric CAMBRA Protocols. Journal of California Dental Association, 39(10):723-733.

Raudenbush S. W. & Bryk A. S. (2002). Hierarchical linear models: Applications and data analysis method. (2nd ed). Newbury Park, CA: Sage.

Ribelles L. M., Guinot J. F., Mayné A. R., & Bellet D. L. (2010). Effects of xylitol chewing gum on salivary flow rate, pH, buffering capacity and presence of Streptococcus mutans in saliva. European Journal of Paediatric Dentistry, 11(1), 9-14.

Seki M., Yamashita Y., Shibata Y., Torigoe H., Tsuda H., & Maeno M. (2006). Effect of mixed mutans streptococci colonization on caries development. Oral Microbiology Immunology, 21(1), 47-52.

Shemesh M., Tam A., & Steinberg D. (2007). Expression of biofilm-associated genes of Streptococcus mutans in response to glucose and sucrose. Journal of Medical Microbiology, 56(Pt 11), 1528-1535.

Skrondal A. & Rabe-Hesketh S. (2004). Generalized latent variable modeling: Multilevel, longitudinal and structural equation models. Boca Raton, FL: Chapman & Hall/CRC.

Socransky S. S. & Haffajee A. D. (2005). Periodontal microbial ecology. Periodontology 2000, 38:135-87.

Söderling E. M. (2009). Xylitol, mutans streptococci, and dental plaque. Advances in Dental Research, 21(1), 74-78.

Söderling E. M., Ekman T. C., & Taipale T. J. (2008). Growth inhibition of Streptococcus mutans with low xylitol concentrations. Current Microbiology, 56(4), 382-385.

Söderling E., Isokangas P., Pienikakkinen K., & Tenovuo J. (1996). Xylitol vs. chlorohexidine as reducers of mother-child transmission of mutans streptococci. Journal of Dental Research, 75 Abstract 1384.

Söderling E. & Trahan L. (1992). Altered agglutination pattern of xylitol-resistant S. mutans 10449 cells. Journal of Dental Research, 71:734.

Söderling E., Trahan L., Tammiala-Salonen T., & Hakkinen L. (1997). Effects of xylitol, xylitol-sorbitol, and placebo chewing gums on the plaque of habitual xylitol consumers. European Journal of Oral Sciences, 105(2), 170-177.

Stookey G. K. (1990). Critical evaluation of the composition and use of topical fluorides. Journal of Dental Research, 69, Spec No. 805-812.

Svensater G., Larsson U. B., Greif E. C., Cvitkovitch D. G., & Hamilton I. R. (1997). Acid tolerance response and survival by oral bacteria. Oral Microbiology and Immunology, 12(5), 266-273.

Tabchoury C. P. M., Sousa M. C. K., Arthur R. A., Mattos-Graner R. O., Del Bel Cury A. A., & Cury J. A. (2008). Evaluation of genotypic diversity of Streptococcus mutans using distinct arbitrary primers. Journal of Applied Oral Science, 16(6), 403-407.

Tanaka K., Miyake Y., Sasaki S., & Hiroka Y. (2013). Infant feeding practices and risk of dental caries in Japan: the Osaka Maternal And Child Health Study. Pediatric Dentistry, 35(3), 267-271.

Tassery H., Levallois B., Terrer E., Manton D. J., Otsuki M., Koubi S., Gugnani N., Panayotov I., Jacquot B., Cuisinier F., & Rechmann P. (2013). Use of new minimum intervention dentistry technologies in caries management. Australian Dental Journal, 58(Supp 1), 40-59.

Ten Cate J. M. & Featherstone J. D. (1991). Mechanistic aspects of the interactions between fluoride and dental enamel. Critical Reviews in Oral Biology and Medicine, 2(2), 283-296.

Trahan L., Bourgeau G., & Breton R. (1996). Emergence of multiple xylitol-resistant (fructose PTS-) mutants from human isolates of mutans streptococci during growth on dietary sugars in the presence of xylitol. Journal of Dental Research, 75(11), 1892-1900.

Trahan L. & Mouton C. (1987). Selection for Streptococcus mutans with an altered xylitol transport capacity in chronic xylitol consumers. Journal of Dental Research, 66(5), 982-988.

Trahan L., Soderling E., Dréan M. F., Chevrier M. C., & Isokangas P. (1992). Effect of xylitol consumption on the plaque-saliva distribution of mutans streptococci and the occurrence and long-term survival of xylitol-resistant strains. Journal of Dental Research, 71(11), 1785-1791.

Waler S. M. & Rølla G. (1990). Xylitol, mechanisms of action and uses. Nor Tannlaeqeforen Tid, 100(4), 140-143.

Wen Z. T. & Burne R. A. (2004). LuxS-mediated signaling in Streptococcus mutans is involved in regulation of acid and oxidative stress tolerance and biofilm formation. Journal of Bacteriology, 186(9), 2682–2691.

Woo PC-Y., Fung AM-Y., Lau SK-P., Chan BY-L., Chiu S-K., Teng JL-L., Que T-L., Yung RW-H., & Yuen K-Y. (2003). Granulicatella adiacens and Abiotrophia defectiva bacteraemia characterized by 16S rRNA gene sequencing. Journal of Medical Microbiology, 52(Pt 2), 137-140.

Yoon R. K., Smaldone A. M., & Edelstein B. L. (2012). Early childhood caries screening tool. A comparison of four approaches. Journal of American Dental Association, 143(7), 756-763.

Zafar S., Harnekar S. Y., & Siddiqi A. (2009). Early childhood caries: etiology, clinical considerations, consequences and management. International Dentistry SA, 11(4), 24-36.

Zero D., Fontana M., & Lennon A. M. (2001). Clinical applications and outcomes of using indicators of risk in caries management. Journal of Dental Education, 65(10), 1126-1132.

Zero D. T. (2006). Dentrifices, mouthwashes, and remineralization/caries arrestment strategies. BioMed Central Oral Health, 15(6)(Suppl 1), 1:S9.

Zhan L., Cheng J., Chang P., Ngo M., DenBesten P. K., Hoover C. I., & Featherstone J. D. (2012). Effects of xylitol wipes on cariogenic bacteria and caries in young children. Journal of Dental Research, 91(Suppl 5), 85S-90S.

Dietary Evidence from a Dental Practice-based Research Network

Yoko Yokoyama
Japan Society for the Promotion of Science
Graduate School of Media and Governance
Keio University, Japan

Naoki Kakudate
Educational Cooperation Center
Kyushu Dental University, Japan

Futoshi Sumida
Mikami Dental & Orthodontics Clinic, Japan

Yuki Matsumoto
Matsumoto Dental Clinic, Japan

1   Introduction

According to both the Centers for Disease Control and Prevention (CDC) and the World Health Organization (WHO), dental caries is the most common chronic disease affecting children and adolescents (World Health Organization, 2012; Centers for Disease Control and Prevention, 2012). Indeed, dental caries affects 60–90% of school-aged children and almost 100% of adults. As oral health is essential for general health and quality of life, the high prevalence of this disease is concerning, and highlights the importance of applying public health approaches to the prevention of dental caries.

Dietary factors are important and modifiable factors in the prevention of dental caries. The potential public health role of general dental practitioners in providing lifestyle advice to their patients has also been recognized as an important factor (Dyer & Robinson, 2006). Previous studies have provided evidence that one-to-one dietary interventions in the dental setting can change the dietary behavior of practitioners and patients (Harris, Gamboa, Dailey, & Ashcroft, 2012). The American Dietetic Association recommends collaboration between dietitians and dental professionals for oral health promotion and disease prevention and intervention (Touger-Decker & Mobley, 2007). However, the evidence regarding the association between diet and dental caries is limited. One possible reason is the private nature of most dental practices, which creates a barrier to the collection of large-scale data.

In overcoming this barrier, the new research model, termed the dental practice-based research network (Dental PBRN), holds great potential in enabling larger-scale clinical research. Dental practice-based research is a form of research conducted in clinical practices by dental practitioners and their staff. It is designed to resolve the issues faced by dental clinicians during the routine care of their patients. This chapter aims to describe and explore this new research model by 1) reviewing the current dietary evidence collected from clinical epidemiology research, 2) describing the Dental PBRN, and 3) presenting the results from research conducted using the Dental PBRN model.

2   Review of Evidence Regarding Dietary Intake and Dental Caries

This section provides an overview of the evidence regarding an association between dietary/nutritional patterns and the development of dental caries, which is largely a preventable disease (Balakrishnan, Simmonds, & Tagg, 2000; Rank, Julien, & Lyman, 1983; Reich, Lussi, & Newbrun, 1999). According to Zero *et al.*, dental caries development is a dynamic dietomicrobial disease involving cycles of demineralization and remineralization (Zero *et al.*, 2009). The early stages of this process are reversible by modifying or eliminating etiologic factors (e.g., modifying diet and/or removing plaque biofilm), and increasing exposure to protective factors (e.g., fluoride) and/or salivary flow (Zero, *et al.*, 2009). This chapter focuses on the role of dietary factors in dental caries development.

Table 1 shows the results of a WHO analysis of the evidence linking diet to dental caries development (Moynihan, 2005). As can be observed, the factors with the strongest evidence for a link to an increase in caries development are frequent intake of free sugars and intake of a high amount of free sugars, followed by undernutrition. The factor with the strongest evidence for a link to a decrease in caries development is fluoride exposure, followed by consumption of hard cheese and chewing of sugar-free gum. Further, there may be a link between a decrease in caries development and consumption of xylitol, milk, and dietary fiber. When focusing on food, intake of sugars (increased caries development), dairy foods (decreased caries development), and dietary fiber (decreased caries development) might relate to dental caries development. This section briefly reviews the findings which WHO's report focused on regarding these dietary factors although association between dental caries and other dietary factors such as vitamin D (Hujoel PP, 2013; Grant WB, Boucher BJ, 2011; Grant WB, 2011) were pointed out.

Evidence[*]	Convincing	Probable	Possible
Increased caries risk	Sugars (intake amount and frequency)		Undernutrition
Decreased caries risk		Dairy (hard cheese)	Dairy (milk) Dietary fiber

Table 1: Summary of the strength of evidence regarding the link between dietary factors and dental caries development (the modified WHO report;(Moynihan, 2005))

2.1   Intake of Sugars

Here, the term "sugars" refer to all monosaccharides and disaccharides, while the term "sugar" refers only to sucrose. The WHO report pointed out the existence of a wealth of evidence from many different types of investigations, including human studies, animal experiments, and experimental studies both in vivo and in vitro, showing the role of dietary sugars in the etiology of dental caries (Moynihan, 2005).

Several randomized controlled trials (RCTs) have been conducted to clarify the amount and frequency of consumption of sugars that affects the development of dental caries. The Vipeholm study, which was conducted in an adult mental institution in Sweden between 1945 and 1953 (Gustafsson, 1952), revealed that increased frequency of consumption of sugars between meals is associated with higher risk of dental caries, and suggested that an increase in dental caries development disappears upon a decrease in consumption of sugar-rich foods. The Turku RCT, a study of adults in Finland in the 1970s, found that an almost total substitution of sucrose in the diet with xylitol, a non-cariogenic sweetener, resulted in an 85% reduction in dental caries over a 2-year period (Scheinin, Makinen, & Ylitalo, 1976). Several animal studies and longitudinal studies have also indicated a relationship between amount of sugars consumed and dental caries development (Burt *et al.*, 1988; Hefti & Schmid, 1979; Kleemola-Kujala & Rasanen, 1982). Nevertheless, whether the frequency or amount of sugars consumed is a stronger factor in dental caries development remains unclear: both factors appear to be important (Moynihan, 2005).

One limitation while comparing the results of RCTs conducted several decades ago to the results of recent studies is that a proportion of the current population has adequate exposure to fluoride (Burt &

---

[*] Evidence level is defined by WHO as follows: **Convincing evidence**: Evidence based on epidemiological studies showing consistent associations between exposure and disease, with little or no evidence to the contrary. The available evidence is based on a substantial number of studies including prospective observational studies and where relevant, randomized controlled trials of sufficient size, duration and quality showing consistent effects. The association should be biologically plausible. **Probable evidence**: Evidence based on epidemiological studies showing fairly consistent associations between exposure and disease, but where there are perceived shortcomings in the available evidence or some evidence to the contrary, which precludes a more definite judgement. Shortcomings in the evidence may be any of the following: insufficient duration of trials (or studies); insufficient trials (or studies) available; inadequate sample sizes; incomplete follow-up. Laboratory evidence is usually supportive. Again the association should be biologically plausible. **Possible evidence**: Evidence based mainly on findings from case--control and cross-sectional studies. Insufficient randomized controlled trials, observational studies or non-randomized controlled trials are available. Evidence based on non-epidemiological studies, such as clinical and laboratory investigations, is supportive. More trials are required to support the tentative associations, which should also be biologically plausible.

Pai, 2001). Since it would not be possible to conduct RCTs to investigate how consumption of sugars affects dental caries today because of ethical issues, Burt and Pai conducted a systematic review that investigated the importance of intake of sugars in caries etiology in populations exposed to fluoride. Based on their findings, they concluded that consumption of sugars is a moderate risk factor for caries development in most people who have adequate exposure to fluoride, and a more powerful risk factor in people who do not have regular exposure to fluoride (Burt & Pai, 2001). Thus, restriction of the consumption of sugars remains a factor in the prevention of caries in situations where there is widespread exposure to fluoride, although it is not as strong a factor as where there is not widespread exposure to fluoride (Burt & Pai, 2001).

2.2   Hard Cheese Intake

The WHO report categorizes hard cheese intake as a "probable" factor in decreasing caries development (Moynihan, 2005). Stimulation of salivary flow, inhibition of plaque bacteria, and delivery of high amounts of calcium and inorganic phosphate have been suggested as the possible mechanisms by which hard cheese intake reduces cariogenicity (Kashket & DePaola, 2002). To explore the in-situ rehardening effect of hard cheese, Gedalia et al. and Sela et al. (Gedalia, Davidov, Lewinstein, & Shapira, 1992; Sela et al., 1994) intraorally exposed vitro-etched enamel slabs prepared from human teeth to 1 of 2 substances for 5 minutes: 1) parafilm-stimulated salivary secretions or 2) cheese compounds and saliva resulting from mastication of 20 g of hard cheese (Sela, et al., 1994). Their results suggested a significantly higher level of rehardening in the group that consumed cheese.

Only a few clinical studies have attempted to clarify the association between hard cheese intake and dental caries development. In a 2-year observational study in the United Kingdom comparing 65 children who developed no caries with 71 children with the highest 2-year caries increment ($\geq$7 decayed missing filled teeth: DMFS), Rugg-Gunn et al. found that mean daily cheese intake was not associated with dental caries development (Rugg-Gunn, Hackett, Appleton, Jenkins, & Eastoe, 1984). The relationship between hard cheese intake and dental caries development reached statistical significance when they limited 19 children who had been caries-free at the beginning of the study and had developed no caries lesions during the study and the 23 children who had the highest caries experience ($\geq$ 20 DMFS). Moreover, the researchers did not adjust for possible demographic and behavioral confounders such as tooth brushing frequency, use of fluoride, and between-meal snack frequency (Rugg-Gunn, et al., 1984). In addition, because they did not present the data regarding other categories, the existence of a dose-response relationship cannot be determined from a review of the findings. The results of a recent observational study of 2,058 Japanese children aged 3 years who participated in the Fukuoka Child Health Study (Tanaka, Miyake, & Sasaki, 2010) suggest no association between hard cheese intake and the prevalence of dental caries when the results are adjusted for sex, tooth brushing frequency, use of fluoride, between-meal snack frequency, maternal smoking during pregnancy, environmental tobacco smoke exposure at home, and paternal and maternal education levels (Tanaka, Miyake, & Sasaki, 2010). Therefore, the evidence that hard cheese intake has a protective effect on dental caries development in children is scarce.

The evidence suggesting the protective effects of hard cheese intake on dental caries development in adults is also scarce. In a study of the association between both root and coronal caries development and hard cheese intake in an aging population in the United States (Papas, Joshi, Palmer, Giunta, & Dwyer, 1995), Papas et al. found that high intake of cheese was negatively associated with caries development, independent of sugar consumption. However, they focused only on the lower quartile of adults with root caries and filled surfaces (DFS)/100 teeth (N = 13) and the upper quartile of adults with root

DFS/100 teeth (N = 16) (Papas, *et al.*, 1995). Therefore, the evidence regarding a linear relationship between the frequency of cheese intake and dental caries development in adults is weak.

In summary, the evidence regarding the preventive effects of hard cheese intake on dental caries development is weak and scarce in both children and aging adults. Further studies must examine this relationship using a prospective design, larger sample size, and adjusted with confounder.

2.3   Dietary Fiber Intake

According to the WHO report, intake of dietary fiber is categorized as a possibly preventive factor in decreasing caries development (Moynihan, 2005). In a survey of the association between dietary fiber and dental experience in 12- and 13-year-old participants (N = 592) in South Korea, Kwon *et al.* examined (Kwon *et al.*, 1997) the effect of nutrient intake on dental caries development by logistic regression analysis while controlling for other variables such as sex, pit and fissure retentiveness, resazurin disk test results, and intake of other dietary factors (Kwon, *et al.*, 1997). They found that both total caries development and occlusal caries development are significantly negatively correlated with the amount of daily dietary fiber intake (Kwon, *et al.*, 1997). However, stronger evidence of the association between dietary fiber intake and caries development, ideally from a prospective cohort study, is required to confirm this correlation.

2.4   Dietary Patterns

We reviewed the associations between dietary intake of individual foods or nutrients and dental caries. However, Hu et al. pointed out that the results of such analysis can be difficult to interpret because people do not consume nutrients in isolation; hence, strong correlations between various foods and nutrients may be identified (Hu, 2002). In contrast, the collinearity of nutrients or foods can be an advantage in dietary pattern analysis because patterns are characterized on the basis of habitual food use (Hu, 2002). In addition, dietary interventions may be easier to implement and more comprehensive when initiated as changes in the overall dietary pattern (Hu, 2002).

Component	Examples	Direction
Nutrient	Carbohydrates, protein, fat, vitamin, etc.	
Food	Whole grains, dairy, fruits, vegetables, beans, etc.	
Dietary pattern	"The Mediterranean diet," "the prudent diet," "the Dietary Approach to Stop Hypertension (DASH)," a "plant-based diet," a "vegetarian diet," etc.	Closer to real-world pattern of combined consumption of nutrients and foods, allowing for investigation of their synergetic effects

Table 2: Level of exposure in nutritional epidemiology

Using data from the US Third National Health and Nutrition Examination Survey (NHANES III) Nunn et al. attempted to clarify the relationship between dietary patterns and caries experience (Nunn *et al.*, 2009). When they examined the relationship between dietary quality as measured by the Healthy Eating Index (HEI) and the prevalence of early childhood caries (ECC) in 2- to 5-year-old children (N = 3,912), they found that children with the best dietary practices were 44% less likely to exhibit severe

ECC than children with worst dietary practices when the results were adjusted by demographic and be-havioral characteristics (Nunn *et al.*, 2009). A healthy diet has also been linked to improvements in con-ditions such as hypertension (Chobanian *et al.*, 2003), diabetes (Alhazmi *et al.*, 2012), cardiovascular disease (Mente, de Koning, Shannon, & Anand, 2009; Yang *et al.*, 2012), and cancer (Doll & Peto, 1981; Kushi *et al.*, 2012; Palacios, Joshipura, & Willett, 2009). Use of an approach analyzing dietary patterns may allow for clarification of the associations between dietary intake and development of dental caries as well as other chronic diseases. As the dietary advice provided regarding general development and well-being needs to be integrated into oral health counseling (Nunn, *et al.*, 2009), further studies are needed to clarify the relationship between dietary patterns and dental caries.

2.5   Summary of Evidence Regarding Diet and Caries

In summary, this section reviewed the evidence regarding the association between caries development and diet, nutrition, and dietary patterns. Except for the amount and frequency of intake of sugars, little evidence exists based on which recommendations for the intake of particular foods or use of dietary pat-terns can be made to prevent caries development. Further research using a well-designed epidemiological research design and a dietary pattern-level approach that approximates "real-world" dietary patterns is required. Also, since caries is multifactorial disease (Bratthall D, *et al.*, 2005), further research on interac-tion between dietary factors and other factors is needed.

3   The Practice-based Research Network: A New Research Model

3.1   Practice-based Research

Practice-based research is a form of research conducted in clinical practices by practitioners and their staff that is designed to answer the questions that clinicians face in the routine care of their patients (Kakudate N, in press). Practice-based research holds great potential for answering clinical questions and expediting the translation of research findings into clinical practice. In conducting such research, the study of PBRNs offers unique advantages in fostering both research and quality improvement and infor-mation sharing among practitioners (Gilbert GH. & for the DPBRN Collaborative Group, 2009).

3.2   Dental Practice-based Research Networks

Since 2000, the Agency for Healthcare Research and Quality (AHRQ) has devoted funding to support primary care PBRNs in the United States. Currently, more than 150 PBRNs other than dental networks are operating in the United States (AHRQ Website). In the dental research area, the National Institute for Dental and Craniofacial Research (NIDCR) has funded 3 dental PBRNs in the United States since 2005 with approximately $75 million: the Dental Practice-Based Research Network (DPBRN), Practitioners Engaged in Applied Research and Learning PEARL (PEARL), and the Northwest Practice-based Re-search Collaborative in Evidence-based Dentistry (PRECEDENT). In 2012, the NIDCR decided to pro-vide a new grant that consolidates its dental practice-based research network. Upon receiving funding of approximately $66.8 million, the DPBRN established the National Dental Practice-Based Research Net-work (the National Dental PBRN) (National Dental PBRN Website), which has been headquartered at the University of Alabama at the Birmingham School of Dentistry for 7 years. According to its website, the National Dental PBRN plans to expand the number of participating practitioners to 5,000 and welcomes the greater participation of practitioners in the various dental subspecialties to develop innovative, low-cost techniques to improve the oral health of all Americans (National Dental PBRN Website). Since 2005, the National Dental PBRN has conducted more than 20 research studies, generating more than 70 peer-reviewed journal articles on topics ranging from preventive and restorative dentistry to temporo-mandibular muscle and joint disorders.

In 2010, we established the Dental PBRN Japan (JDPBRN; Kakudate N, in press; Kakudate *et al.*, 2012; Dental PBRN Japan Website). Currently, the only network in an Asian country, our network has been acknowledged by the US AHRQ as an international network. The aims of the JDPBRN include the following: 1) building research networks in which dental practitioners are the main actors, 2) sharing information on clinical research that will have a beneficial impact on routine dental practice, 3) participating in international collaborative research and presenting evidence globally, 4) enabling dental professionals to participate in clinical studies to solve their clinical questions, 5) changing dental professionals' views of their daily dental practice and making their practice more interesting, and 6) contributing to the overall health of patients globally by improving the quality of dental practice (Kakudate N, in press). The JDPBRN is a consortium of dental practices with a broad representation of practice types, treatment philosophies, and patient populations that share the DPBRN's mission (Gilbert *et al.*, 2008) that is now called the National Dental PBRN (National Dental PBRN Website). The network regions of the JDPBRN represent all 7 districts in Japan (Hokkaido, Tohoku, Kanto, Chubu, Kansai, Chugoku-Shikoku, and Kyushu). In 2011, we initiated the first international collaborative study with the US National Dental PBRN entitled "Assessment of Caries Diagnosis and Caries Treatment." Our previous research results had revealed country-based variations in the proportion of dentists who indicated surgical intervention in patients at high risk of caries development when the interproximal cavity was located within the enamel. Specifically, we found that the proportion of dentists who indicated surgical intervention in the enamel lesions was as follows: Scandinavia, 21%; the United States, 75%; and Japan, 74%. Thus, most JDPBRN dentists indicated that they would restore lesions within the enamel in individuals at high risk of caries. As a first step to improve clinical decision-making, the results of our studies should be reported to the dentists for the purpose of self-assessment of their daily dental practice. Comparison of dental practice patterns will also promote the assessment of each country's dental health care system and dental education.

Through these research activities, we aim to achieve the following goals: 1) contribute to evidence construction by collaboration with dental clinicians and clinical epidemiologists, 2) improve health care system and policies, 3) create a community of clinicians with a research inclination, and 4) establish a new style of continuing education with the objectives of self-assessment of individual practices and presentation of updates regarding the latest dental information. We anticipate that the achievement of these goals will lead to dietary behavioral modification among the clinicians and improvements in the quality of dental care using feedback from the research results.

3.3   Research Steps in Dental Practice-based Research Networks

The PBRN is a new model of epidemiological research. Figure 1 shows that the following steps were used in introducing the research steps in the Dental PBRN in Japan: 1) proposal of a research question based on dental practice; 2) preparation of a protocol and application for approval from the Ethical Review Board; 3) officially beginning data collection within the entire network upon approval of the Ethical Review Board; 4) obtaining of data collected from patients or medical records from each dental clinic for data analysis by the Data Analysis Staff of Research Committee of the JDPBRN; 5) upon completion of data analysis, collection of the results for presentation at conferences at local, national, or international scientific societies by the principal investigator (PI) or the writing of papers by the PI for eventual publication; and 6) presentation of the results to the network members for improving their daily dental practice. By completing these steps, research data are produced that each member can compare with data from his or her own clinic to develop routine practice, which will generate additional ideas for further research as part of a research cycle.

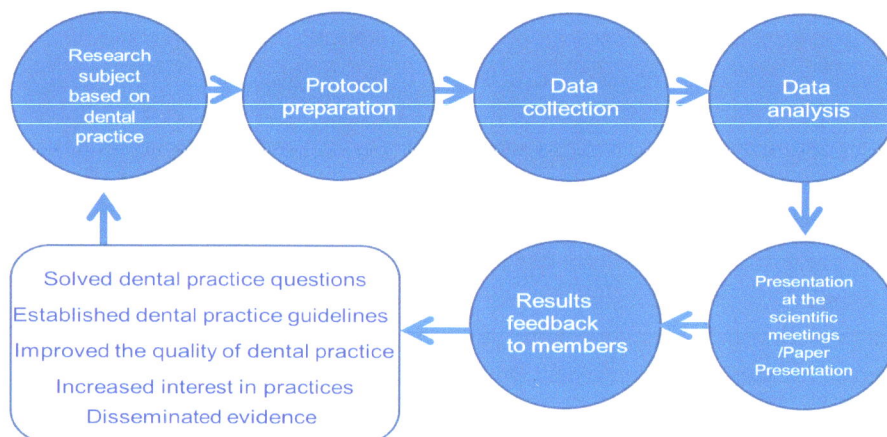

Figure 1: JDPBRN Research Cycle (http://www.dentalpbrn.jp/category/1445790.html)

4   Practice Patterns Regarding Dental Caries Prevention and Dietary Counseling

This section provides an overview of the evidence regarding the practice patterns and practitioner's overall perceptions of dental caries prevention as well as dietary counseling based on the new PBRN research model.

4.1   Practice Patterns in Dental Caries Prevention

Dentists' practice patterns and perceptions regarding caries prevention and dietary counseling and the factors that affect these patterns remain unclear. Fortunately, the recent establishment of the JDPBRN created an opportunity to conduct international comparisons of these patterns and perceptions. To assess dentists' perceptions of the importance of diet and their practice patterns regarding dietary counseling as well as collect patient, practice, and dentist background data, we conducted a cross-sectional survey in Japan between May 2011 and February 2012 (Kakudate, *et al.*, 2012). We used the same questionnaire as that used in the US DPBRN Study, "Assessment of Caries Diagnosis and Caries Treatment" (Gordan *et al.*, 2009), and the DPBRN Enrollment Questionnaire (Makhija *et al.*, 2009). Table 3 shows the variables examined and the questionnaire items used to collect data regarding the variables.

Variable	Questionnaire item
Prevalence of preventive dentistry	What percentage of patient contact time do you (not your hygienist or other office staff) spend performing prevention-related care (i.e., sealant adhesion, periodic and hygiene examination, diagnostic procedures, and other preventive dentistry procedures)?
Perception of preventive dentistry	How strongly do you agree with the following statement: "A dentist's assessment of caries risk for an individual patient can predict whether or not that patient develops new caries in the future"? (1) strongly disagree, (2) somewhat disagree, (3) neither agree nor disagree, (4) somewhat agree, (5) strongly agree
Factors associated with promoting preventive dentistry	(1) dentists' individual characteristics, (2) practice setting, (3) patients' characteristics, (4) procedure-related characteristics
Prevalence of dietary counseling	What is the percentage of patients to whom you or your staff provided dietary counseling at some time?
Perception of dietary counseling	For patients aged more than 18 years, how important is consideration of diet when you decide on a treatment plan? (1) not at all important, (2) slightly important, (3) moderately important, (4) very important, (5) extremely important
Factors associated with promoting dietary counseling	(1) dentists' individual characteristics, (2) practice setting, (3) patients' characteristics, (4) procedure-related characteristics

Table 3: Variables examined and questionnaire items used to collect data in the JDPBRN study

4.2   Practice Patterns Regarding Dental Caries Prevention

We conducted research to (1) clarify dentists' practice patterns regarding caries-preventive dentistry, (2) clarify dentists' perceptions of caries-preventive dentistry, and (3) test the hypothesis that certain dentists' characteristics are associated with these practice patterns (Yokoyama *et al.*, 2013a). According to the study results, 72 (38%) participants reported that they provide individualized caries prevention to 50% or more of their patients ("more preventive group"). Overall, the participants reported that they spend 10% of daily practice time on prevention-related care. In a survey using the same questionnaire by the US DPBRN, 52% of patients reported receiving individualized caries prevention (Gordan *et al.,* 2011; Riley *et al.*, 2011). The results of this study suggest that dentists in the US DPBRN (52%) and JDPBRN (41.3%) have similar tendencies in providing individualized caries prevention, but the proportion of those who do so is lower in Japan than that in the United States. Additionally, they revealed that Japanese dentists spend 10% of their daily practice time on prevention-related care, a percentage that is lower than that reported among Northern European dentists. Specifically, a previous study conducted in Norway reported that the mean percentage of time devoted to caries prevention is 16.6% of the total treatment time (dentists who did not treat adult patients were excluded;(Haugejorden & Nielsen, 1987) and 22% of the total time for pediatric patients (Wang & Aspelund, 2010).

In Denmark, Iceland, and Norway, providing caries prevention treatment constitutes 18–50% of the dentist's total time in providing dental care to children and adolescents (Wang, Kalletstal, Petersen, & Arnadottir, 1998). In the United States, the average percentage of total time that general practitioners spend performing preventive procedures increased from 9.4% in 1981 to 12.4% in 1993 (Brown & Lazar, 1998). The lower percentage of time devoted to preventive treatment in Japan may be due to differences between the health care systems of Northern Europe and Japan. In Finland, all inhabitants aged less than

19 years have been entitled to free comprehensive public dental care since 1999, resulting in a utilization rate of approximately 95% (Helminen & Vehkalahti, 2003). In contrast, as the Japanese dental insurance system mainly covers dental treatment (Miyazaki & Morimoto, 1996), the percentage of time spent on providing preventive treatment in Japan might be restricted for economic reasons.

The majority of participants (67%) in our study agreed that performing caries risk assessment is effective for prediction of future caries increment (Yokoyama *et al.*, 2013a). This percentage is consistent with those reported by previous studies, including a study by the US DPBRN using the same questionnaire, which reported that 77% of dentists agree with the effectiveness of caries risk assessment. The results of multiple logistic regression analysis suggest that following variables are associated with whether or not dentists provide individualized caries prevention to 50% or more of their patients (Yokoyama *et al.*, 2013a). Specifically, we found that the percentage of patients interested in caries prevention and the percentage of patients who receive hygiene instruction are significantly associated with a high percentage of patients who receive individualized caries prevention. Our study clarified that a high percentage of patients with a positive perception of preventive dentistry (as measured by the percentage interested in caries prevention) and a high percentage who receive hygiene instruction in a practice are associated with the use of individualized caries prevention by a higher percentage of patients. In a study using the same questionnaire, the US DPBRN found that dentists' individual characteristics, practice settings, and dental procedures are associated with providing individualized caries prevention to a greater percentage of patients. These findings concur with those of Brennan *et al.*, who noted that dentists' individual characteristics, dentists' practice settings, and patient characteristics influence the pattern of preventive care delivered (Brennan & Spencer, 2005). Our model also revealed that dentists' individual characteristics, their practice settings, the dental procedures that they perform, and their perceptions of their patients' preference for preventive care are more strongly related to the pattern of preventive care delivered than those factors. A previous systematic review noted that potential barriers to adherence to physicians' guidelines included dentists' and patients' preferences (Cabana *et al.*, 1999; Cochrane *et al.*, 2007). As Cabana *et al.* noted, potential barriers to adherence to physicians' guidelines vary according to the topic (Cabana, *et al.*, 1999), and it is possible that dentists' ratings of patient preferences are strongly related to the practice of preventive dentistry.

We also identified substantial variation in dentists' practice patterns regarding caries preventive dentistry in our study population. Specifically, we found that the provision of individualized caries prevention is significantly related to a dentist's provision of other preventive services and to a high percentage of patients interested in prevention, but not to a dentist's beliefs regarding the effectiveness of caries risk assessment.

Variable	Summary
Prevalence of preventive dentistry	1) 38% of dentists surveyed (N = 72) reported providing individualized caries prevention care to 50% or more of their patients. 2) The dentists surveyed spend a mean of 10% of the total daily practice time in providing prevention-related care.
Perception of preventive dentistry	Among dentists, 67% agree that caries risk assessment is effective.
Factors associated with promoting preventive dentistry	1) Percentage of dental patients interested in receiving caries prevention care 2) Percentage of dental patients who receive hygiene instruction

Table 4: Summary of evidence (Yokoyama, et al., 2013a)

4.3   Practice Patterns in Dietary Counseling

Previous studies have provided evidence that one-to-one dietary interventions in the dental setting can change the dietary behavior of practitioners and patients (Harris, *et al.*, 2012). In accordance, the American Dietetic Association recommends collaboration between dieticians and dental professionals for oral health promotion and disease prevention and intervention (Touger-Decker & Mobley, 2007). Kakudate *et al.* showed that administering dietary counseling is significantly associated with appropriate interproximal enamel surgical intervention: specifically, that dentists who provide dietary counseling tend not to intervene surgically into enamel carious lesions, an approach that is consistent with evidence-based dental treatment (Kakudate, *et al.*, 2012). Although Kelly *et al.* reported that few dentists or other dental professionals conduct dietary counseling as a key component of regular patient care (Kelly & Moynihan, 2008), dentists' dietary perceptions and practice patterns regarding dietary counseling remain unclear.

To clarify Japanese dentists' perceptions and practices, we conducted a cross-sectional survey of the JDPBRN (Yokoyama, *et al.*, 2013b) to identify dentists' practice patterns regarding dietary counseling, dentists' perceptions of dietary counseling, and characteristics associated with dentists' provision of dietary counseling. We found that the majority of the participants (n = 116, 63%) categorized into "more important" group when they decide on a caries treatment plan. However, less than half (n = 56, 48%) who indicated that diet is "more important" reported that they provide dietary counseling to more than 20% of their patients.

The proportion of Japanese dentists who reported placing high value on the importance of diet when deciding on a treatment plan (63%) in our study is consistent with that found in previous studies. According to the results of a study conducted by the US DPBRN using the same questionnaire, 67% of male and 72% of female dentists agree that consideration of a patient's diet is very or extremely important when deciding on a treatment plan (Riley, Gordan, Rouisse, McClelland, & Gilbert, 2011). In a United Kingdom study, Kelly *et al.* noted that 66% of British dentists agree that nutrition plays an important role in the maintenance of periodontal health (Kelly & Moynihan, 2008). These studies revealed that over 60% of dentists in the United States, the United Kingdom, and Japan recognize the importance of diet.

However, only about 20% of patients would receive diet counseling in this study (Yokoyama, *et al.*, 2013b). This low rate of dietary counseling practice patterns in dental clinics. This low percentage is consistent with that reported by other studies, including a study conducted by Kelly *et al.*, which found that only 14% of dentists or other dental professionals provided dietary advice as a regular part of patient care (Kelly & Moynihan, 2008). In accordance, Touger-Decker *et al.* reported that perceived needs for nutrition education in dental school are high, with most respondents in their study indicating a need for graduates of dental school programs to know how and when to conduct a nutritional assessment (Touger-Decker, Barracato, & O'Sullivan-Maillet, 2001). These findings indicate that increasing the administration of dietary counseling in dental settings depends on the provision of appropriate education to dentists.

The results of multiple logistic regression analysis in our study suggest that several variables are associated with a dentist's tendency to provide dietary counseling (Yokoyama, *et al.*, 2013b). Specifically, the sex of the dentist, the level of practice activity (i.e., the dentist's "busyness"), whether the dentist performs caries risk assessment, the perceptions of the dentist regarding patient interest in preventive programs, the percentage of the dentist's patients interested in caries prevention, and the percentage of the dentist's patients receiving blood pressure screening were all found to be significantly associated with providing dietary counseling. Previous studies reported that lack of willingness of a patient to undergo screening, the costs of screening in term of money and time, and the liability associated with screening are perceived barriers to the performance of medical screening in dental practices (Greenberg, Glick, Frantsve-Hawley, & Kantor, 2010). In our study, over half of the participants (51%, n = 96) reported that they considered >25% of their patients to be interested in participating in preventive programs. However, a previous study of patient attitudes toward preventive programs reported that the majority of patients expressed willingness to undergo screening for heart disease, high blood pressure, and diabetes by a dentist (Greenberg, Kantor, Jiang, & Glick, 2012). Increasing understanding of the role of preventive care in dental practice and improving its provision requires providing education to both patients and dentists. It also requires gaining a better understanding of patients' and dentists' agreement regarding the need for communication of preventive care, an issue that should be further explored (Riley *et al.*, 2012).

Variable	Summary
Prevalence of dietary counseling	21% of patients receive dietary counseling
Perception of dietary counseling	63% agree that dietary counseling is important
Factors associated with promoting dietary counseling	1) Female sex 2) Level of practice activity (i.e., "busyness") 3) Percentage of patients interested in caries prevention 4) Percentage of patients who undergo caries risk assessment 5) Percentage of patients who undergo blood pressure screening

Table 5: Summary of evidence (Yokoyama, et al., 2013b)

4.4   Summary

Studies using the new Dental PBRN model have revealed that more than 60% of the dentists surveyed reported that the provision of both dental preventive care and dietary counseling is important. However, a low percentage of the same dentists also reported actually providing dental preventive care and dietary counseling in their practice. The results of the present study indicate that this discordance between dentists' perceptions of the importance of providing preventive care and their actual provision of preventive care is related to whether they believe that their patients are interested in caries prevention. To increase patients' interest in caries prevention, well-designed studies that can collect strong evidence regarding the factors affecting caries prevention, such as diet, are needed.

5   Conclusions

Our review of the evidence of a link between dietary intake and dental caries development revealed that few observational studies have explored this association. To fill this research gap, we need well-designed prospective studies that can investigate this link and provide strong evidence of its existence or lack thereof. Our study and previous studies exploring practice patterns in dental caries prevention and dietary counseling in dental clinics also suggest that although most dentists are interested in providing preventive care and/or dietary counseling, relatively few do so in practice.

Our review also suggests a continuing deficiency of evidence regarding the effect of dietary factors on dental caries development. Overcoming this deficiency requires nutritional epidemiology research to provide findings that can promote provision of dietary counseling in dental clinics. Such research should take the form of practice-based research, a new epidemiology study model that collects real-world data, using the Dental PBRN model. Use of the Dental PBRN model has been found to be an effective means of exploring the evidence and producing feedback that can be rapidly and effectively disseminated throughout practitioner networks. This new research model has great potential to change practice patterns and the provision of health guidance in dental settings. As such, the development of clinical practice guidelines based on evidence obtained from practice-based research in dental settings is expected in the future.

Acknowledgements

The authors would like to thank the US National Dental PBRN members, especially the Director, Dr. Gregg H Gilbert, who is a professor at and chair of the Department of Clinical and Community Sciences, School of Dentistry, University of Alabama at Birmingham, and Dr. Valeria V Gordan, who is a professor at the Department of Restorative Dental Sciences, University of Florida College of Dentistry.

References

AHRQ PBRN Website. http://pbrn.ahrq.gov/ Accessed 2013 Oct 27.

Alhazmi, A., Stojanovski, E., McEvoy, M., Garg, M. L. (2012). The association between dietary patterns and type 2 diabetes: a systematic review and meta-analysis of cohort studies. J Hum Nutr Diet. 2014, 27(3), 251-60. doi: 10.1111/jhn.12139.

American Diabetes Association. (2012). Standards of medical care in diabetes--2012. Diabetes Care, 35 Suppl 1, S11-63. doi: 10.2337/dc12-s01135/Supplement_1/S11 [pii]

Balakrishnan, M., Simmonds, R. S., & Tagg, J. R. (2000). Dental caries is a preventable infectious disease. Aust Dent J, 45(4), 235-245.

Bratthall D, Hänsel Petersson G. (2005). Cariogram--a multifactorial risk assessment model for a multifactorial disease. Community Dent Oral Epidemiol, 33(4), 256-64.

Brennan, D. S., & Spencer, A. J. (2005). The role of dentist, practice and patient factors in the provision of dental services. Community Dent Oral Epidemiol, 33(3), 181-195. doi: COM207 [pii]10.1111/j.1600-0528.2005.00207.x

Brown, L. J., & Lazar, V. (1998). Dental procedure fees 1975 through 1995: how much have they changed? J Am Dent Assoc, 129(9), 1291-1295.

Burt, B. A., Eklund, S. A., Morgan, K. J., Larkin, F. E., Guire, K. E., Brown, L. O., & Weintraub, J. A. (1988). The effects of sugars intake and frequency of ingestion on dental caries increment in a three-year longitudinal study. J Dent Res, 67(11), 1422-1429.

Burt, B. A., & Pai, S. (2001). Sugar consumption and caries risk: a systematic review. J Dent Educ, 65(10), 1017-1023.

Cabana, M. D., Rand, C. S., Powe, N. R., Wu, A. W., Wilson, M. H., Abboud, P. A., & Rubin, H. R. (1999). Why don't physicians follow clinical practice guidelines? A framework for improvement. JAMA, 282(15), 1458-1465. doi: jrv90041 [pii]

Centers for Disease Control and Prevention (2012) Preventing Chronic Diseases: Investing Wisely in Health, Preventing Dental Caries. Available: http://dental.ufl.edu/files/2012/06/PreventingDentalCaries.pdf. Accessed 2013 Oct 27.

Chobanian, A. V., Bakris, G. L., Black, H. R., Cushman, W. C., Green, L. A., Izzo, J. L., Jr., Roccella, E. J. (2003). Seventh report of the Joint National Committee on Prevention, Detection, Evaluation, and Treatment of High Blood Pressure. Hypertension, 42(6), 1206-1252. doi: 10.1161/01.HYP.0000107251.49515.c201.HYP.0000107251.49515.c2 [pii]

Cochrane, L. J., Olson, C. A., Murray, S., Dupuis, M., Tooman, T., & Hayes, S. (2007). Gaps between knowing and doing: understanding and assessing the barriers to optimal health care. J Contin Educ Health Prof, 27(2), 94-102. doi: 10.1002/chp.106

Dental PBRN Japan Website. http://www.dentalpbrn.jp/category/1445788.html Accessed 2013 Oct 27.

Doll, R., & Peto, R. (1981). The causes of cancer: quantitative estimates of avoidable risks of cancer in the United States today. J Natl Cancer Inst, 66(6), 1191-1308.

Dyer, T. A., & Robinson, P. G. (2006). General health promotion in general dental practice--the involvement of the dental team Part 2: A qualitative and quantitative investigation of the views of practice principals in South Yorkshire. Br Dent J, 201(1), 45-51; discussion 31. doi: 4813774 [pii]10.1038/sj.bdj.4813774

Gedalia, I., Davidov, I., Lewinstein, I., & Shapira, L. (1992). Effect of hard cheese exposure, with and without fluoride prerinse, on the rehardening of softened human enamel. Caries Res, 26(4), 290-292.

Gilbert, G. H., Williams, O. D., Rindal, D. B., Pihlstrom, D. J., Benjamin, P. L., & Wallace, M. C. (2008). The creation and development of the dental practice-based research network. J Am Dent Assoc, 139(1), 74-81. doi: 139/1/74 [pii]

Gilbert G. H., & for the DPBRN Collaborative Group.. (2009). The role of practice-based research networks in improving clinical care: The Dental PBRN" example. Dental Abstracts, 54(6), 284-285.

Gordan, V. V., Garvan, C. W., Heft, M. W., Fellows, J. L., Qvist, V., Rindal, D. B., & Gilbert, G. H. (2009). Restorative treatment thresholds for interproximal primary caries based on radiographic images: findings from the Dental Practice-Based Research Network. Gen Dent, 57(6), 654-663; quiz 664-656, 595, 680.

Gordan, V. V., Riley, J. L., 3rd, Carvalho, R. M., Snyder, J., Sanderson, J. L., Anderson, M., & Gilbert, G. H. (2011). Methods used by Dental Practice-based Research Network (DPBRN) dentists to diagnose dental caries. Oper Dent, 36(1), 2-11. doi: 10.2341/10-137-CR

Grant WB, Boucher BJ. (2011). Are Hill's criteria for causality satisfied for vitamin D and periodontal disease? Dermatoendocrinol, 2(1), 30-36.

Grant WB. (2011). A review of the role of solar ultraviolet-B irradiance and vitamin D in reducing risk of dental caries. Dermatoendocrinol, 3(3), 193-198.

Greenberg, B. L., Glick, M., Frantsve-Hawley, J., & Kantor, M. L. (2010). Dentists' attitudes toward chairside screening for medical conditions. J Am Dent Assoc, 141(1), 52-62. doi: 141/1/52 [pii]

Greenberg, B. L., Kantor, M. L., Jiang, S. S., & Glick, M. (2012). Patients' attitudes toward screening for medical conditions in a dental setting. J Public Health Dent, 72(1), 28-35. doi: 10.1111/j.1752-7325.2011.00280.x

Gustafsson, B. (1952). [Summary of findings in the Vipeholm studies to date]. Odontol Tidskr, 60(5), 338-345.

Harris, R., Gamboa, A., Dailey, Y., & Ashcroft, A. (2012). One-to-one dietary interventions undertaken in a dental setting to change dietary behaviour. Cochrane Database Syst Rev, 3, CD006540. doi: 10.1002/14651858.CD006540.pub2

Haugejorden, O., & Nielsen, W. A. (1987). Experimental study of two methods of data collection by questionnaire. Community Dent Oral Epidemiol, 15(4), 205-208.

Hefti, A., & Schmid, R. (1979). Effect on caries incidence in rats of increasing dietary sucrose levels. Caries Res, 13(5), 298-300.

Helminen, S. K., & Vehkalahti, M. M. (2003). Does caries prevention correspond to caries status and orthodontic care in 0- to 18-year-olds in the free public dental service? Acta Odontol Scand, 61(1), 29-33.

Hu, F. B. (2002). Dietary pattern analysis: a new direction in nutritional epidemiology. Curr Opin Lipidol, 13(1), 3-9.

Hujoel PP.(2013). Vitamin D and dental caries in controlled clinical trials: systematic review and meta-analysis. Nutr Rev, 71(2), 88-97.

Kakudate N, Sumida. F., Matsumoto Y, Yokoyama Y. (in press). The Development of the Japanese Dental Practice-Based Research Network. Journal of the Pakistan Dental Association.

Kakudate, N., Sumida, F., Matsumoto, Y., Manabe, K., Yokoyama, Y., Gilbert, G. H., & Gordan, V. V. (2012). Restorative treatment thresholds for proximal caries in dental PBRN. J Dent Res, 91(12), 1202-1208. doi: 10.1177/0022034512464778002203451246478 [pii]

Kashket, S., & DePaola, D. P. (2002). Cheese consumption and the development and progression of dental caries. Nutr Rev, 60(4), 97-103.

Kelly, S. A., & Moynihan, P. J. (2008). Attitudes and practices of dentists with respect to nutrition and periodontal health. Br Dent J, 205(4), E9; discussion 196-197. doi: sj.bdj.2008.655 [pii]10.1038/sj.bdj.2008.655

Kleemola-Kujala, E., & Rasanen, L. (1982). Relationship of oral hygiene and sugar consumption to risk of caries in children. Community Dent Oral Epidemiol, 10(5), 224-233.

Kushi, L. H., Doyle, C., McCullough, M., Rock, C. L., Demark-Wahnefried, W., Bandera, E. V., Gapstur, S., Patel, A. V., Andrews, K., Gansler, T.; American Cancer Society 2010 Nutrition and Physical Activity Guidelines Advisory Committee. (2012). American Cancer Society Guidelines on nutrition and physical activity for cancer prevention: reducing the risk of cancer with healthy food choices and physical activity. CA Cancer J Clin, 62(1), 30-67. doi: 10.3322/caac.20140

Kwon, H. K., Suh, I., Kim, Y. O., Kim, H. J., Nam, C. M., Jun, K. M., & Kim, H. G. (1997). Relationship between nutritional intake and dental caries experience of junior high students. Yonsei Med J, 38(2), 101-110.

Makhija, S. K., Gilbert, G. H., Rindal, D. B., Benjamin, P. L., Richman, J. S., & Pihlstrom, D. J. (2009). Dentists in practice-based research networks have much in common with dentists at large: evidence from the Dental Practice-Based Research Network. Gen Dent, 57(3), 270-275.

Mente, A., de Koning, L., Shannon, H. S., & Anand, S. S. (2009). A systematic review of the evidence supporting a causal link between dietary factors and coronary heart disease. Arch Intern Med, 169(7), 659-669. doi: 169/7/659 [pii]10.1001/archinternmed.2009.38

Miyazaki, H., & Morimoto, M. (1996). Changes in caries prevalence in Japan. Eur J Oral Sci, 104(4 (Pt 2)), 452-458.

Moynihan, P. J. (2005). The role of diet and nutrition in the etiology and prevention of oral diseases. Bull World Health Organ, 83(9), 694-699. doi: S0042-96862005000900015 [pii]/S0042-96862005000900015

National Dental PBRN Website. http://nationaldentalpbrn.org/ Accessed 2013 Oct 27.

Nunn, M. E., Braunstein, N. S., Krall Kaye, E. A., Dietrich, T., Garcia, R. I., & Henshaw, M. M. (2009). Healthy eating index is a predictor of early childhood caries. J Dent Res, 88(4), 361-366. doi: 88/4/361 [pii]10.1177/0022034509334043

Palacios, C., Joshipura, K., & Willett, W. (2009). Nutrition and health: guidelines for dental practitioners. Oral Dis, 15(6), 369-381. doi: 10.1111/j.1601-0825.2009.01571.xODI1571 [pii]

Papas, A. S., Joshi, A., Palmer, C. A., Giunta, J. L., & Dwyer, J. T. (1995). Relationship of diet to root caries. Am J Clin Nutr, 61(2), 423S-429S.

Rank, P., Julien, J. H., & Lyman, D. O. (1983). Preventable dental disease. West J Med, 139(4), 545-546.

Reich, E., Lussi, A., & Newbrun, E. (1999). Caries-risk assessment. Int Dent J, 49(1), 15-26.

Riley, J. L., 3rd, Gordan, V. V., Ajmo, C. T., Bockman, H., Jackson, M. B., & Gilbert, G. H. (2011). Dentists' use of caries risk assessment and individualized caries prevention for their adult patients: findings from The Dental Practice-Based Research Network. Community Dent Oral Epidemiol, 39(6), 564-573. doi: 10.1111/j.1600-0528.2011.00626.x

Riley, J. L., 3rd, Gordan, V. V., Rindal, D. B., Fellows, J. L., Qvist, V., Patel, S., Gilbert, G. H. (2012). Components of patient satisfaction with a dental restorative visit: results from the Dental Practice-Based Research Network. J Am Dent Assoc, 143(9), 1002-1010. doi: 143/9/1002 [pii]

Riley, J. L., 3rd, Gordan, V. V., Rouisse, K. M., McClelland, J., & Gilbert, G. H. (2011). Differences in male and female dentists' practice patterns regarding diagnosis and treatment of dental caries: findings from The Dental Practice-Based Research Network. J Am Dent Assoc, 142(4), 429-440. doi: 142/4/429 [pii]

Rugg-Gunn, A. J., Hackett, A. F., Appleton, D. R., Jenkins, G. N., & Eastoe, J. E. (1984). Relationship between dietary habits and caries increment assessed over two years in 405 English adolescent school children. Arch Oral Biol, 29(12), 983-992.

Scheinin, A., Makinen, K. K., & Ylitalo, K. (1976). Turku sugar studies. V. Final report on the effect of sucrose, fructose and xylitol diets on the caries incidence in man. Acta Odontol Scand, 34(4), 179-216.

Sela, M., Gedalia, I., Shah, L., Skobe, Z., Kashket, S., & Lewinstein, I. (1994). Enamel rehardening with cheese in irradiated patients. Am J Dent, 7(3), 134-136.

Tanaka, K., Miyake, Y., & Sasaki, S. (2010). Intake of dairy products and the prevalence of dental caries in young children. J Dent, 38(7), 579-583. doi: 10.1016/j.jdent.2010.04.009S0300-5712(10)00089-8 [pii]

Touger-Decker, R., Barracato, J. M., & O'Sullivan-Maillet, J. (2001). Nutrition education in health professions programs: a survey of dental, physician assistant, nurse practitioner, and nurse midwifery programs. J Am Diet Assoc, 101(1), 63-69.

Touger-Decker, R., & Mobley, C. C. (2007). Position of the American Dietetic Association: oral health and nutrition. J Am Diet Assoc, 107(8), 1418-1428.

Wang, N. J., & Aspelund, G. O. (2010). Preventive care and recall intervals. Targeting of services in child dental care in Norway. Community Dent Health, 27(1), 5-11.

Wang, N. J., Kalletstal, C., Petersen, P. E., & Arnadottir, I. B. (1998). Caries preventive services for children and adolescents in Denmark, Iceland, Norway and Sweden: strategies and resource allocation. Community Dent Oral Epidemiol, 26(4), 263-271.

World Health Organization (2012) Oral health. Fact sheet Nu318. Available: http://www.who.int/mediacentre/factsheets/fs318/en/index.html. Accessed 2013 Oct 27.

Yang, Q., Cogswell, M. E., Flanders, W. D., Hong, Y., Zhang, Z., Loustalot, F., Hu, F. B. (2012). Trends in cardiovascular health metrics and associations with all-cause and CVD mortality among US adults. JAMA, 307(12), 1273-1283. doi: 10.1001/jama.2012.339jama.2012.339 [pii]

Yokoyama, Y., Kakudate, N., Sumida, F., Matsumoto, Y., Gilbert, G. H., & Gordan, V. V. (2013a). Dentists' practice patterns regarding caries prevention: results from a dental practice-based research network. BMJ Open, 3(9), e003227. doi: 10.1136/bmjopen-2013-003227bmjopen-2013-003227 [pii]

Yokoyama, Y., Kakudate, N., Sumida, F., Matsumoto, Y., Gilbert, G. H. & Gordan, V. V. (2013b) Dentists' Dietary Perception and Practice Patterns in a Dental Practice-Based Research Network. PLoS One, 8, e59615.

Zero, D. T., Fontana, M., Martinez-Mier, E. A., Ferreira-Zandona, A., Ando, M., Gonzalez-Cabezas, C., & Bayne, S. (2009). The biology, prevention, diagnosis and treatment of dental caries: scientific advances in the United States. J Am Dent Assoc, 140 Suppl 1, 25S-34S. doi: 140/suppl_1/25S [pii]

Skin Cancer Prevention and Sun Protection Habits in Children

Maria Saridi
Faculty of Social Sciences
University of PCeloponnese, Greece

Maria Rekleiti
Faculty of Nursing
University of Peloponnese, Greece

Aikaterini Toska
Faculty of Social Sciences
University of Peloponnese, Greece

Greta Wozniak
School of Medicine
University of Thessaly, Greece

Ioannis Kyriazis
1st Internal Medicine Department Diabetes & Obesity Outpatient Clinic
General Hospital "Asclepeion" Voulas, Athens, Greece

Athena Kalokerinou
Faculty of Nursing
University of Athens, Greece

Kyriakos Souliotis
Faculty of Social Sciences
University of Peloponnese, Greece

1 Introduction

Epidemiological studies in the last two decades have shown that at least two-thirds of cutaneous melanomas seen worldwide are attributable to sun exposure. Harmful effects of UVR solar radiation occupy a good part of the international literature (Hoang & Eichenfield, 2000). Today, climatic conditions can allow ultraviolet radiation to affect skin and eyes and consequently to increase the risk for serious health conditions like skin cancer (Armstrong & Kricker, 2001).

The alarming fact is that Malign Melanoma (MM) cases, perhaps the most aggressive type of cancer, are increasing and so are other skin cancer types at increasingly younger ages. As it seems from the SEER research (SEER Program, 2007a) the incidence of MM in US population, increased over the course of a decade from 16.38/100000 in 1995 to 21.25/100000 in 2005. It is estimated that 90% of non-melanoma and 65% of melanoma skin cancers worldwide are associated with UVR exposure (Garbe & Blum, 2001; Jemal *et al.,* 2001; Nikolaou & Stratigos, 2013).

The effects of sun exposure during early life are important because most of an individual's exposure occurs during childhood and adolescence. Childhood exposure to UVR increases the risk for skin cancer as an adult. Children are at a higher risk of suffering damage from exposure to UVR than adults, in particular because their skin is thinner and more sensitive and even being outdoors for a short time in the midday sun can result in serious sunburns. Children have also a less developed pigmentation system that does not have a self-defence system and consequently, children have a risk of developing skin cancer later in life (Bleyer et al., 2006; Linabery & Ross, 2008; Wong et al., 2013).

Sun protection of children is a national priority. Individuals receive a substantial proportion of lifetime exposure to ultraviolet radiation (UVR) during childhood and severe sunburns in this age may increase lifetime risk of developing melanoma. Blistering sunburns between 15 and 20 years of age are significantly associated with increased skin cancer risk (Strouse et al., 2005; Purdue et al., 2008).

Public health advisors now recommend that the adoption of sun protection behaviours, including limiting sun exposure, using sunscreens and protective clothing, minimizing sunburns, avoiding tanning beds and wearing sunglasses to prevent eye damage, should best start in childhood. Many sun-awareness programs and resources for school-aged children have been reported in Australia, Canada, the USA and Europe (British Association of Dermatologists, 1995; Peiper, 1999; Harris & Alberts, 2004; Cancer Society of New Zealand, 2006; Purdue et al., 2008; US-EPA, 2013).

Knowledge levels, attitudes, and behaviour patterns of children and teenagers have already been discussed in various international studies. Countries with high rates of melanoma incidence have launched targeted studies and prevention-oriented interventions. Most of those studies have shown that more knowledge entails better attitudes and wiser behaviours. Knowledge of how behaviours vary among children can provide health promotion planners with insight (Piperakis et al., 2003; Buller et al., 2006; Dadlani & Orlow, 2008).

Primary prevention strategies for skin cancer include increasing knowledge and awareness in individuals, changing sun protection behaviours and implementing policy and environmental interventions. These strategies in childhood can contribute to higher knowledge levels and adoption of healthier behaviours regarding sun protection habits (Whiteman et al., 1997; Hicke et al., 2008).

2   Ultraviolet Radiation

Ultraviolet radiation (UVR) is part of the electromagnetic spectrum emitted from the sun, ranging from cosmic radiation to radio-electric waves. UVR can be divided into three types according to wavelength: UVA (400 - 315 nm), UVB (315 - 280 nm) and UVC (280 - 100 nm). Most UVA radiation and 10% of UVB can reach the Earth's surface, while UVC is absorbed by atmospheric ozone, vapors, oxygen and carbon dioxide (Armstrong, 1994; Zerefos et al., 2000; Armstrong & Kricker, 2001).

UVA is known as a long-wavelength, low-energy radiation. It is able to reach the Earth's surface, it remains practically steady throughout the year and it doesn't decrease while latitude increases. This type of radiation can penetrate the skin to deeper layers reaching the dermis, where it causes damage to collagen tissues leading to low skin elasticity and skin aging (Table 1).

UVR TYPES	UVA	UVB	UVC
WAVELENGTH	400 - 315 nm	315 - 280 nm	280 - 100 nm
ENERGY	low	average	high
SKIN PENETRATION	Severe-Hypodermis	Average-Dermis	Low-epidermis
EXISTENCE ON THE EARTH'S SURFACE	Relatively stable throughout the year	Reaching its peak in the summer at noon hours.	None. It is absorbed by the ozone layer.
MAIN EFFECTS	Activates melanin pigment. Causes skin aging.	Causes redness. (sunburns)	Can cause severe sunburns on humans.

Table 1: Types and characteristics of UVR (Rhodes, 1999).

UVB is a short-wavelength, high-energy radiation, but a big part of it gets absorbed by the ozone layer. UVB reaches its peak in the summer at noon-hours, and it can reach the epidermis. It can cause sunburns, skin reactions and activates melanin and stimulates tanning (Gies et al., 1998; Armstrong & Kricker, 2001; TOMS, 2005). UVC is a high-energy radiation that can trigger chemical and genetic alterations in living organisms. It plays no role regarding melanin activation, and it is absorbed by stratospheric ozone. UVR intensity varies according to several factors, such as latitude, season of the year, time of day, altitude, reflection, skin phototype, etc (Albert & Ostheimer, 2003; NASA, 2010).

2.1   Ozone as a Natural Protection Mechanism

The ozone layer that surrounds the Earth is a vital shield against the devastating effects UVR can have. A relatively significant proportion of atmospheric oxygen makes up stratospheric ozone (15-50km), which absorbs most of UVB and all of UVC. It is also present in lower layers, i.e. the troposphere, 0-10 km from the Earth's surface, being the by-product of pollution and solar radiation. In this case, it is considered as a pollutant, it is linked to photochemical smog and can cause problems to both humans and nature when above a certain limit.

In 1985, British scientist Joe Farman discovered a hole in the ozone layer above Antarctica, which is still under close observation. The ozone hole of the southern hemisphere varies in size, since it reaches its peak around mid-September and then shrinks and disappears around mid-December.

The stratospheric ozone layer depletion because of the use of chlorofluorocarbons in the late 20th century is a global problem that worries not only the scientific community, but governments and the public as well. It has been estimated that if 1% of the ozone layer is depleted, 2% more UVB can reach the Earth, something that entails an 1-3% increase in basal cell carcinoma, squamous-cell carcinoma and melanoma cases. Countries such as Australia or New Zealand have significant variations of the ozone layer, something that has lead to high skin cancer incidence, given that UVC is able to reach the Earth's surface more easily (Isaksen et al., 2005; Andersson & Engardt, 2010; Stevenson et al., 2013).

2.2 UV Index

The ultraviolet index is used globally as a measurement of UVR intensity. It is used in daily forecasts available in the Media and online in almost any country, including Greece. The UV index has specific values and standard colors that make it easier for anyone to understand the forecast and the recommended protection measures. Table 2 illustrates that when anyone knows their local UV index, they are able to understand if sun exposure may be dangerous on a particular day. The higher the index value, the higher the risk for UVR-related negative effects (Corrêa et al., 2010; Nikolaou & Stratigos, 2013).

Description	UV Index Value	Color
Low danger	$0-2$	green
Moderate risk	$3-5$	yellow
High risk	$6-7$	orange
Vey high risk	$8-10$	red
Extreme risk	≥ 11	purple

*Source: Global Solar UV Index: A Practical Guide. A joint recommendation of the World Health Organization, World Meteorological Organization, United Nations Environment Program, and the International Commission on Non-Ionizing Radiation Protection

Table 2: UV Index descriptions and colors

3   Biological Effects of Solar Radiation

Moderate sun exposure can have several positive effects on human health and mood. The sun is vital for life on Earth. It activates provitamin D_3, which exists in the skin, to vitamin D_3 which regulates calcium and phosphorus metabolism; D_3 deficiency can cause rickets, especially in children. Solar radiation can also ameliorate some skin diseases, such as psoriasis and acne, and it also activates the synthesis of melanin, a procedure that thickens the keratin layer and consequently is seen as the most important protection mechanism against sunburns (Haake & Holbrook, 1999; Rhodes, 1999). Sun exposure can also affect in a positive way the autonomic nervous system by activating several vitamins, hormones and enzymes. It stimulates blood circulation, boosts hemoglobin synthesis and lowers blood pressure. It also makes the body less prone to some bacterial and fungal infections because of its drying effects on the skin. Moderate sun exposure improves mood and creates positive and optimistic feelings (Stolz et al., 2002; Lucas, 2010; Zepp et al., 2011).

The sun is also a well-known heat source and an exploitable source of energy; it also is a key-factor for photosynthesis, a process vital for plants and animals and for the water cycle, the procedure responsible for the continuous movement of water on the Earth and provides fresh water to rivers, lakes and underground water reservoirs. Consequently, running water can be used as a source of hydroelectric energy, and solar radiation may be used as a sustainable alternative source of energy (photovoltaic systems) (Eide & Weinstock, 2006; Zepp et al., 2011).

The organs most exposed to sun rays are the skin and the eyes. Exposure to solar radiation could result in direct or chronic disorders of the skin, the eyes and the immune system (Haake & Holbrook, 1999; Canadian Cancer Statistics, 2008; Lucas, 2010). Exposure to solar radiation may have sunburns or photokeratitis as a direct impact. Cancer and premature skin aging are among the chronic effects. UVA affects the subcutaneous tissue and can alter collagen and elastin structure. Cataract, pterygium and keratopathy are also among chronic conditions due to exposure to solar radiation.

UVR can lead to the restructuring of DNA, which in its turn can lead to mutations. The ability of the human body to heal and restore solar radiation-induced damages decreases by age. As a rule of thumb, the shorter the wavelength, the higher the risks associated with UVR exposure (Haake & Holbrook, 1999; Stolz et al., 2002). The reactions of the skin after prolonged sun exposure are acute or chronic. Acute or direct effects are noticeable within hours or days after exposure; chronic effects are usually the result of sun exposure for prolonged periods of time (Eide & Weinstock, 2006; Canadian Cancer Statistics, 2008; Zepp et al., 2011).

Skin redness, Sunburn, Photo-ageing, Actinic Hyperkeratosis, Basal Cell Carcinoma (BCC), Squamous Cell Carcinoma (SCC) and Malign Melanoma (MM) are the most common effects of UVR on the human skin. Epidemiological studies focus regularly on melanomas because of their exceptional interest. The fact that melanoma affects more and more white persons and its relation to solar radiation, has attracted scientific interest. According to epidemiological studies, melanoma is an extraordinary neoplasm, of rapidly increasing incidence in Western countries, and some authors suggest that it is an epidemiological phenomenon (Haake & Holbrook, 1999; Lucas, 2010).

3.1   Skin Cancer Incidence and Mortality Rates

In the last decades, many countries have witnessed an alarming increase of melanoma cases in people under the age of 40. In 2004, the WHO highlighted the impact of increasing melanoma incidence as a major concern worldwide. It has been estimated that since 1940 MM and other types of skin cancer have soared by 600%, while almost a million new cases of skin cancer other than melanoma are being diagnosed each year. Australia, New Zealand and the USA are among the countries with the highest melanoma incidence. Australia has the highest melanoma incidence, with 4 800 new cases and 600 deaths each year and the average age of emergence was 40.51 years, while 155 000 new cases of skin cancer are diagnosed each year. New Zealand has the highest death rate from MM among OECD countries and 45 000-70 000 new cases of skin cancer are identified each year. In the US in the past 20 years MM incidence and mortality have soared, and more than 1 000 000 new cases of MM emerge each year (Hoang & Eichenfield, 2000; Garbe & Blum, 2001; Jemal et al., 2001; Nikolaou & Stratigos, 2013).

In Canada, in the last 20-30 years melanoma-related mortality rates have increased and the incidence of other types of skin cancer has doubled in the last 15 years. Melanoma incidence continues to increase in men and women (by 1.8% and 1.0% per year, respectively).

Mortality rates were stable in men but decreased in women (0.8% per year) (EUROSKIN, 2008). In Europe, almost 26 000 males and 33 300 females are diagnosed each year with melanoma and 8 300 males and 7 600 females die from it. Northern and Western Europe have the highest rates; mortality rates do not vary according to geographical position, but melanoma incidence tends to get lower in Southern Europe for both men and women. In Greece, few studies about malign melanoma have taken place. Cases that are diagnosed in healthcare institutions are not recorded in a coordinated manner. Nevertheless, from 2 000 onwards Greece participates in the 'Euromelanoma' campaign, which has lead to new initiatives for educating the public and recording new cases of skin cancer; so far, it has been shown that there is a general increase in skin cancer incidence and a more prominent one in younger ages (Krüger et al., 1992).

3.2   Risk Factors for Melanoma

There are several risk factors for melanoma both environmental and biological ones (Table 3). The most significant ones are: skin complexion in combination with many moles or dysplastic nevi, excessive sun exposure during childhood and adolescence, and the existence of at least one sunburn in the said stages of life (Hoang & Eichenfield, 2000; Garbe & Blum, 2001; Bleyer et al., 2006).

Risk Factors	Relative Risk
History of previous melanoma	9
Dysplastic nevi and family history of melanoma	148
Dysplastic nevi without a melanoma history in first-degree relatives	2 - 8
Melanoma in first-degree relatives	2 - 8
Immunosuppression	4
Large number of nevi	5 - 20
Large number of ephelides on the hands	2 - 4
Sunburn-proneness	2 - 5
Blonde or ginger hair color	1.5 - 5
Blue eyes	0.8 - 2.5
Socio-economical factors (high standard of living)	2 - 3
Other risk factors	
Excessive sun exposure	2 - 3
History of sunburns (at least one)	1.5 - 3
5 or more painful sunburns by age 15	2 - 6
Outdoor activities (sports, hobbies)	1 - 2
Factors that their riskiness has not been established	
Fluorescent lamps	No data available
Contraceptive pills	No data available
Factors that have not been studied thoroughly yet	
Artificial tanning	Found dangerous by recent studies

*Information provided by A. Rhodes, as modified Rhodes et al., in 5th edition of Fizpatrick's Dermatology in General Medicine, p 1026, table 90-1(Rhodes, 1999)

Table 3: Melanoma risk factors.

Skin phototype describes the reaction of the skin to the initial sun exposure, according to one's hair and eye color and skin complexion. There are six phototypes for white persons (Table 4). Sunburns in childhood and adolescence are a risk factor for developing MM later in adulthood. Minimum erythema dose (MED) has been used as a measure of sunburns (Table 5); MED is the minimum UVR exposure that can cause an erythema on the skin after just one exposure. It is expressed as amount of energy per amount of skin surface, mJ/cm^2 (UVB) or J/cm^2 (UVA). UVB minimum erythema dose for white people is 20-40 mJ/cm^2 for skin phototypes I and II, in northern latitudes after 20 minutes of exposure at noon in June.

The erythema caused by UVB develops within 6-24 hours and disappears within 72-120 hours. The erythema caused by UVA reaches its peak within 4-16 hours and disappears within 48-120 hours (Strouse et al., 2005; Bleyer et al., 2006; Linabery & Ross, 2008).

Several studies have concluded that a large number of nevi can be a risk factor for melanoma. Estimates vary, but the risk has been found to increase 10-60 times, according to the individuals and the size of the pigmented/dysplastic nevi. Any changes regarding pigmented nevi do not necessarily mean that they will become malignant (Tucker et al., 1983; Krüger et al., 1992; WHO, 2013). However, in such cases not only a thorough medical examination is necessary, but the individuals should monitor themselves those changes according to the ABCDE rule (Table 6). According to several studies, for the nevi to become malignant both genetic and environmental factors, e.g. solar radiation, are involved (Task Force on Community Preventive Services, 2004; Dummer et al., 2005).

Phototype	Skin complexion	Reaction to sun exposure
I	Pale white skin	Does not tan, burns easily
II	Fair white skin	Hard to tan, burns easily
III	Darker white skin	Tans after initial burn
IV	Light brown	Tans easily
V	Brown	Tans easily
VI	Black	Tans darker

Table 4: Skin phototypes (Rhodes, 1999).

Skin phototype	Tan	Sunburn	Hair color	Eye color	1 MED
I	never	always	ginger	blue	200 J m^{-2}
II	sometimes	sometimes	blonde	Blue-green	250 J m^{-2}
III	always	rarely	brown	Gray-brown	350 J m^{-2}
IV	always	never	black	black	450 J m^{-2}

Table 5: European skin types (Krüger et al., 1992).

A (Asymmetry)	Asymmetrical skin lesion. Half of a mole does not match the other.
B (Border irregularity)	The edges are blurred, irregular, ragged or notched. Pigmentation tends to expand to the surrounding skin.
C (Color)	The color is uneven with different shades of black and brown, with patches of white, grey, red, pink or blue.
D (Diameter >6 mm)	Diameter is greater than 6 mm. Usually the lesion becomes larger regarding the size.
E (Evolution/Elevation)	The mole is raised above the surface and has an uneven surface and it looks different from the rest or changing in size, shape, color

Table 6: The ABCDE rule for monitoring nevi (Stolz et al., 2002).

3.3   Sun protection measures

Obviously, the main measure for the prevention of skin cancer is as little as possible exposure to the sun. The WHO has issued guidelines regarding protection measures especially for children and adolescents that are exposed to the sun (Dummer et al., 2005; WHO, 2008).

Clothes also play an important role. Light-coloured, dry, long-sleeved shirts and long pants made of tightly woven fabric can protect significantly from the sun. Hats with a brim all around that shades face, ears and the back of the neck can reduce by 50% the UVR that reaches the head and are highly recommended for children. Sunglasses protect the eyes from UVA and UVB. Also clouds can reduce the UVR amount but the shade of the trees absorbs a bigger part of UVR and thus is an important protection factor.

The UVR intensity varies throughout the day. In the summer, it reaches its peak between 10a.m. and 16 p.m. and prolonged exposure to the sun should be discouraged.

Sun blockers aim at protecting the skin from UVR and their efficiency regarding protection from UVA and UVB has been established. The Sun Protection Factor (SPF) is the most important factor regarding choosing the right sunscreen. SPF denotes the minimum amount of time that a dose of UVR reaching skin surface that was covered by the sun-blocker needs to cause an erythema, compared to the time needed without the sunscreen lotion. According to the WHO, an SPF around 15-30 provides medium protection, while for children sunscreens with SPF 50 are recommended. It should be noted that sunscreens work best in combination with the above-mentioned protection measures (Fry & Verne, 2003; WHO, 2008).

Finally, the efficiency of a sunscreen is linked to the way it is used. Sunscreens should be applied 20-30 minutes before one leaves the house on any part of the body that will be directly exposed to the sun. Special attention should be given to areas such as ears, nose, lips, palms, the "V" of the neck, elbows and head for bald people. Reapplication should take place every 2 hours for as long the exposure to the sun continues, even after 16 p.m. For adults, the recommended amount of lotion is about 30-40 gr (about a handful) and for children half this amount for achieving a desirable outcome (Laughlin-Richard, 2000; Fry & Verne, 2003; Dummer et al., 2005; WHO, 2008).

4   Attitudes and Knowledge of Children and Adolescents

Knowledge, behaviours and attitudes of children and adolescents have been studied thoroughly in the recent years, mainly because these age groups are in high risk because of frequent and prolonged exposure to the sun. There is some evidence that the annual received UV dose is independent of age and remains constant throughout life. Children spend an estimated 2.5–3 hours outdoors each day and may receive three times more UVB rays annually than adults, because they have a greater opportunity for midday sun exposure during the summer months (Masso, 2006; Lawler et al., 2007; MacNeal & Dinulos, 2007).

Consequently, providing information to younger people via coordinated educational programs is an essential priority especially for countries that have high skin cancer rates (Marks, 2004; Buller et al., 2006).

Studies published in the last decades have shown that educational programs regarding sun protection measures should adapt to the specific needs of each age group and can contribute to the adoption of healthier behaviours that could reduce short and long-term damage due to solar radiation (WHO, 2003; Lawler *et al.,* 2007; MacNeal & Dinulos, 2007).

In the last two decades, several international studies have investigated knowledge levels of children and adolescents by using questionnaires about solar radiation. Those questionnaires may not be the same every time but they share many common items, since they are based on the guidelines issued by the WHO, CDC and other scientific institutions (CDC, 2003; Livingston et al., 2007).

Studies from Australia, a country with extremely high melanoma incidence rates, have shown that 80% of young people are aware of sun-related risks and protection measures. Recently the knowledge level has risen even more since educational programs have been implemented targeting the general public (Fisher et al., 1996; Dixon et al., 1999; Cokkinides et al., 2006).

Relevant studies from the USA, a country with increasing melanoma incidence in younger people, have shown a fairly high knowledge level ($\approx$65%), albeit slightly lower than the Australian one (Anthony et al., 2002; Geller et al., 2005; LaBat et al., 2005; Yurtseven et al., 2012).

In the last years, in Europe the official authorities have shown awareness regarding solar radiation and its impact. According to several studies, children and teenagers have a fairly good knowledge level ($\approx$50%-60%), with southern countries scoring higher than northern ones, perhaps because of more hours of sunshine annually. Because of a recent increase in skin cancer rates in northern Europe, educational programs and campaigns have been launched throughout Europe (EUROMELANOMA), that seem to have improved knowledge levels and thus promote the prevention of melanoma (Bandura, 1986; Horsley et al., 2002; Aquilina et al., 2004; Kristjánsson et al., 2004; Savona et al., 2005; Vries *et al.,* 2005; Reinau et al., 2010; Dupont & Pereira, 2012).

Numerous studies have correlated knowledge with attitude and behaviour. In other words, the higher the knowledge levels, the healthier the behaviours. The socio-cognitive approach holds that both behaviourist and cognitive methods should be used within educational programs in order for healthier behaviours to be adopted (Bandura, 1997; Elder et al., 1999).

Of course, attitude change will not emerge after individual, one-off interventions. For instance, a program about sun protection aimed at school-age children should also take into account that children usually follow and copy their parents and family, and can be influenced by school, the media and the current trends regarding any subject (Doré & Chignol, 2011). Adolescents, on the other hand, although they have satisfactory knowledge levels regarding sun-related risks, nevertheless they do not seem to take the necessary protection measures. Appearance and beauty standards, along with beach sports, are two factors that seem to stop teenagers from adopting protection measures, such as applying sunscreen or wearing appropriate cloths, etc. Being tan is promoted as something positive and several teenagers expose themselves to the sun especially at noon in order to get tan (Saridi et al., 2012).

Several studies about younger people have also found a paradox, namely that although most of them know that sunscreens can protect their skin, nevertheless they do not know what the correct sun protection factor is for them or how to apply the sunscreen correctly.

Sunburn incidence has also been the subject of many studies, especially since it has been established that the occurrence of even one sunburn during childhood or adolescence can increase the risk for melanoma later in life. Naturally, high sunburn incidence means poor sun protection measures (CDC, 2003; Fry & Verne, 2003; Livingston et al., 2007).

Finally, providing information about the way the (dysplastic) nevi can change and the way to monitor such changes has also been the subject of several studies. Mole mapping and annual monitoring through campaigns such as the EUROMELANOMA, have promoted the prevention, early diagnosis and successful treatment of malign melanomas (Krüger *et al.,* 1992).

4.1   Knowledge and Attitudes of Young People in Greece

There are few studies about knowledge and attitudes of children and adolescents regarding sun protection in Greece (Katsambas & Nicolaidou, 1996; Stratigos et al., 1996; Roussaki-Schulze et al., 2005; EPA, 2008). Naturally, investigating knowledge and attitudes cannot lead to the adoption of healthier behaviours. But it can assess the weak points and knowledge deficits, highlight negative behaviours and perceptions, focus on specific targets, and implement targeted interventions. Thus, knowledge and attitudes of adolescents and primary education students was investigated from 2007 to 2011 (Stratigos et al., 1996).

Regarding adolescents, a study took place including 801 high-school students aged 15-18 years from a coastal area in Greece. The study investigated knowledge, attitudes and perceptions of the participants regarding the impact of solar radiation on the human body as well as sun protection measures. After a double pilot standardization, an anonymous questionnaire was used as the study instrument (Figure 1).

According to the findings, only 37.9% of the adolescents knew what a melanoma was, 29.7% knew what UVR was and less than 50% knew something about SPF. On the other hand, 85% of the adolescents knew when the intensity of the sun reached its peak and that sun exposure should be avoided. Similarly, 73.5% were aware of protection measures, e.g. staying in the shade. Regarding sunburns, 55% of the participants reported more than one in the summer prior to the study, and 66.7% of the sunburns were on the back. Being tan was attributed to style (41.9%), or beauty-related reasons (67.7%). Mole mapping revealed that more than 60% had had 1-20 moles on their bodies, 77.8% had never visited a doctor to have their moles checked and 62.7% did not know how to monitor any changes in the moles. An alarming finding was that 77.5% of the participants are usually exposed to the sun between 10 a.m. and 16 p.m., when sun radiation is at its peak, and only 40% said they used sunscreen –but most of them did not know how to apply it correctly.

Two years later another study took place in the same area, but this time the participants were students aged 8-12 years (n = 2163). The children had to complete an anonymous, standardized questionnaire. It was found that children wear hats (40.6%) and sunglasses (36.3%), use sunscreen (72.1%), but 34.5% of them did not know what the sunscreen SPF was. Only 46.3% of the children stayed in the shade when at the beach, 32.5% liked to be tan, and sunburn incidence was found to be 32%. The correlation between protection measures and sunburns showed that children who took less protection measures had had higher sunburn incidence. Similar negative results have been found by many studies from several countries, but recent studies from Australia, New Zealand and the US have shown some encouraging findings. This can be attributed to the fact that for at least a decade these countries have been implementing education and prevention programs for the entire population, but mainly targeted on children and adolescents. These interventions are combined with relevant advertising campaigns and efforts to change beauty standards. Teachers and parents participate actively in such programs and consequently the information is transmitted to other age groups as well.

The correlation between behaviours and gender in the Greek study showed that females have a more cautious behaviour than males, a common finding in many international studies. The main reason for this, is probably the social culture regarding female appearance and the fact that younger females usually adopt easier the current beauty standards.

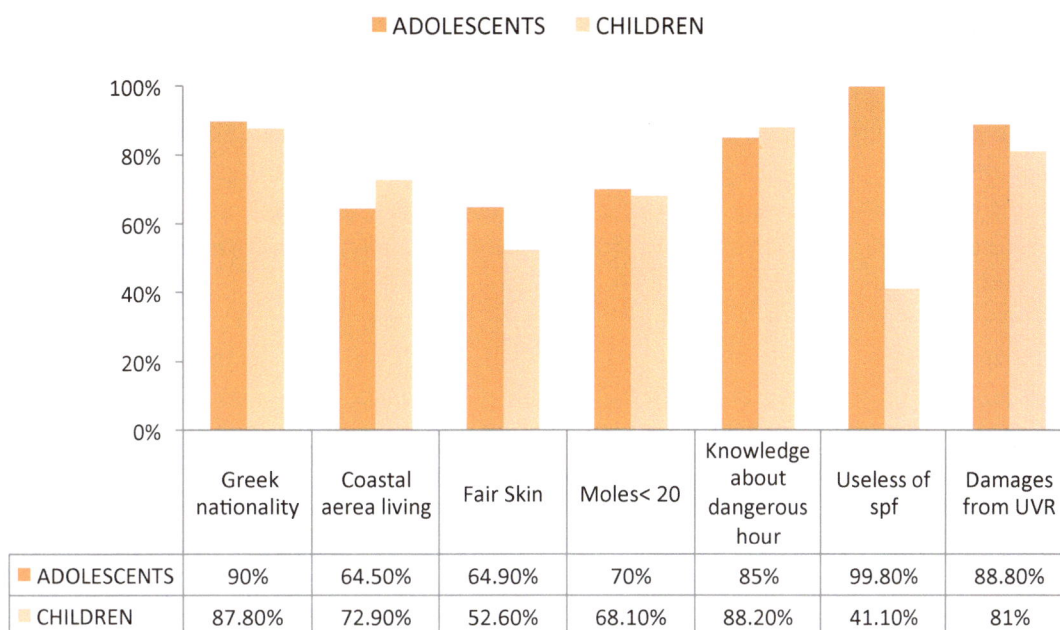

ADOLESCENTS   **CHILDREN**

	Greek nationality	Coastal aerea living	Fair Skin	Moles< 20	Knowledge about dangerous hour	Useless of spf	Damages from UVR
ADOLESCENTS	90%	64.50%	64.90%	70%	85%	99.80%	88.80%
CHILDREN	87.80%	72.90%	52.60%	68.10%	88.20%	41.10%	81%

Figure 1: The findings of two studies from Greece.

This study also showed that students of non-Greek nationality fail to adopt healthy behaviours compared to Greek students, something that may be attributed to lower educational level or cultural differences.

Finally, older students were found to adopt more protection measures, also a common finding in many studies. It seems that (cognitive and social) maturity brings along the adoption of a more cautious behaviour.

4.2 Intervention Programs

In an attempt to prevent further deterioration, some countries with high melanoma incidence rates have launched targeted studies and educational campaigns. The majority of those studies have shown that the higher the knowledge levels, the better the attitudes and behaviours. Although these interventions have been partially successful in improving knowledge regarding sun exposure and skin cancer, they have failed to elicit behavioural changes (CDC, 2003).

At the United Nations Conference on Environment and Development (UNCED) in 1992 it was declared under Agenda 21 that there should be more activities about UVR effects. The World Health Organization's Intersun program, collaborates with specialist agencies to implement key research activities that fill the gaps in knowledge, identify and quantify health risks from UV radiation, provide practical advice and information to national authorities on health and environmental effects of UV exposure, focus on sun protection for children and education in schools, promote the UV Index as an educational tool for sun protection etc. Many collaborating centers such as the Australian Radiation Protection and Nuclear Safety Agency and the Health Protection Agency of the United Kingdom are key contributors to Intersun's activities (SunSmart, 2008).

School and daycare administrators and personnel can implement a variety of policies to minimize harmful sun exposure and promote skin cancer prevention. Examples of school initiatives include the promotion of wearing hats and protective clothing, seeking shade when outdoors, wearing sunglasses for eye protection and using sunscreen with the proper sun protection factor. Several national health authorities have provided information about best practices for skin cancer prevention in schools. For example, as part of its Healthy School Initiative, the Government of Queensland in Australia has published guidelines for developing a curriculum and a strategy to address skin cancer prevention and sun safety in primary and secondary schools. Many governments and health authorities have developed policies and programs to promote sun-safe education and behaviour in schools.

Australia has a long history of sun safety initiatives operating at the national and state levels. The most prominent targeting schoolchildren, is the Anti-Cancer Council of Victoria's (ACCV) SunSmart Schools program (part of the larger SunSmart initiative) which was created in 1988 to provide professional support to schools and early childhood centres for the implementation of sun protection practices (SunWise, 2008).

SunSmart is a not-for-profit health promotion intervention in Australia that aims to minimise the human cost of skin cancer and takes a leading role in promoting a balance between the benefits and harms of ultraviolet radiation exposure and the benefits of vitamin D. SunSmart recommends that all schools implement a SunSmart policy to ensure a healthy UV exposure balance – one that minimises skin cancer risk and helps with vitamin D. This also helps address the duty of health and safety responsibilities for staff and students. SunSmart has a number of resources, sample policies, family notes and online curriculum support to help share the SunSmart message. The majority of Victorian primary schools and over half of special education schools are registered members of the SunSmart schools program.

The SunWise is a health and environmental education program in the USA, that teaches children ages 5-15 and their caregivers how to protect themselves from overexposure to the sun. Through the use of classroom, school, and community components, SunWise develops sustained sun-safe behaviors. Intervention participants receive free materials that facilitate cross-curricular learning about sun safety, UVR, and ozone science (Gilaberte et al., 2008; ACS, 2010).

In the United States, the SunSafe Project, was supported by the National Cancer Institute to enhance and promote sun protection behaviour of children ages 2–9 and of teenagers through interventions in several settings including preschools, schools, sports facilities, and recreational environments. SunSafe for the middle years provides teachers with curriculum materials to incorporate UV radiation and sun protection into class curriculums, and also recommends specific school policy changes that support sun safety during school outings and sports events (ACS, 2010).

Environment is a program also based on Intersun which encourages schools to develop policies that ensure that teachers, parents and students are aware of the risks of being over- exposed to the solar radiation, organize outdoor activities but not during the peak hours between 11 a.m. to 4 p.m., and if possible try to keep children entirely way from the sun from noon to 2 p.m., educate children and youth about the benefits of wearing protective clothing, sunglasses and sunscreen with a sun protection factor (SPF) of 15 or higher and have shade structures on playgrounds and at sport fields. This can also include creating a sun-safe environment by encouraging kids to seek shade from trees, awnings, umbrellas or buildings (SunSmart, 2008).

SolSano is the first Spanish health education intervention, created in 2001, for sun safety targeted at elementary schoolchildren. The objective was to evaluate SolSano's effects on students' knowledge, attitudes and practices about sun safety. This intervention involved over 5,000 students from 215

Aragonese primary schools (grades 1–2). The health authority provided schools with an educational package including an activity guide to teachers for teachers, a workbook for each student, a poster and an informative pamphlet for families (Gilaberte et al., 2008).

5   Conclusions

The impact of UVR on the human body combined with ozone layer depletion has lead to a significant increase in skin cancer and melanoma incidence rates. There is a worldwide concern for the fact that melanoma occurs at ever younger ages in the last years.

Important risk factors for skin cancer include also excessive sun exposure during childhood and adolescence, the existence of dysplastic nevi, occurrence of sunburns and lack of sun-protection measures.

Investigating knowledge levels and attitudes of different age groups can help us identify the information deficits and design efficient educational interventions. Such programs have been implemented in several countries and have contributed in the adoption of healthier behaviours regarding sun protection.

Most public health authorities conclude that continuing education from an early age combined with keeping parents, teachers and the society in general well-informed, can contribute to the adoption of healthier behaviours regarding sun exposure. States have to design well-coordinated programs with the participation of all relevant health, education and information agencies, aiming at the adoption of wiser behaviours and keeping the public's knowledge up- to-date.

References

Albert, M. R. & Ostheimer, K. G. (2003). The evolution of current medical and popular attitudes toward ultraviolet light exposure: part 2. Journal of American Academy Dermatology, 48(6), 909–918.

American Cancer Society. Cancer Facts and Figures. (2010). Available from: http//:www.cancer.org/acs/groups/content/@nho/documents/document/acspc-024113.pdf (PDF)

Anthony, J., Alberg Herbst, R.M., Genkinger, J.M., & Duszynski, K.R.(2002). Knowledge, attitudes, and behaviours towards skin cancer in Maryland youths. Journal of Adolescent Health, 31, 372-377.

Armstrong, B.K. (1994). Stratospheric ozone and health. International Journal of Epidemiology, 23(5), 873–885.

Armstrong, B. K. & Kricker, A. (2001). The epidemiology of UV induced skin cancer. Journal of Photochemistry and Photobiology B, 63(1–3), 8–18.

Arola A., Lakkala K., Bais A., Kaurola J., Meleti C., & Taalas P. (2003). Factors affecting short- and long-term changes of spectral UV irradiance at two European stations. Journal of Geophysical Research D, 108(17), 9-11.

Aquilina, S., Amato Gauci, A., Ellul, M., & Scerri, L. (2004). Sun awareness in Maltese secondary school students. Journal of the European Academy of Dermatology and Venereology, 18, 670–6.

Bandura, A. (1986). Social foundations of thought and action. A social cognitive theory. Englewood Cliffs, N.J.: Pienctice-Hall.

Bandura, A. (1997). Self-efficacy: The exercise of control. W.H. USA: Freeman and Company Pbl.

Bleyer, A., O'Leary, M., Barr, R., Ries, L.A.G. (2006). eds. Cancer Epidemiology in Older Adolescents and Young Adults 15 to 29 Years of Age, Including SEER Incidence and Survival: 1975–2000 (NIH Pub. No. 06-5767). Bethesda, MD: National Cancer Institute.

Buller, D.B., Buller, M.K., & Reynolds, K.D. (2006). A survey of sun protection policy and education in secondary schools. Journal of the American Academy of Dermatology, 54(3), 427–432.

Canadian Cancer Statistics. (2008). Canadian Cancer Society et al. Available from: http://www.cancer.ca/vgn/images/portal/cit_86751114/10/34/614137951cwlibrary_WYNTK_Bladder_Punjabi2005.pdf

Cancer Society of New Zealand. Sample Sun Protection Policy for Primary Schools. (2006). Cancer Society of New Zealand, Wellington, New Zealand.

CDC. (2003). Counseling to prevent skin cancer: recommendations and rationale of the US Preventive Services Task Force. Morbidity and Mortality Weekly Report, 52(No.RR-15), 13–17.

Cokkinides, V., Weinstock, M., Glanz, K., Albano, J., Ward, E., & Thun, M. (2006). Trends in sunburns, sun protection practices, and attitudes toward sun exposure protection and tanning among US adolescents, 1998-2004. Pediatrics, 118(3), 853-64.

Dadlani, C. & Orlow, S. J. (2008). Planning for a brighter future: a review of sun protection and barriers to behavioral change in children and adolescents. Dermatology Online Journal, 14(9), article 1.

Dixon, H., Borland, R., & Hill, D. (1999). Sun protection and sunburn in primary school children: the influence of age, gender and coloring. Preventive Medicine, 28, 119–130.

Doré, J. F. & Chignol, M. C. (2011). Tanning salons and skin cancer.. Photochemical and Photobiological Sciences, 11, 30.

Dummer, R., Panizzon, R., Bloch, P.H., & Burg, G. (2005). Updated Swiss Guidelines for the Treatment and Follow-Up of Cutaneous Melanoma. Dermatology, 210, 39–44.

Dupont, L. & Pereira, D.N. (2012). Sun exposure and sun protection habits in high school students from a city south of the country. Anais Brasileiros de Dermatologia, 87(1), 90-95.

Eide, M., & Weinstock, M. (2006). Public Health Challenges in Sun Protection. Dermatologic Clinics, 24, 119–124.

Elder, J.P., Ayala, G.X., & Harris, S. (1999). Theories and intervention approaches to health-behavior change in primary care. American Journal Preventive Medicine 17, 275–284.

Environmental Protection Agency (EPA). (2008). EPA SunWise. Available from: http://www.epa.gov/sunwise/

European Society of Skin Cancer Prevention (EUROSKIN). (2008). Sunbeds and Solaria [webpage]. Available from: http://www.euroskin.eu/238d7297f20aa420b/index.html

Fisher, K.J., Lowe, J.B., Gillespie, A.M., Balanda, K.P., Baade, P.D., & Staton, W.R. (1996). The relationship between Australian students' perceptions of behaviour, school policies and sun protection behaviors. Journal of Health Education, 27, 242–247.

Fry, A., & Verne, J. (2003). Preventing skin cancer: Messages should emphasise the need to cover up and stay out of the sun. British Medical Journal, 326, 114–115.

Garbe, C. & Blum, A. (2001). Epidemiology of cutaneous melanoma in Germany and worldwide. Skin Pharmacology and Applied Skin Physiology, 14(5), 280-90.

Geller, A.C., Shamban, J., O'Riordan, D.L., Slygh, C., Kinney, J.P., & Rosenberg, S. (2005). Raising Sun Protection and Early Detection Awareness among Florida High Schoolers. Pediatric Dermatology, 22(2), 112–118.

Gies, P.H., Roy, C.R., Toomey, S., & McLennan, A. (1998). Protection against solar UV radiation. Mutation Research, 422(1), 15–22.

Gilaberte, Y., Alonso, J.P., Teruel, M.P., Granizo, C., & Gallego, J. (2008). Evaluation of a health promotion intervention for skin cancer prevention is Spain: the SolSano program. Health Promotion International, 23(3), 209–219.

Haake, A. R. & Holbrook, K. (1999). The structure and development of skin: In: Freedberg, I.M., Eisen, A.Z., Wolff, K., Austen, K.F., Goldsmith, L.A., Katz, S.I., Fitzpatrik, T.B., eds. Dermatology in General Medicine. 1999 New York: McGraw-Hill (pp. 70–114).

Harris, R. B. & Alberts, D. S. (2004). Strategies for skin cancer prevention. International Journal of Dermatology, 43(4), 243–251.

Health Education Authority/Department of Health/British Association of Dermatologists. Sun Awareness and Protection Guidelines for Schools. (1995). Health Education Authority, London, UK.

Hicke, J.A., Slusser, J., Lantz, K., & Pascual, F.G. (2008). Trends and interannual variability in surface UVB radiation over 8 to 11 years observed across the United States. Journal of Geophysical Research, 113, D21302.

Hoang, M. T. & Eichenfield, L. F. (2000). The rising incidence of melanoma in children and adolescents. Dermatology Nursing, 12(3), 188–192.

Horsley, L., Charlton, A., & Waterman, C. (2002). Current action for skin cancer risk reduction in English schools: pupils' behaviour in relation to sunburn. Health education Research, Theory & Practice, 17(6), 715–731.

Jemal, A., Devesa, S.S., Hartge, P., & Tucker, M.A. (2001). Recent trends in cutaneous melanoma incidence among whites in the United States. Journal of the National Cancer Institute, 93(9), 678-83.

Incidence of childhood and adolescent melanoma in the United States: 1973-2009. Pediatrics, 131(5), 846-54. doi: 10.1542/peds.2012-2520.

Isaksen, I.S.A., Zerefos, C., Kourtidis, K. Meleti, C., Dalsøren, S.B., Sundet, J.K., et al. (2005). Tropospheric ozone changes at unpolluted and semipolluted regions induced by stratospheric ozone changes. Journal of Geophysical Research D, 110(2), 1–15.

Katsambas, A. & Nicolaidou, E. (1996). Cutaneous malignant melanoma and sun exposure. Recent developments in epidemiology. Archives of Dermatology, 132(4), 444-450.

Kristjánsson, S., Ullén, H., & Helgason, A.R. (2004). The importance of assessing the readiness to change sun-protection behaviours: a population-based study. European Journal of Cancer, 40(18), 2773-80.

Krüger, S., Garbe, C., Büttner, P., Stadler, R., Guggenmoos-Holzmann, I., & Orfanos, C.E. (1992). Epidemiologic evidence for the role of melanocytic nevi as risk markers and direct precursors of cutaneous malignant melanoma: Results of a case control study in melanoma patients and nonmelanoma control subjects. Journal of the American Academy of Dermatology, 26(6), 920–926.

LaBat, K., De Long, M., & Gahring, S.A. (2005). A Longitudinal Study of Sun-Protective Attitudes and Behaviors. Family and Consumer Sciences Research Journal, 33(3), 240-254.

Laughlin-Richard, N. (2000). Sun exposure and skin cancer prevention in children and adolescents. Journal of School Nursing, 16(2), 20–26.

Lawler, S., Spathonis, K., Eakin, E., Gallois, C., Leslie, E., & Owen, N. (2007). Sun exposure and sun protection behaviours among young adult sport competitors. Australia and New Zealand Journal of Public Health, 31(3), 230–234.

Linabery, A. M. & Ross, J. A. (2008). Trends in childhood cancer incidence in the U.S. (1992–2004). Cancer, 112(2), 416–432.

Livingston, P.M., White, V., Hayman, J., & Dobbinson, S. (2007). Australian adolescents' sun protection behavior: who are we kidding? Preventive Medicine, 44(6), 508-12.

Lucas, R. M. (2010). Solar Ultraviolet Radiation: Assessing the Environmental Burden of Disease at National and Local Levels. Environmental Burden of Disease Series 17. World Health Organization, Geneva, Switzerland.

MacNeal, R., & Dinulos, J. (2007). Update on sun protection and tanning in children. Current Opinion in Pediatrics, 19, 425–429.

Marks, R. (2004). Campaigning for melanoma prevention: a model for a health education program. Journal of the European Academy of Dermatology and Venereology, 18, 44–47.

Masso, M. (2006). Policy and Practice for Preventing Skin Cancer in Children. Public Health Nursing, 23(4), 361–365.

NASA's Total Ozone Mapping Spectrometer. (2005). TOMS. Avaliable from: http://ozoneaq.gsfc.nasa.gov/

NASA. UV exposure has increased over the last 30 years, but stabilized since the mid-1990s. (2010). Available from: www.nasa.gov/topics/solarsystem/features/uv-exposure.html

Nikolaou, V. & Stratigos, A. J. (2013). Emerging trends in the epidemiology of melanoma. British Journal of Dermatology. doi: 10.1111/bjd.12492.

Peiper A. (1999). National Sun Smart Schools Program. Australian Cancer Society, Sydney, Australia.

Piperakis, S.M., Papadimitriou, V., Piperakis, M.M., & Zisis, P. (2003). Understanding Greek primary school children's comprehension of sun exposure. Journal of Science Education and Technology, 12(2), 135–142.

Purdue, M.P., Freeman, L.E., Anderson, W.F., & Tucker, M.A. (2008). Recent trends in incidence of cutaneous melanoma among US Caucasian young adults. Journal of Investigative Dermatology, 128(12), 2905–2908.

Reinau, D., Meier, C., Gerber, N., Hofbauer, G.F., & Surber, C. (2010). Sun protective behaviour of primary and secondary school students in North-Western Switzerland. Swiss Medical Weekly, 142, w13520. doi: 10.4414/smw.2012.13520

Rhodes, A.R. (1999). Benign neoplasias and hyperplasias of melanocytes. In: Freedberg IM, Eisen AZ, Wolff K, Austen KF, Goldsmith LA, Katz SI, et al. editor. Fitzpatrick's dermatology in general medicine. 5th ed. New York: McGraw-Hill (pp. 1018–1059).

Roussaki-Schulze, A.V., Rammos, C., Rallis, E., Terzis, A., Archontonis, N., Sarmanta, A., et al. (2005). Increasing incidence of melanoma in central Greece: a retrospective epidemiological study. International Journal of Tissue Reactions, 27(4), 173-179.

Saridi, M., Toska, A., Rekleiti, M., Wozniak, G., Liachopoulou, A., Kalokairinou, A., et al. (2012). Sun-protection habits of primary students in a coastal area of Greece. Journal of Skin Cancer, 629652. doi: 10.1155/2012/629652

Savona, M.R., Jacobsen, M.D., James, R., & Owen, M.D. (2005). Ultraviolet radiation and the risks of cutaneous malignant melanoma and non-melanoma skin cancer: perceptions and behaviours of Danish and American adolescents. European Journal of Cancer Prevention, 14(1), 57-62.

SEER Program (2007a) Surveillance, Epidemiology, and End Results (SEER) Program (www.seer.cancer.gov) SEER*Stat Database: Incidence—SEER 9 Regs Limited-Use, November 2006 Sub (1973–2004)—Linked To County Attributes—Total US, 1969–2004 Counties, National Cancer Institute, DCCPS, Surveillance Research Program, Cancer Statistics Branch, released April 2007, based on the November 2006 submission

Stevenson, D.S., Young, P.J., Naik, V. Lamarque, J.F, Shindell, D.T., Voulgarakis, A., et al. (2013). Tropospheric ozone changes, radiative forcing and attribution to emissions in the Atmospheric Chemistry and Climate Model Intercomparison Project (ACCMIP). Atmospheric Chemistry and Physics, 13, 3063–3085.

Strouse, J.J., Fears, T.R., Tucker, M.A., & Wayne, A.S. (2005). Pediatric melanoma: risk factor and survival analysis of the surveillance, epidemiology and end results database. Journal of Clinical Oncology, 23(21), 4735–4741.

Stolz, W., Braun-Falco, O., Bilek, P., Landthaler, M., Burgdorf, W.H.C., & Cognetta, A.B. (2002). Color atlas of dermatoscopy. 2nd ed. Berlin: Blackwell Wessenschafts-Verlag.

Stratigos, J.D., Katsambas, A., Christofidou, E., Hasapi, V., Katoulis, A., Stratigos, A., et al. (1996). Non-melanoma skin cancer in Greece - A clinico-epidemiological profile, Greece. Skin Cancer, 11(1), 9-17.

SunSmart Victoria. (2008). How to become a SunSmart school. Available from: http://www.sunsmart.com.au/browse.asp?ContainerID=1545

Sun Wise programme. (2008). Available from: http://www2.epa.gov/sunwise/join-sunwise

Task Force on Community Preventive Services. (2004). Recommendations to Prevent Skin Cancer by Reducing Exposure to Ultraviolet Radiation. American Journal of Preventive Medicine, 27(5), 467–470.

Tucker, M.A., Greene, M.H., Clark, W.H. Jr., Kraemer, K.H., Fraser, M.C., & Elder, D.E. (1983). Dysplastic nevi on the scalp of prepubertal children from melanoma-prone families. The Journal of Pediatrics, 103(1), 65–69.

United States Environmental Protection Agency. Sunwise Program. (2013). Available from: http://www.epa.gov/sunwise/

Vries, H., de Lezwijn, J., Hol, M., & Honing, C. (2005). Skin cancer prevention: behaviour and motives of Dutch adolescents, European Journal of Cancer Prevention, 14(1), 39-50.

Whiteman, D.C., Valery, P., McWhirter, W., & Green, A.C. (1997). Risk factors for childhood melanoma in Queensland, Australia. International Journal of Cancer, 70(1), 26–31.

Wong, J.R., Harris, J.K., Rodriguez-Galindo, C., & Johnson, K.J. (2013). Andersson, C. & Engardt, M. (2010). European ozone in a future climate: Importance of changes in dry deposition and isoprene emissions, Journal of Geophysical Research: Atmospheres, 115, D02303. doi:10.1029/2008JD011690, 2010

World Health Organization. Sun Protection and schools. How to make a difference. (2003). Available from: http://www.who.int/phe/uv.

World Health Organization (WHO). (2008). Protecting Children from ultraviolet radiation. Available from: http://www.who.int/mediacentre/factsheets/fs261/en/

World Health Organization (WHO). (2008). Ultraviolet Radiation. Available from http://www.who.int/uv/en/

World Health Organization. Adolescent health. (2013). Available from: www.who.int/topics/adolescent_health/en/

Yurtseven, E., Ulus, T., Vehid, S., Köksal, S., Bosat, M., & Akkoyun, K. (2012). Assessment of Knowledge, Behaviour and Sun Protection Practices among Health Services Vocational School Students. Int J Environ Res Public Health, 9(7), 2378–2385.

Zepp, R.G., Erickson, D.J. III, Paul, N.D., & Sulzberger B. (2011). Effects of solar UV radiation and climate change on biogeochemical cycling: interactions and feedbacks. Photochemical & Photobiological Sciences, 6, 286-300.

Zerefos, C.S., Meleti, C., Balis, D.S., Bais, A.F., & Gillotay, D. (2000). On changes of spectral UV-B in the 90's in Europe. Advances in Space Research, 26(12), 1971–1978.

Zerefos, C. S. (2002). Long-term ozone and UV variations at Thessaloniki, Greece. Physics and Chemistry of the Earth, 27(6–8), 455–460.

Basal Cell Carcinomas: An Epidemiologic Analysis

Ozan Luay Abbas

Plastic, Reconstructive and Aesthetic Surgery
Ahi Evran University, Kırsehir, Turkey

Huseyin Borman

Plastic, Reconstructive and Aesthetic Surgery
Baskent University, Ankara, Turkey

1   Introduction

The incidence of skin cancer has markedly increased over the past few decades. Basal cell carcinoma (BCC), Squamous cell carcinoma (SCC), and malignant melanoma are grouped under the term "skin cancer". BCCs and SCCs are distinctly labelled as non-melanoma skin cancers (NMSC). NMSCs are the most common forms of cancer and account for 90% of all skin cancer diagnosed in the world (Garner & Rodney, 2000). Basal cell carcinoma (BCC) is a malignant epithelial neoplasm that originates from the pluripotential cells in the epidermis and hair follicles (Pinkus, 1953). It is the most common skin cancer seen in human population (Jemal *et al.*, 2003). It is often slow growing and may take years to enlarge significantly. But it can cause extensive local tissue destruction and slow death if inadequately treated or left untreated. The mortality rates associated with this cancer is low. However, it causes considerable functional and cosmetic deformity and cost of treatment is significant (Housman *et al.*, 2003).

2   Methods

Our BCC database was reviewed between 1994 and 2012. Variables collected by operating surgeon were the patient's age, sex, tumor site, size, histologic subtype, surgical margin of excision, multiplicity of lesions, presence of involved margins, recurrence during follow up and the presence of metastasis. All of the pathology specimens were examined and reported by the Department of Pathology at our centre.

3   Results

3.1   Age and Gender

From January 1994 to May of 2012, 518 BCCs were excised from 486 patients. The median age was 65.6 (range, 20 to 93 years), 182 patients were women (37.4%) and 304 were men (62.55%) (Figure 1).

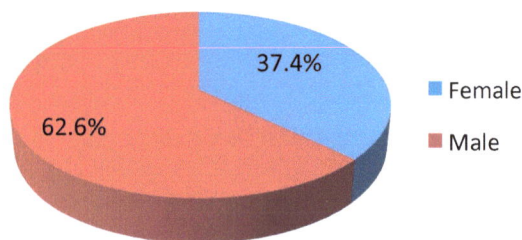

Figure 1: Gender percentages in BCC patients.

3.2   Anatomical Site

Most basal cell carcinomas were located on the head region (83.8 %). Anatomical distribution were as follows: the nose (25.09%), scalp (15.44%), periorbital region (10.03%), cheek (10.42%), periauricular area (9.65%), forehead (6.17%), upper lip (3.86 %), lower lip (1.15 %), chin (1.15 %) and neck (0.77 %) (Figure 2).

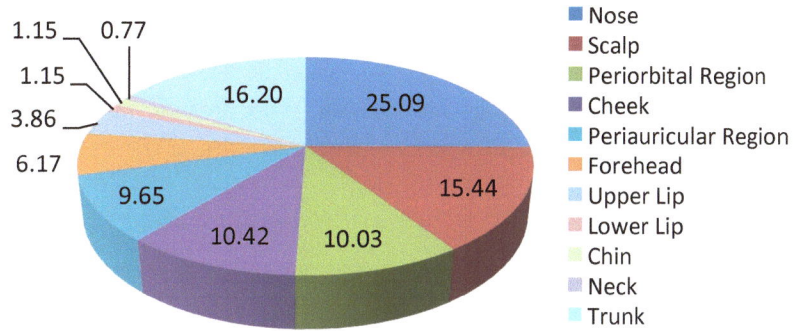

Figure 2: Anatomic distribution of the lesions.

3.3   Diameter of Lesion

294 lesions were smaller than 10 mm (56.7%), 196 lesions were between 10 and 20 mm (37.8%) and 28 lesions were bigger than 20 mm (5.4%). (Figure 3).

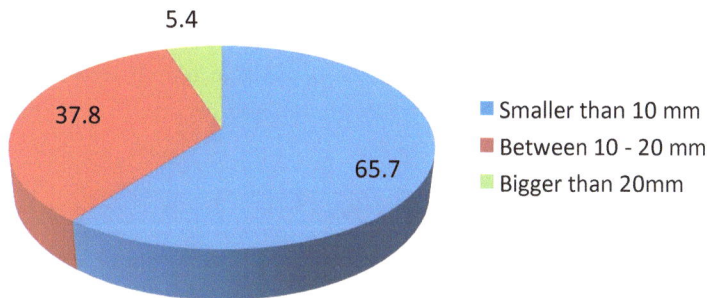

Figure 3: Lesion diameter.

3.4   Histologic Subtypes

Among 518 diagnosed BCCs; 358 were nodular (69.11%), 94 were superficial (18.14%), 36 were pigmented (6.94), 18 were morphea like (3.74%) and 12 were basosquamous (2.3%). (Figure 4).

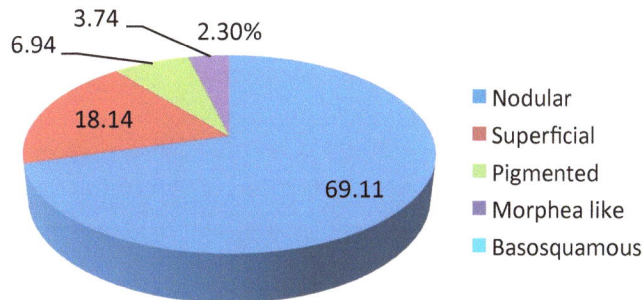

Figure 4: Histologic subtypes.

3.5   Tumor Excision

Only 18 patients (3.7 percent) had more than one lesion excised at the same operation. For lesions smaller than 1 cm in diameter we used a 3 mm margin for excision. We increased the excision margin 1 mm for every increase of 1 cm in diameter. We used a safety margin of 4 mm for morpheaform BCC and 5 mm for recurrent BCC. 12 BCCs (2.3%) required re-excision because of involved margins. During follow up we observed recurrence in 16 cases (3.08%). All occurred during the first four years. 8 were in the nose, 4 were in the periauricular area and 4 were in the periorbital area.

4   Discussion

The American Cancer Society reports skin cancers as being the most common cancer in the United States, with over 1 million new cases diagnosed and more than 10,000 deaths estimated yearly. The Skin Cancer Foundation currently estimates that one in every five Americans will develop skin cancer in their lifetime. Basal cell carcinoma incidence increases roughly by 3 to 6% per year (Bastiaens *et al.*, 1998). BCC accounts for 80% of all skin cancers but is the least likely cancer to behave in a malignant fashion and metastasize (Garner & Rodney, 2000). The mortality estimate from BCC is extremely low, with total 5 year survival rate of greater than 95% (Gloster & Brodland, 1996).

The majority of BCCs occur in men, the ratio of male to female in our series is 1.6:1. The higher incidence in men is probably due to increased recreational and occupational exposure to the sun. However, the incidence in women is increasing because of changing fashions in lifestyle. The likelihood of developing BCC increases with age, it is rarely found in patients younger than 40 years. The mean age of our patients is 65.6. The damaging effects of the sun begin at an early age. The results may not appear for 20 – 30 years. Unfortunately, BCCs is no longer exclusively associated with elderly population. It has been encroached upon younger age groups because of the unprotected levels of sun exposure.

Although the exact etiology of BCC is unknown, a well-established relationship exists between BCC and the pilosebaceous unit, as tumors are most often discovered on hair-bearing areas. Many believe that BCCs arise from pluripotential cells in the basal layer of the epidermis or follicular structures. These cells form continuously during life and can form hair, sebaceous glands, and apocrine glands. Tumors usually arise from the epidermis and occasionally arise from the outer root sheath of a hair follicle, specifically from hair follicle stem cells residing just below the sebaceous gland duct in an area called the bulge.

Several factors are believed to predispose the patient to basal cell carcinoma. Exposure to sunlight is the most frequent association. Cumulative exposure to sunlight over years is necessary for tumor development (Blum, 1948). There are three types of UV radiation: UVA (320-400 nm), UVB (290 – 320 nm), and UVC (200 – 280 nm). UVB rays are the most carcinogenic, triggering skin cancer via photochemical damage to DNA, injury to DNA repair mechanisms, and partial suppression of cell-mediated immunity (Gloster & Brodland, 1996). Patients often have a history of chronic sun exposure. Those at high risk for developing basal cell carcinoma are Fitzpatrick skin types I and II (A. J. J. Emmett, 1988). Because of the climate in our region, most of our patients had a history of chronic sun exposure.

Ionizing radiation exposure may generate BCC by two mechanisms. The first entails the initiations of prolonged cellular proliferation, thereby increasing the likelihood of transcription errors that can lead to cellular transformation. The second mechanism is direct damage of DNA replication, leading to cellular mutation that may activate proto-oncogenes or deactivate tumor suppressor genes. The minimum reported radiation dosage for inducing skin cancer is 4,6 grays (Modan, Baidatz, Mart, Steinitz, & Levin, 1974).

A modest increase in the lifetime risk of basal cell carcinoma has been noted in chronically immunosuppressed patients, such as recipients of organ or stem cell transplants. Immunosuppression alters the immune surveillance mechanism that destroys potentially malignant cells (Strom & Yamamura, 1997). Six of our patients were immunosuppressed after renal transplantation. Organ transplant patients must be instructed to limit sun exposure and alerted that skin cancer is a serious problem for them. In fact, immunosuppression and sun damage may cooperate to cause skin cancer. The skin cancer incidence is 10-fold higher in transplant patients than in the general population; up to 65-75% of patients with long-term immunosuppression develop skin cancer. Skin cancers can significantly alter and reduce the transplant recipients' quality of life; some patients may develop more than 100 skin cancers per year.

The vast majority of Basal cell carcinomas occur sporadically, but patients with the rare heritable disorder basal cell nevus syndrome (also known as Gorlin Syndrome) have marked susceptibility to develop BCCs. In sporadic BCCs, p53 mutation was essentially the only known molecular abnormality (Ling et al., 2001). However, family based linkage studies of kindreds with basal cell nevus syndrome identified the patched 1 (PTCH1) gene, an inhibitor of the hedgehog signaling, as being mutated (Hahn et al., 1996; Johnson et al., 1996; Klein, Dykas, & Bale, 2005). Biallelic inactivation of PTCH1results in upregulation of hedgehog signaling, which in turn leads to uncontrolled cell growth and proliferation. Because UV irradiation is a significant risk factor for BCC development, mutations in genes that control the extent of UV-induced DNA damage are associated with an increased risk of developing BCCs. Mutations of the melanocortin 1 receptor gene (MC1R) result in the production of pheomelanin (Rees, 2004). These people with fair pigment are at increased of BCCs.

The anatomic distribution of BCCs correlates with embryonic fusion planes. Recent data indicate that after adjusting for surface area, BCC occurrence is greater than 4 times more likely on embryonic fusion planes than on other regions of the midface, a finding that supports the possibility of an embryologic role for BCC pathogenesis.

The distribution of basal cell carcinoma across the body varies. Most of these carcinomas occur on sun exposed areas (Shanoff, Spira, & Hardy, 1967). In our series, 84 percent of basal cell carcinomas are found on head and 16 percent are found on trunk and extremities. The most common site for occurrence is the nose (25.09%)

Patients presenting with basal cell carcinoma (BCC) often report a slowly enlarging lesion that does not heal and that bleeds when traumatized. As tumors most commonly occur on the face, patients often give a history of an acne bump that occasionally bleeds. Patients often have a history of chronic sun exposure, including recreational sun exposure and occupational sun exposure. BCC usually appears as a flat, firm, pale area that is small, raised, pink or red, translucent, shiny, and waxy, and the area may bleed following minor injury. BCCs may have one or more visible and irregular blood vessels, an ulcerative area in the center that often is pigmented, and black-blue or brown areas. Large BCCs may have oozing or crusted areas. The lesion grows slowly, is not painful, and does not itch

Several histologic types of BCC exist. Histological diagnostics and classification of basal cell carcinomas (BCCs) are essential for an assessment of the percentage proportions of particular histological groups, risk determination of the recurrence of this illness, and comparison of treatment results. There is no unified and generally accepted classification of BCCs. When classifying BCCs, most authors start from the growth pattern, which gives more information about bio-behavior, and less often from the differentiation of tumors. Usually, BCCs are well differentiated and cells appear histologically similar to basal cells of the epidermis. BCCs can be divided into several subtypes: superficial, nodular, pigmented, morphea-like and basosquamous.

Nodular BCC is the most common type. It represents 69.11% of our series. It generally consists of large, round or oval tumor islands within the dermis, often with an epidermal attachment. Artificial retraction of the tumor islands from the surrounding stroma is commonly seen. Clinically it presents as well defined translucent pearly nodule that is either round or oval with rolled border and occasional ulceration. Telangiectasias are commonly seen coursing through the lesion. (Figure 5) Most tumors of this kind are observed on the face.

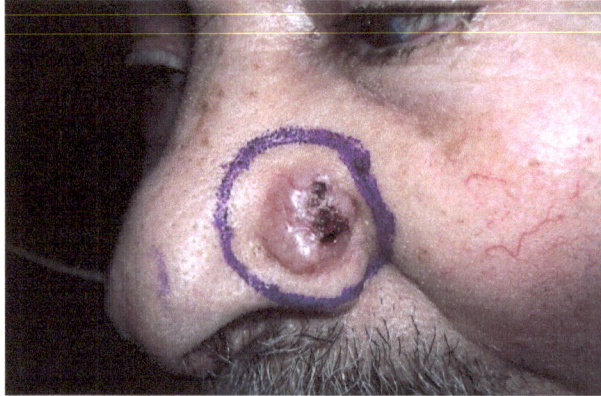

Figure 5: Nodular BCC presents as well defined translucent pearly nodule that is either round or oval with rolled border and occasional ulceration. Telangiectasias are commonly seen coursing through the lesion.

Superficial BCC is the second most common subtype in our series (18%). It is characterized by numerous small nests of tumor cells usually attached to the undersurface of the epidermis by a broad base. Clinically, it presents as slightly elevated plaque or discrete macule that may be scaly (Wade & Ackerman, 1978). (Figure 6) Most often developing on the upper trunk or shoulders. Superficial BCC had the lowest percentage of positive margins after excision (3.6%) (Sexton, Jones, & Maloney, 1990). None of our recurrent BCCs were superficial type.

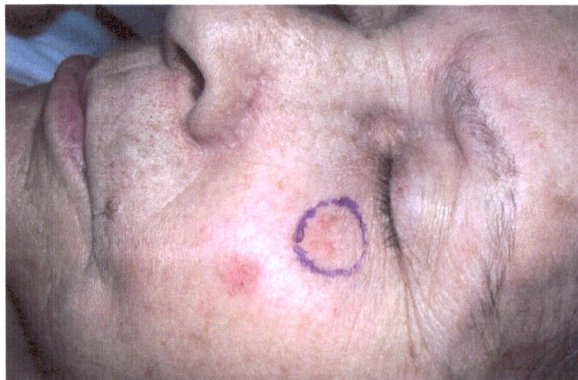

Figure 6: Superficial BCC presents as slightly elevated plaque or discrete macule that may be scaly.

Pigmented BCC is a rare variant (6.9%). Benign melanocytes in and around the tumor produce large amounts of melanin. These melanocytes contain many melanin granules in their cytoplasm and dendrites. It ranges from brown to blue black and can be mistaken for melanoma (Figure 7). Telangiectases that are typical of a nodular basal cell carcinoma can be observed. This aids clinically in differentiating this tumor from a melanoma.

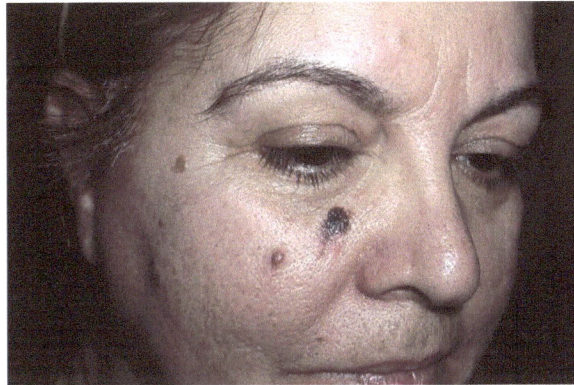

Figure 7: Pigmented BCC

Basosquamous carcinomas have both basal and squamous cell differentiations. It has been defined as a basal cell carcinoma with differentiation towards squamous cell carcinoma. It is made up of basaloid cells that are a larger, paler, and rounder than those of a solid BCC. It also consists of squamoid cells and intermediate cells. Some consider the diagnosis of this type most appropriate when one evaluates a tumor with contiguous areas of BCC and SCC. This type is considered to have metastatic potential and is considered an aggressive skin cancer. They have a higher growth rate as well as higher metastatic potential than do other BCCs. It represents 2.3% of all our series.

Morphea like BCC is an aggressive rare variant accounting for 3.7% of all our BCCs. It presents as firm plaques that is yellow or white with ill-defined border (Figure 8). Tumor cells induce a proliferation of fibroblasts within the dermis and an increased collagen deposition (sclerosis) that clinically resembles a scar. The extent of the tumor is usually not apparent on clinical examination. Morphea form BCCs had the highest percentage of positive margins after excision. Thirty three percent of our morphea form BCCs had involved margins after excision. Mohs micrographic surgery is valuable in the management of these lesions.

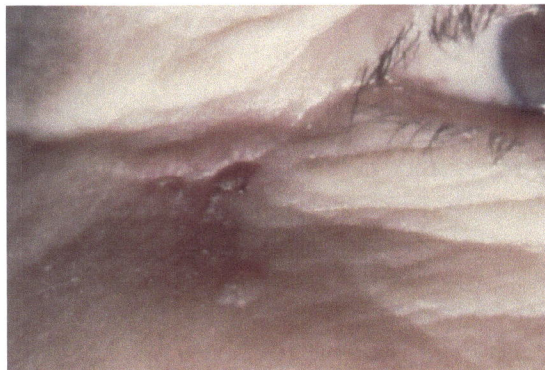

Figure 8: Morphea–form BCC

Regardless of the appearance of the lesion, we perform a histologic confirmation and typing. The histologic characteristics influence clinical behaviour, recurrence, and metastatic potential. Shave biopsy with a scalpel is a simple method removing the epidermis and a portion of the dermis. Since this tumor arises from the basal layer of the epidermis, shave biopsy will provide sufficient material for histological diagnosis and classification. Approximately 75.9% accuracy rate has been found with shave biopsy (Russell, Carrington, & Smoller, 1999). We don't prefer this type of biopsy in pigmented BCC's that are difficult to differentiate from the melanomas. Punch biopsy garners a full-thickness specimen. The punched out defect may be sutured or may heal secondarily. The accuracy rate with punch biopsy is 80.7% (Russell *et al.*, 1999). We only prefer using this type of biopsy when a large lesion of uncertain diagnosis exists. Excisional biopsy, is the biopsy type that we usually prefer. We advise excisional biopsy for small lesions that enable primary closure afterwards that does not cause distortion of the environmental tissues. Otherwise, an incisional biopsy may be done before the definitive treatment.

Once the pathologic diagnosis of BCC is confirmed, the next step is to plan for tumor eradication by correlating tumor characteristics with patient's age, skin history, medical history, social history, and cosmetic expectations. Treatment options include standard surgical excision, Mohs micrographic surgery, nonsurgical ablation and topical chemotherapy.

Surgical excision is the preferred method in our centre. We generally perform excision under local anaesthesia or in the outpatient surgery settings. Our excision margins usually change according to the size, type and location of the lesions. We use the minimal safety margins in areas like the periorbital region and send the tumor for frozen section examination during the operation to ensure complete removal of the tumour. For lesions less than 1 cm in diameter we use a 3mm margin for excision. We increase the excision margin 1 mm for every increase of 1 cm in tumor diameter. We use a safety margin of 4 mm for morpheaform BCC and 5 mm for recurrent BCC. The safety margins may well be increased according to the degree of destruction of tissues in recurrent BCCs. In areas where there is no delicate structure nearby such as the back region, we prefer to use a wider excision margin in our excision spectrum. It is certainly better not to leave any residual tumour after the first operation as long as the surgical result is not compromising the aesthetic result. Frozen section examination or Mohs surgery may be used anywhere any suspicion about the completeness of removal arises. Proper curettage to better define the BCC's border prior to excision may increase the cure rate for primary lesions (Telfer, Colver, Morton, & British Association of, 2008). The wound may be left for secondary healing, closed primarily, skin grafted or closed using a flap. The specimen is sent to the pathology laboratory with results transmitted within a few days. The final surgical decision is made on the basis of these results. A flap is used only after the final margins are negative.

Mohs micrographic surgery aims to completely remove the tumor via consecutive excision of the tumor, spatially orienting the specimen, histologically examining the margins, re-excising the residual tumor, and repeating the cycle until the area is tumor free. It is based on the principle that the tumor spreads by contiguous growth. The cure rates for primary BCCs < 2 cm treated with MMS approach 99%.[14,15] Recurrent BCC cure rates range from 94 to 96% (Lawrence, 1999; Shriner, McCoy, Goldberg, & Wagner, 1998). Mohs micrographic surgery is indicated for the treatment of recurrent BCC, primary BCC occurring at sites with high rates of recurrence (e.g., periorbital, periauricular and nasolabila areas), histologically difficult BCC (i.e., morphelike), and BCCs in which conservation of tissue is critical (e.g., on the nose and ear).

Destructive methods like curettage and electrodesiccation (C&E), cryosurgery and laser are appropriate methods for the management of smaller lesions that have low recurrence rates. Due to unacceptably high recurrence rates, poor cosmetic outcomes and lack of histological control, it is generally not accepted as a first line therapy for BCC in our centre.

Curettage refers to the use of a curet for separating and cutting the tumor from the skin. Electrodesiccation refers to the use of electrocautery, in which a high-frequency electrical current is directly applied to the tissue. The current destroys tumor cells and obtains hemostasis. During the curetting, the physician should feel the difference between tumor and normal skin. Tumor tissue feels soft and easily breakable, whereas normal dermis is difficult to scrape and feels coarse. After curettage, electrocautery is applied to the entire curetted area. This cycle can repeated in a single visit (Orengo, Katta, & Rosen, 2002). C&E is an easy technique to learn and requires only minimal equipment's. However, the wound may take 6 weeks to heal leaving a hypopigmented or hypertrophic scar. Recurrence rates can be as high as %13 depending on BCC subtype, anatomic location and tumor diameter (Rowe, Carroll, & Day, 1989; Silverman, Kopf, Grin, Bart, & Levenstein, 1991). We recommend avoiding C&E in BCCs along the embryonic fusion lines.

Cryosurgery uses various mechanisms to treat carcinoma by forming crystals, demonstrating recrystallization patterns as the cells thaw, exposing cells to electrolyte concentrations in adjacent thawing and nonfrozen fluids, causing ischemic damage from vascular destruction (Giuffrida, Jimenez, & Nouri, 2003). Liquid nitrogen is the most common used cryogen. High risk BCCs with aggressive histologic subtype or BCCs in critical facial sites are not appropriate for cryosurgery. The recurrence rate for primary BCCs treated with cryosurgery is 4.3% (Thissen, Neumann, & Schouten, 1999). Immediately after application, pain, redness and edema are observed at the treated site. Within the first days after cryosurgery blisters may develop. It may take several weeks for wounds to heal. Cryosurgery may produce permanent hyperpigmentation or hypopigmentation.

Laser therapy is a novel option for the treatment of BCCs. However, long term results have not been determined yet and more clinical studies are warranted. Treatment with a combined 585 nm pulsed dye laser (PDL) and 1,064 nm Neodymium Yttrium Aluminum Garnet (Nd:YAG) laser was found effective in reducing tumor burden in patients with BCC (Jalian, Avram, Stankiewicz, Shofner, & Tannous, 2013). Lasers are still not well accepted primary treatment of BCCs.

Photodynamic (PTD) therapy is administered by application of photosensitizer to the target area. When these molecules are activated by light, they become toxic, therefore destroy the target cells. Long-term cure rates for PDT have been disappointing, and treatment may require multiple sessions to increase the clearance rate. This modality may still prove to be a good option for select patients. Since the photosensitizers may have limited penetration and diffusion, BCCs should be of the superficial subtype and less than 2-mm thick to increase the chances of successful tumor treatment.

Most BCCs are sensitive to doses of radiation therapy (RT) that can be endured by normal surrounding skin. RT of tumors < 2 mm has a cure rate of 90% for BCC (Leshin, Yeatts, Anscher, Montano, & Dutton, 1993). However, larger lesions have a much lower success rate. We reserve radiation for elderly patients who are poor surgical candidates or for patients having residual or recurrent tumors. RT is contraindicated in young patients because of the high risk of radiodermatitis and scars; in lesions on the trunk and extremities; and in delayed cancer recurrence. RT requires multiple visits. Treatment results in radiation damage and, therefore, should be reserved for older patients. RT is less effective for nonfacial tumors. RT also is contraindicated in patients with connective tissue diseases or genetic conditions predisposing to skin cancer (e.g., xeroderma pigmentosum, epidermodysplasia verruciformis, and basal cell nevus syndrome.) This histologic type in conjunction with RT may induce more tumors in the treated area. Radiation adverse effects include dermatitis, keratinization of the conjunctiva, and chronic keratitis.

Topical treatment using 5-fluorouracil may be used to treat small, superficial BCCs in low-risk areas. It interferes with DNA synthesis by blocking methylation of deoxyuridylic acid and inhibiting thymidylate synthetase and, subsequently, cell proliferation. In properly selected tumors, cure rates of approximately 80% have been obtained. The recurrence rate is very high. It is not in our routine. Retinoids are derivatives of vitamin A, and are essential to maintaining cellular differentiation. When present in physiologic to supra-physiological levels, retinoids can impede the progression of epithelial carcinogenesis. Oral retinoids may be indicated for multiple BCCs, such as basal cell nevus syndrome. Others include organ transplant recipients and patients with greatly sun-damaged skin.

Although the results of primary excision are excellent, recurrences can occur. Recurrence rates are higher in the inner canthus, base of the nostril and preauricular and postauricular areas (A. J. Emmett & Broadbent, 1981). This can be attributed to the scarcity of tissue, proximity to vital structures and cosmetic considerations that must be taken into account in treating lesions on these locations. Recurrence rates are also increasing with increasing lesion size. We observed recurrence in 16 cases (3.08%). All occurred during the first four years. 8 were in the nose (Figure 9), 4 were in the periauricular area and 4 were in the periorbital area.

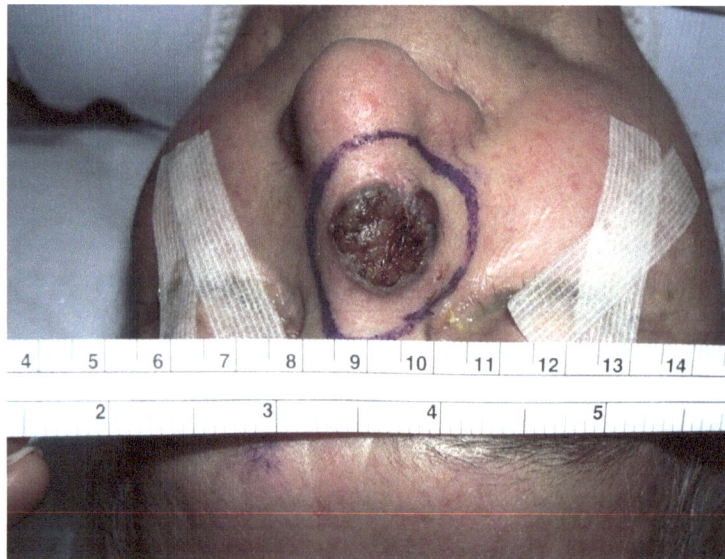

Figure 9: Recurrent BCC in the nose

The incidence of incomplete excision of BCC reported in retrospective studies is in the range of 6.3 to 25 percent (Bogdanov-Berezovsky *et al.*, 2001; Dieu & Macleod, 2002; Griffiths, 1999; Hauben, Zirkin, Mahler, & Sacks, 1982; Hussain & Earley, 2003; Mak *et al.*, 1995; Richmond & Davie, 1987; Rippey & Rippey, 1997; Schreuder & Powell, 1999; Sussman & Liggins, 1996). In our series, 12 BCCs (2.3%) reported to have involved margins. The anatomic distribution of lesions with involved surgical margins were as follows; 6 lesions in the nose, 4 in the periauricular area and 2 in the periorbital area. In these cases, we prefer re-excision because reported recurrence rates for incompletely excised basal cell carcinomas can be as high as 86% (Pascal, Hobby, Lattes, & Crikelair, 1968). The hedgehog pathway inhibitor, Vismodegib, represents a new opportunity for the treatment of such patients with involved margins. Vismodegib has approval from the United States Food and Drug Administration for treatment of metastatic BCC, locally advanced BCC recurring after surgery, and BCC that is not treatable via surgery or radiation (Bayers, Kapp, Beer, & Slavin, 2013; Sobanko, Okman, & Miller, 2013).

The prognosis for patients with BCC is excellent, with a 100% survival rate for cases that have not spread to other sites. Nevertheless, if BCC is allowed to progress, it can result in significant morbidity, and cosmetic disfigurement is not uncommon.

Although basal cell carcinoma is a malignant neoplasm, it rarely metastasizes. The rate of metastasis is below 0.1% (Goldberg, 1997).This low rate can be explained by BCCs connective tissue stroma dependent growth. Experimentally transplanted BCCs will not survive without dermal tissue (Grimwood, Ferris, Mercill, & Huff, 1986). Size, depth of invasion and histological type are important predictors for metastasis (Randle, 1996). Favoured sites of metastasis include regional lymph nodes, liver, lung, bone and skin. This rare metastasis is twice as common in males as in females.

Adequate patient education is essential in the prevention of recurrence of basal cell carcinoma. Avoiding extreme sun exposure is imperative. Wearing sunscreen, with a protective factor index of at least 30 or higher may decrease the chance of BCCs. Presently, sunscreen manufacturers are including protection against both types of rays. Whenever possible, one should wear long sleeves and long pants while outdoors. Wide-brimmed hats are also advised Patients should avoid other possible potentiating factors. Patients should be educated on how to recognize any unexplained changes in their skin, especially changes that last for more than 3-4 weeks.

For those without a history of skin cancer, a dermatologic examination is recommended every 3 years for persons aged 20-40 years and every year for persons older than 40 years. The American Cancer Society recommends a dermatologic examination every 3 years for people aged 20-40 years and every year for people older than 40 years.

5   Conclusion

BCC is by far the most common cancer in the world and is the main cause of the skin cancer epidemic we are now facing. Fortunately, the majority of BCC cases are also preventable due to the chief etiologic factor, UV radiation. An ever increasing amount of evidence, linking the dangers of UV radiation to cancer, is discovered and imposed upon the health care field and the general public. With this evidence in hand, it is the job of physicians to reinforce and educate patients until the message is understood. Many treatment modalities are also becoming available, including topical regimens. It is necessary to explore these newer agents with large clinical trials to prove their efficacy to have them available in the near future for our patients. A large body of information serves as a foundation for oncologic principles, diagnosis methods, surgical excisions, follow up protocols and reconstructive methodologies that are currently in use. Surgical ablation remains the mainstay of treatment.

References

Bastiaens, M. T., Hoefnagel, J. J., Bruijn, J. A., Westendorp, R. G., Vermeer, B. J., & Bouwes Bavinck, J. N. (1998). Differences in age, site distribution, and sex between nodular and superficial basal cell carcinoma indicate different types of tumors. J Invest Dermatol, 110(6), 880-884. doi: 10.1046/j.1523-1747.1998.00217.x

Bayers, S., Kapp, D. L., Beer, K. R., & Slavin, B. (2013). Treatment of margin positive Basal cell carcinoma with vismodegib: case report and consideration of treatment options and their implications. J Drugs Dermatol, 12(10 Suppl), s147-150.

Blum, H. F. (1948). Sunlight as a casual factor in cancer of the skin of man. J Natl Cancer Inst, 9(3), 247-258.

Bogdanov-Berezovsky, A., Cohen, A., Glesinger, R., Cagnano, E., Krieger, Y., & Rosenberg, L. (2001). Clinical and pathological findings in reexcision of incompletely excised basal cell carcinomas. Ann Plast Surg, 47(3), 299-302.

Czajkowski, K., Fitzgerald, S., Foster, I., & Kesselman, C. (2001). Grid information services for distributed resource sharing. In 10th IEEE International Symposium on High Performance Distributed Computing (pp. 181–184).

Dieu, T., & Macleod, A. M. (2002). Incomplete excision of basal cell carcinomas: a retrospective audit. ANZ J Surg, 72(3), 219-221.

Emmett, A. J., & Broadbent, G. G. (1981). Basal cell carcinoma in Queensland. Aust N Z J Surg, 51(6), 576-590.

Emmett, A. J. J. (1988). The bare facts : the effect of sun on skin. Sydney ; Baltimore: Williams & Wilkins and Associates.

Foster, I., Kesselman, C., Nick, J., & Tuecke, S. (2002). The Physiology of the Grid: an Open Grid Services Architecture for Distributed Systems Integration. Technical report, Global Grid Forum.

Garner, K. L., & Rodney, W. M. (2000). Basal and squamous cell carcinoma. Prim Care, 27(2), 447-458.

Giuffrida, T. J., Jimenez, G., & Nouri, K. (2003). Histologic cure of basal cell carcinoma treated with cryosurgery. J Am Acad Dermatol, 49(3), 483-486.

Gloster, H. M., Jr., & Brodland, D. G. (1996). The epidemiology of skin cancer. Dermatol Surg, 22(3), 217-226.

Goldberg, D. P. (1997). Assessment and surgical treatment of basal cell skin cancer. Clin Plast Surg, 24(4), 673-686.

Griffiths, R. W. (1999). Audit of histologically incompletely excised basal cell carcinomas: recommendations for management by re-excision. Br J Plast Surg, 52(1), 24-28. doi: 10.1054/bjps.1998.3018

Grimwood, R. E., Ferris, C. F., Mercill, D. B., & Huff, J. C. (1986). Proliferating cells of human basal cell carcinoma are located on the periphery of tumor nodules. J Invest Dermatol, 86(2), 191-194.

Gusfield, D. (1997). Algorithms on Strings, Trees and Sequences: Computer Science and Computational Biology. Cambridge: Cambridge University Press.

Hahn, H., Wicking, C., Zaphiropoulous, P. G., Gailani, M. R., Shanley, S., Chidambaram, A., . . . Bale, A. E. (1996). Mutations of the human homolog of Drosophila patched in the nevoid basal cell carcinoma syndrome. Cell, 85(6), 841-851.

Hauben, D. J., Zirkin, H., Mahler, D., & Sacks, M. (1982). The biologic behavior of basal cell carcinoma: analysis of recurrence in excised basal cell carcinoma: Part II. Plast Reconstr Surg, 69(1), 110-116.

Hern'andez, M. A. & Stolfo, S. J. (1995). The merge/purge problem for large databases. SIGMOD Record, 24(2), 127–138.

Housman, T. S., Feldman, S. R., Williford, P. M., Fleischer, A. B., Jr., Goldman, N. D., Acostamadiedo, J. M., & Chen, G. J. (2003). Skin cancer is among the most costly of all cancers to treat for the Medicare population. J Am Acad Dermatol, 48(3), 425-429. doi: 10.1067/mjd.2003.186

Hussain, M., & Earley, M. J. (2003). The incidence of incomplete excision in surgically treated basal cell carcinoma: a retrospective clinical audit. Ir Med J, 96(1), 18-20.

Jalian, H. R., Avram, M. M., Stankiewicz, K. J., Shofner, J. D., & Tannous, Z. (2013). Combined 585 nm pulsed-dye and 1,064 nm Nd:YAG lasers for the treatment of basal cell carcinoma. Lasers Surg Med. doi: 10.1002/lsm.22201

Jemal, A., Murray, T., Samuels, A., Ghafoor, A., Ward, E., & Thun, M. J. (2003). Cancer statistics, 2003. CA Cancer J Clin, 53(1), 5-26.

Johnson, R. L., Rothman, A. L., Xie, J., Goodrich, L. V., Bare, J. W., Bonifas, J. M., . . . Scott, M. P. (1996). Human homolog of patched, a candidate gene for the basal cell nevus syndrome. Science, 272(5268), 1668-1671.

Klein, R. D., Dykas, D. J., & Bale, A. E. (2005). Clinical testing for the nevoid basal cell carcinoma syndrome in a DNA diagnostic laboratory. Genet Med, 7(9), 611-619. doi: 10.109701.gim.0000182879.57182.b4

Lawrence, C. M. (1999). Mohs' micrographic surgery for basal cell carcinoma. Clin Exp Dermatol, 24(2), 130-133.

Leshin, B., Yeatts, P., Anscher, M., Montano, G., & Dutton, J. J. (1993). Management of periocular basal cell carcinoma: Mohs' micrographic surgery versus radiotherapy. Surv Ophthalmol, 38(2), 193-212.

Ling, G., Ahmadian, A., Persson, A., Unden, A. B., Afink, G., Williams, C., . . . Ponten, F. (2001). PATCHED and p53 gene alterations in sporadic and hereditary basal cell cancer. Oncogene, 20(53), 7770-7778. doi: 10.1038/sj.onc.1204946

Mak, A. S., Poon, A. M., Leung, C. Y., Kwan, K. H., Wong, T. T., & Tung, M. K. (1995). Audit of basal cell carcinoma in Princess Margaret Hospital, Hong Kong: usefulness of frozen section examination in surgical treatment. Scand J Plast Reconstr Surg Hand Surg, 29(2), 149-152.

Modan, B., Baidatz, D., Mart, H., Steinitz, R., & Levin, S. G. (1974). Radiation-induced head and neck tumours. Lancet, 1(7852), 277-279.

Orengo, I., Katta, R., & Rosen, T. (2002). Techniques in the removal of skin lesions. Otolaryngol Clin North Am, 35(1), 153-170, vii.

Pascal, R. R., Hobby, L. W., Lattes, R., & Crikelair, G. F. (1968). Prognosis of "incompletely excised" versus "completely excised" basal cell carcinoma. Plast Reconstr Surg, 41(4), 328-332.

Pinkus, H. (1953). Premalignant fibroepithelial tumors of skin. AMA Arch Derm Syphilol, 67(6), 598-615.

Randle, H. W. (1996). Basal cell carcinoma. Identification and treatment of the high-risk patient. Dermatol Surg, 22(3), 255-261.

Rees, J. L. (2004). The genetics of sun sensitivity in humans. Am J Hum Genet, 75(5), 739-751. doi: 10.1086/425285

Richmond, J. D., & Davie, R. M. (1987). The significance of incomplete excision in patients with basal cell carcinoma. Br J Plast Surg, 40(1), 63-67.

Rippey, J. J., & Rippey, E. (1997). Characteristics of incompletely excised basal cell carcinomas of the skin. Med J Aust, 166(11), 581-583.

Rowe, D. E., Carroll, R. J., & Day, C. L., Jr. (1989). Mohs surgery is the treatment of choice for recurrent (previously treated) basal cell carcinoma. J Dermatol Surg Oncol, 15(4), 424-431.

Russell, E. B., Carrington, P. R., & Smoller, B. R. (1999). Basal cell carcinoma: a comparison of shave biopsy versus punch biopsy techniques in subtype diagnosis. J Am Acad Dermatol, 41(1), 69-71.

Schreuder, F., & Powell, B. W. (1999). Incomplete excision of basal cell carcinomas: an audit. Clin Perform Qual Health Care, 7(3), 119-120.

Sexton, M., Jones, D. B., & Maloney, M. E. (1990). Histologic pattern analysis of basal cell carcinoma. Study of a series of 1039 consecutive neoplasms. J Am Acad Dermatol, 23(6 Pt 1), 1118-1126.

Shanoff, L. B., Spira, M., & Hardy, S. B. (1967). Basal cell carcinoma: a statistical approach to rational management. Plast Reconstr Surg, 39(6), 619-624.

Shriner, D. L., McCoy, D. K., Goldberg, D. J., & Wagner, R. F., Jr. (1998). Mohs micrographic surgery. J Am Acad Dermatol, 39(1), 79-97.

Silverman, M. K., Kopf, A. W., Grin, C. M., Bart, R. S., & Levenstein, M. J. (1991). Recurrence rates of treated basal cell carcinomas. Part 2: Curettage-electrodesiccation. J Dermatol Surg Oncol, 17(9), 720-726.

Smith, T. F. & Waterman, M. S. (1981). Identification of common molecular subsequences. Journal of Molecular Biology, 147, 195–197.

Sobanko, J. F., Okman, J., & Miller, C. (2013). Vismodegib: a hedgehog pathway inhibitor for locally advanced and metastatic Basal cell carcinomas. J Drugs Dermatol, 12(10 Suppl), s154-155.

Strom, S. S., & Yamamura, Y. (1997). Epidemiology of nonmelanoma skin cancer. Clin Plast Surg, 24(4), 627-636.

Sussman, L. A., & Liggins, D. F. (1996). Incompletely excised basal cell carcinoma: a management dilemma? Aust N Z J Surg, 66(5), 276-278.

Telfer, N. R., Colver, G. B., Morton, C. A., & British Association of, D. (2008). Guidelines for the management of basal cell carcinoma. Br J Dermatol, 159(1), 35-48. doi: 10.1111/j.1365-2133.2008.08666.x

Thissen, M. R., Neumann, M. H., & Schouten, L. J. (1999). A systematic review of treatment modalities for primary basal cell carcinomas. Arch Dermatol, 135(10), 1177-1183.

Wade, T. R., & Ackerman, A. B. (1978). The many faces of basal-cell carcinoma. J Dermatol Surg Oncol, 4(1), 23-28.

Potential Risks of Indiscriminate Medicated Soaps Usage: Toxicity and Antimicrobial Resistance

Kennedy D. Mwambete

Department of Pharmaceutical Microbiology, School of Pharmacy
Muhimbili University of Health & Allied Sciences, Tanzania, Africa

1 Introduction

1.1 Background ofAntimicrobial Resistance

Antimicrobial resistance is a serious and growing phenomenon in contemporary medicine and has emerged as one of the important public health concerns of the 21st century, because of its association with both human and animal diseases-causing microorganisms (Sharma *et al.*, 2005; Russell, 2003). Each year, innumerable antibiotics are prescribed by physicians and patients are self-medicated for health problems against which antimicrobial agents are useless or the patient does not complete treatment; these have been attributed to the development of antimicrobial resistance. Indiscriminate use of consumer products–containing antimicrobial agents (biocides), such as medicated soaps and other personal care products, also runs the risk of creating resistant microorganisms. Additionally, because of globalization (easy travel around the world), the potential of creating pandemics isalarming and evident (Rolain *etal.*, 2010; Harbarth & Samore, 2005).

Constant exposure of microorganisms to sub-lethal concentrations of biocides such as chlorahexidine gluconate (CHG) and Triclosan[5-chloro-2-(2, 4-dichlorophenoxy) phenol)]-(TCS) also popular as *Irgasan*® DP 300tends to decrease microbial susceptibility over hundred folds (McBain *et al.*, 2004). Biocides and antibiotics have so many in common regarding their mechanisms of action; hence similar mechanisms of bacterial insusceptibility may apply, though major differences are also noticeable (Gilbert & Moore, 2005; Poole, 2002). Most of the antimicrobial agents used in medicated soaps and other consumer products, contain TCS, CHG and quaternary ammonium compounds (QACs), which are used as antiseptic, disinfectant, and preservative while others such as chlorine dioxide, glutaraldehyde, orthophthalaldehyde are used predominantly as disinfectants (Russell, 2003).As some of these biocides have wide antimicrobial spectra, thus have multiple antimicrobial targets that might have similarities to those of antibiotics.

Evidences exist that naturally occurring antimicrobial resistance is inevitable, because of microbial evolution through constant mutations (Davies & Davies, 2010; Silbergeld *et al.*, 2008; Wright, 2007; Walsh, 2000). Therefore, antimicrobial resistance is a continually evolving and perilous problem that requires urgent attention and well-planned measures to impede a global health crisis.Since microorganisms thrive on mutations; therefore removal of selective pressures can significantly slow mutational rates (Davies & Davies, 2010).

1.2 Current Uses of Soaps and Medicated Soaps

1.2.1 Prevention of Microbial Infections

Microbial infections such as tuberculosis, pneumonia, strep throat, food borne and meningitis: these are just a few of the stubborn diseases caused by bacteria, which have ever since been prevented by adopting appropriate hygienic measures, including the use of plain soaps. Hygiene is one of the best ways to curb the development and spread of microbial infections, but lately consumers are "misinformed" that washing with regular soap is insufficient. Antibacterial products have never been so popular. Body soaps, household cleaners, sponges, even mattresses and lip glosses are now packing microorganism-killing ingredients, and scientists question what place, if any, these antimicrobials have in the daily routines of healthy people. Traditionally, people sweep away bacteria from their bodies and homes using soap and hot water, alcohol, chlorine bleach or hydrogen peroxide. These substances act nonspecifically, meaning they are capable of wiping out almost every type of microorganisms rather than singling out a particular variety.

Aiello *et al.* (2007) showed that TCS-containing medicated soap does not reduce bacterial counts on hands significantly more than plain soap unless used repeatedly and in relatively high concentrations (>1%) compared to the 0.1-0.45% in consumer medicated soaps. Therefore, routine cleaning with or without plain soap is often sufficient, but in cases of household infection, may not adequately reduce environmental contamination. In such circumstances, the use of medicated soaps/biocides is recommended. Nonetheless, the effectiveness of biocides varies considerably and depends on how they are used as well as their intrinsic efficacy (Kagan *et al.*, 2002).

1.2.2   Human Health and Environmental Concerns of Medicated Soap Usage

Many antimicrobial agents/biocides used in everyday household products have never been formally approved by Food and Drug Administration (FDA). That's because many microbial-killing agents were developed decades ago before there were laws requiring scientific review of cleaning ingredients. In 1978, the FDA published its first tentative guidelines for antimicrobial agents used in liquid hand soaps and washes. The draft stated that antimicrobial agents such as TCS was "not generally recognized as safe and effective," because regulators could not find enough scientific proof demonstrating its safety and effectiveness (Larson, 1999).

At this time, FDA does not have evidence that antimicrobial agents added to antibacterial soaps and body washes provides extra health benefits over soap and water. Consumers who are concerned about using hand and body soaps with antimicrobial agents should wash with regular soap and water.The American Medical Association (AMA) took an official stance in 2000 against adding antimicrobials to consumer products. The AMA has repeatedly urged the FDA to better regulate these chemicals, advising that they should be avoided "until the data emerge to show antimicrobials in consumer products are effective at preventing infection." Since 2000, about 1,500 new antibacterial products have hit the market(FDA, 2013).

Halden, an expert in environmental health once pointed out that: "First, to protect our health, we mass-produce and use a toxic chemical which the FDA has determined has no scientifically proven benefit. Second, when we try to do the right thing by recycling bio-solids, we end up spreading a known reproductive toxicant on the soil where we grow our food." He emphasizes the importance of considering the full life cycle of the chemicals we manufacture (Halden & Paull, 2005).

The evolution of drug-resistant bacteria is not just the result of prescription negligence. Domestically used antimicrobial soaps and other cleaning products, are also responsible. Not only antibiotic prescriptions can be misused, but also consumer antimicrobial products. Originally, antimicrobial agents had one main role that is to kill or inhibit the growth of microorganisms and improve human welfare by preventing and controlling microbial-associated infections/diseases (Larson, 1988). Nevertheless, antimicrobial agents are now common ingredients in many everyday household, personal care and consumer products like medicated soaps. Numerous cleaning agents are available in the market, which are presented in various forms with distinct formulations (Ikpoh *et al.*, 2012; Mwambete & Lyombe, 2011).

But the question still is whether medicated soaps actually work any better at killing or inhibiting the spread of infectious microorganisms than plain soap and water, which merely wash away microorganisms before they reach a dangerous level. Several studies suggest that these products may encourage the growth of "superbugs" resistant to antimicrobial agents; a problem when these microorganisms run uncontrolled, turning into a perilous infection that cannot be treated with available medication (Drury*et al.*,

2013; Hegstad *et al.*, 2010; Ahn*et al.*, 2008). By using more antimicrobial products, people may encourage microorganisms to evolve and become more virulent than they were before. Similar growth of antimicrobial-resistant strains has already occurred with antibiotics. The overuse and misuse of antibiotics has led to several antimicrobial-resistant microorganisms, such as *Staphylococcus aureus*, *Streptococcus pneumonia*and*E. coli* as well as *Candida* species (Richter*et al.*, 2005; Sharma *et al.*, 2005).Irrational use of antimicrobial products is now one of the major health concerns that are being addressed in the field of pharmaco-epidemiology (Gilbert & McBain, 2003).

  TCS-an antimicrobial agentwidely used in a variety of consumer products is known to promote the growth of resistant microorganisms, including *E. coli*. Heath and Rock (2000) predicted that "the use of TCS in these household consumer products will lead to the emergence of resistance." "There is no strong rationale for their use' they emphasized. Certainly, introduction of enormousantimicrobial agents into the environment in this way, can results into increasing pathogens' resistance to clinically important antibiotics. It is suggested that, although the practical implications of reduced susceptibility to antimicrobial agents associated with exposure to sub-lethal concentrations of medicated soaps appears to be insignificant; the impact must be balanced against the benefits of such use to consumer health and the environmental impacts:public health and product toxicity. The risks must also be taken into account in relation to interactions of the medicated soap-embedded antimicrobial agents with physical or chemical agents and other living organisms, to which microbial populations are continually exposed. It is well recognized that chemical exposures,such as to consumer products, early in life are significant and preventable causes of non-communicable diseases in children and adults (Landrigan & Goldman, 2011).

Brands	Active ingredient	Expiry date	Indication	Manufacturer
Meditex	PCMX	None	Bactericide	Mukwano Industries Tanzania Ltd
Duru	None	None	Bactericide	Murzar oil mills Ltd
Protex	TCC 0.25% and TCS 0.20%	08/2009	Bactericide	Colgate Palmolive (pty) Ltd
Lifebuoy	TCC 0.06%, DCP 0.02%	06/2010	Bactericide	Unilever Kenya Ltd
Rungu	Irgasan DP 300®	None	Bactericide	HB worldwide Ltd
Roberts	Irgasan DP 300®	None	Bactericide	PZ Cussons East Africa Ltd
Family	TCC, Irgasan DP 300®	None	Bactericide	G & B soap Industries Ltd
Dettol	PCMX 0.5% TCC 0.5%	09/2010	None	Reckitt Benkiser East Africa Ltd
Protector	Irgasan DP 300®	None	None	Showerlux Industries Ltd
Regency neem	Neem	None	Antiseptic	Neem Africa Ltd
Dalan	None	None	Bactericide	
Imperial	None			
Linda	None			SH Amoni Interprise
Mbuni	None			
Liquid soap	None	None	Antiseptic, antibacterial and germicidal effect	Ravino Industries
Tetmesol	Monosulfiram 5% w/w	None	Scabicide	Nicholas Piramal India Ltd /Shelly's Pharmaceuticals.

Key: Irgasan DP 300® identical to Triclosan= TCS; Triclocarban/Trichlorocarbanilide =TCC; Chloroxylenol=PCMX

Table 1: Label disclosure of the assayed medicated soaps available in Tanzania market.

Concerns also have been raised about the biological and toxicological effects of the triclocarban (N-(4-chlorophenyl)-N'-(3, 4-dichlorophenyl) urea) also known as 3, 4, 4'-Trichlorocarbanilide (TCC) and TCS, which are some of the most common antimicrobials in medicated soaps and other personal care products (Table 1). Several studies have evaluated their biological activities in mammalian cells to assess their potential for their adverse effects. These observations have possible implications for human and animal health (Dann & Hontela, 2011; Ahn *et al.*, 2008; Miller *et al.*, 2008; Ying *et al.*, 2007; Haden & Paul, 2005).

2   Definition of Terms and Concepts

Throughout this chapter, the word antimicrobial agent will be used interchangeably with active ingredient contained in medicate soaps, while household consumer products or biocides will refers to medicated soaps, disinfectants, toothpastes, preservatives and other antimicrobial agents incorporated in cosmetics and/or employed for control of microbial infections or proliferation. The term 'biocide' refers to a chemical agent, usually broad-spectrum in nature, which inhibits or kills microorganisms. Biocides are typically used against microorganisms in suspension or on surfaces. Antibiotics refer to chemotherapeutic agents that are used for clinical purposes to treat microbial related infections and diseases. They are natural organic compounds produced by living microorganisms and/or synthetic substances derived from those originally produced by microorganisms (Prescott *et al.*, 2005). Antibiotics are habitually effective at low concentrations, effective against a limited number of microorganisms owing to selectivity of their mode of action, and typically applied on or within living tissues/organisms. The outcome of antibiotic and biocide use is the same: destruction of troublesome microorganisms (Nester *et al.*, 2002). Biocides can be applied at concentrations higher than the minimum inhibitory concentration (MIC) or minimum bactericidal concentration (MBC) that cannot always be achievable with *in vivo*as for the antibiotics. Toxicity and bioavailability are major concerns for antibiotics. Microorganisms, refers to bacteria, fungi and viruses; however the main focus is on bacteria and fungi. Summarily, biocides are generally much broader in their spectrum of activity than are antibiotics (White & McDermott, 2001).The key issues for this chapter are summarized in Figure 1.

Section 2: Provides an overview on soap and medicated soaps uses and defines terms used in the chapter.
Section 3: Briefly describes the wide spread of medicated soaps, particularly in developing countries. It also highlights the potential development of antimicrobial resistance, particularly cross-resistance with clinically used antibiotics.
Section 4: Describes the potential risks associated with indiscriminate and persistent medicated soaps usage: their impact (toxicity) on human health and to environment.
Section 5: Briefly reviews on how to prevent/control the spread and rapid development of antimicrobial resistance. Suggesting rational use of the biocides and control of easy availability of the products.

Figure 1: The key points of this chapter.

2.1   Cleansing Action of Soap

Soaps are useful for cleaning since soap molecules have both a hydrophilic end, which dissolves in water, as well as a hydrophobic end, which is able to dissolve non-polar grease molecules. When applied to a solid surface, soapy water effectively holds particles (dirt) in colloidal suspension and then rinses it off with clean water (Sharma, 2006).

The hydrophobic portion (made up of a long hydrocarbon chain) dissolves dirt and oils, while the ionic end dissolves in water. Therefore, it allows water to liberate insoluble matter by emulsification forming spherical structures called micelles. The cleansing action of soap depends on its physical-chemical properties. Several factors exist, such as adsorption, surface tension, electrostatics forces of the polar soap molecules, its wetting action, emulsifying power, just mentioning a few, which are attributed to the cleansing action of soap (Hassan *et al.*, 2010).

2.2   Uses of Medicated Soaps in Community Settings

Despite some methodological flaws and data gaps, evidence for a causal relationship between hand hygiene and reduced transmission of infections in community is convincing, but frequent hand washing causes skin damage, with resultant changes in microbial flora, increased skin shedding, and risk of transmission of microorganisms. This suggests that some traditional hand hygiene practices warrant re-examination. Some recommended changes in practice include use of waterless alcohol-based products rather than detergent-based antiseptics or medicated soaps, modifications in lengthy surgical scrub protocols could also be important (Larson, 1999).

Equally, the remarkable contributions of disinfection and acceptance of hygienic measures towards advances in public health over the last decades cannot be denied. Certainly, if reductions in the number of infections requiring antibiotic treatment can be achieved through effective hygiene, including the use of antimicrobial agents like medicated soaps and other related products, then this is likely to decrease rather than increase the incidence of antibiotic resistance. Henceforth, it is important to ensure that antimicrobial agents use, as an integral part of good hygiene practice, is not discouraged when there is real benefit in terms of preventing infection transmission. This means that it is also necessary to assess the possibility that the indiscriminate use of antibacterial (biocide)-containing soaps and antibiotics might compromise the in-use effectiveness of such agents in truly hygienic applications (Gilbert & McBain, 2003). Use of such products must be associated with appropriate analyses of added value to the consumer, particularly when there is no apparent gain in public health.

Antimicrobial agents added in soaps, have additional effects on microorganisms and each act differently (Coelho *et al.*, 2013). For instance, TCS exerts its antimicrobial effects by inhibiting the active site of the *enoyl-acyl* carrier protein reductase enzyme (*ENR*), which is involved in fatty acids synthesis in microorganisms. Consequently, TCS prevents the microorganisms from synthesizing fatty acids one of the important constituents of cell membrane (Levy *et al.*, 1999). Human beings have no *ENR* enzyme, and therefore were presumed to be unharmed by TCS. Several biocides have no single target; for instance, polymeric biguanides act via self-promoted uptake, thus destabilize bacterial cell envelope-associated cations to cause a reorganization of the lipopolysaccharide and thereby facilitate their entry (Heath *et al.*, 2000; Wilkinson & Gilbert, 1987).

One previous study conducted in Tanzania showed that label information on packages describes them as efficient agents capable of eradicating several pathogenic microorganisms and thus falsely ensuring healthiness to consumers (Mwambete & Lyombe, 2011). Besides, majority of these products had no expiry dates regardless that being chemical agents, they have specific half-lives (**Table 1**). Such chemicals are incorporated into medicated soaps as active antimicrobial ingredientsthat tend to degrade with time; and the rates of degradation, to a great extent, depend on the storage physicochemical conditions (Reiss *et al.*, 2009). For examples, TCS, CHG, TCC and chloroxylenol/4-chloro-3, 5-dimethylphenol also known as p-chloro-m-xylenol (PCMX) are some of the commonly used antimicrobial agents in medicated soaps and other consumer products, which have different half-lives. Nevertheless, the antimicrobial agents are generally, only contained at preservative levelsalthoughmost of them are clearly marked as antibacterial, antiseptic, or germicidal agents.

This chapter intends to elucidate the long-time existing controversy surrounding the increased use of antimicrobial substances in a wide range of consumer products (medicated soaps) and the possibility that, as with antibiotics, indiscriminate use of biocides might affect the overall antimicrobial susceptibility patterns in the general environment and in the clinic. It highlights mechanisms by which microorganisms may become less sensitive to biocide action and the potential of antibiotics and medicated soap-containing biocide develop cross-resistance, as well as the impacts of medicated soaps on health of consumers and the environment.

3   Medicated Soaps and Development of Antimicrobial Resistance

3.1   Medicated Soaps as Anti-infective Agents

Medicated soaps also commonly known as antibacterial soaps are any cleaning products to which active antimicrobial ingredients have been amalgamated. These chemicals kill bacteria and fungi, but their effectiveness at deactivating viruses are uncertain just like any other regular soaps or detergents. Unfortunately, they also kill human normal flora.

Mahara *et al.* (2002) compared antimicrobial effects of medicated soaps and antibiotics on decolonization of methicillin-resistant *Staphylococcus aureus* (MRSA) carrier status in patients before and after treatment. Swabs were taken from the nasopharynx, axilla, groin and perineum. Results showed that microbial eradication rate after one treatment cycle of 71.4% which is comparable to antibiotic treatment. After two treatment cycles, the rate was 91.4% and came up to 94.2% after a third treatment cycle. However, other researchers reiterate that it cannot be discarded that washing with plain soap and water or doing nothing would not have had a similar effect regarding the eradication of MRSA (Harbarth*et al.*, 1999).

Mwambete & Lyombe (2011) evaluated antimicrobial effect of 16 different brands of the most commonly used medicated soaps, which were randomly collected /purchased from shops, drug stores, and pharmacies in Dar es Salaam, Tanzania. These were subjected to the antimicrobial activity tests. Using a wax marker, a Nutrient agar-plate was divided in four sectors and labeled 1 through 4. Firstly, fingers were rubbed over sector 1 prior to washing hands. Secondly, using a scrub brush, soap, and water, hands were scrubbed for about 2 min, and then the fingers were rubbed over sector 2. The second step was repeated for sectors 3 and 4 (**Table 2**).

The above described technique was performed twice: the first process was conducted in open-air on laboratory bench while the second was aseptically carried out in laminar flow cabin. The aim was to rule out contamination of the agar plates by microorganisms present in the air, which could have been settled onto the agar plates by gravitational force. One un-inoculated agar plate served as negative control. Microbial counts were performed following an incubation of the agar plates for 12 to 42 h at 37° and results are summarized in **Table 2**.

Brand	Sector			
	1st	2nd	3rd	4th
Meditex	+	++	+++	+++
Duru	+	++	+++	+++
Protex	+	++	+	+
Lifebuoy	+	++	+++	+++
Rungu	+	++	+++	+++
Roberts	+	++	+++	+++
Family	+	++	+++	+++
Dettol	+	++	+++	+++
Protector	+	++	+++	+++
Regency neem	+	++	++	++
Dalan	+	++	++	++
Tetmesol	+	++	+++	+++
Linda	+	++	+++	+++
Mbuni	+	+++	++	-
Liquid soap	+	++	+++	+++
Imperial	+	++	+++	++

Key: (-) no growth, (+) <10; (++) <100; (+++) >100 microbial counts/sector.

Table 2: Antimicrobial effects of medicated soaps assayed by hand washing technique.

Results show that in real life: exposure of normal flora to external and extraneous environmental may trigger microbial transformation as they strive to adopt in new micro-environment (Jawetz *et al.*, 2010). Usually potential transient pathogenic microorganisms are the targeted microorganisms that should be removed either by simple scrubbing, hand washing or bathing, if possible with simple soaps, which have proved to be equally effective (Mwambete & Lyombe, 2011).

This can also be justified by the fact that health practitioners routinely wash hands after examining patients and before surgery, in order to remove some potentially harmful transient flora as well as reduce a number of resident flora, which might cause opportunistic infections (Jawetz *et al.*, 2010; Kaiser & Newman, 2006; Nester *et al.*, 2002). Repeated hand washing led to exposure of ''more'' normal skin resident flora (**Table 2**). This is actually what happens when one uses antimicrobial/medicated soaps irrationally, because tends to remove these harmless and protective microorganisms.

3.2   Potential Development of Antimicrobial Resistance

Problems associated with the development and spread of antimicrobial resistance in modern medicine have been increasing since the early 1960s and are currently regarded as one of the major threats to clinical practice (Gilbert & McBain, 2003). Generally, it is postulated that the main cause of this problem has been and still is widespread irrational use and overprescribing of antibiotics in human medicine, animal husbandry, veterinary practice and recently the emergence and wide spread use of medicated soaps may cause an additional threat (Poole, 2002).

Microbial resistance have been attributed to the effects of long term use of antimicrobial agents such as those added in consumer products. For instance, TCS is believed to kill bacteria by the inhibition of the enzyme *ENR*(Heath *et al.*, 1999). This enzyme plays a key role in bacterial and microbial lipid synthesis. Increased resistance to TCS has been recently ascribed to an alteration in the *fabI* gene that codes for *ENR*(Heath *et al.*, 2000). Therefore wide spread use of TCS could cause microbial resistance. The agent being a polychloro phenoxy-phenol can degrade into a large number of other chlorinated aromatic compounds of which their antimicrobial effects and impact on environment are unclear (White & McDermott, 2001; Russell, 1998).

A number of studies have pointed out serious concerns that TCS and other similar products may promote the emergence of bacteria resistant to antimicrobials/antibiotics (Gilbert & McBain, 2003; White & McDermott, 2001; Levy, 2001; Chuanchen *et al.*, 2001). One apprehension is that microorganisms may become resistant to antimicrobial products like TCS, rendering the products useless to those who actually need them, such as people with compromised immune systems.

3.2.1   Bacterial Efflux Pumps: Impact on Antimicrobial Resistance

Efflux pumps consist of either a single component or multiple components. Multi-drug resistance (MDR) efflux pumps confer clinically relevant resistance to antibiotics that are used to treat human diseases. Due to the broad range of substrates of MDR efflux pumps, bacteria that overexpress these pumps can be selected for by numerous antimicrobial agents (Elkins & Mullis, 2006). Mechanisms of drug-resistance for both medicated soaps and other clinically used chemotherapeutic agents (antimicrobials) have so many features in common if not identical. Most of these will involve efflux pumps, which are proteinaceous transporters localized in the cytoplasmic membrane of all kinds of cells.

Drug efflux pumps play a key role in drug resistance and also serve other functions in bacteria. Currently, several multidrug and drug-specific efflux pumps have been identified in bacteria of human, animal, plant and environmental origins. These pumps are mostly encoded on the chromosome although they can also be plasmid-encoded. They are active transporters, which mean they require a source of chemical energy in form of adenosine triphosphate (ATP) to perform their function (Figure 2).

Others are secondary active transporters in which the transport is coupled to an electrochemical potential difference created by hydrogen or/and sodium ions efflux (Li & Nikaido, 2009; Nester *et al.*, 2002). Bacterial efflux transporters are classified into five major super-families (Figure 3), based on the amino acid sequence and energy source used to export their substrates:

- The major facilitator superfamily (MFS)
- The ATP-binding cassette superfamily (ABC)
- The small multidrug resistance family (SMR)
- The resistance-nodulation-cell division superfamily (RND)
- The Multi antimicrobial extrusion protein family (MATE).

Only ABC superfamily is the primary transporters, while others are secondary (Figure 3). RND family has been found in all major Kingdoms (Fangea *et al.*, 2012). Efflux also acts synergistically with other resistance mechanisms to provide higher levels of antimicrobial resistance of clinical significance (Kuroda &Tsuchiya, 2009; Jack *et al.*, 2001).

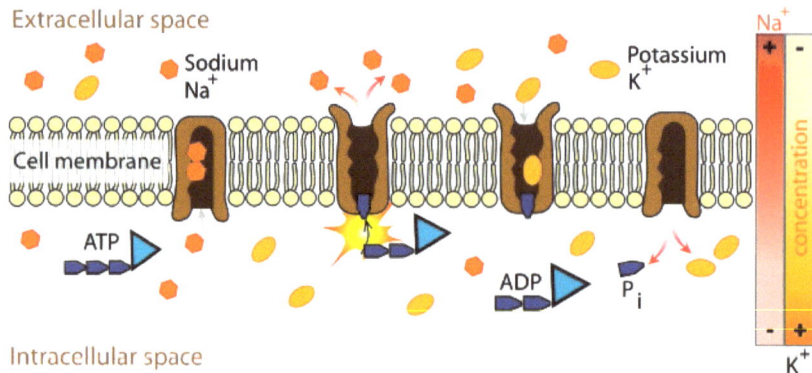

Figure 2: Generalized bacterial efflux pumps as one of the antimicrobial resistance mechanisms.

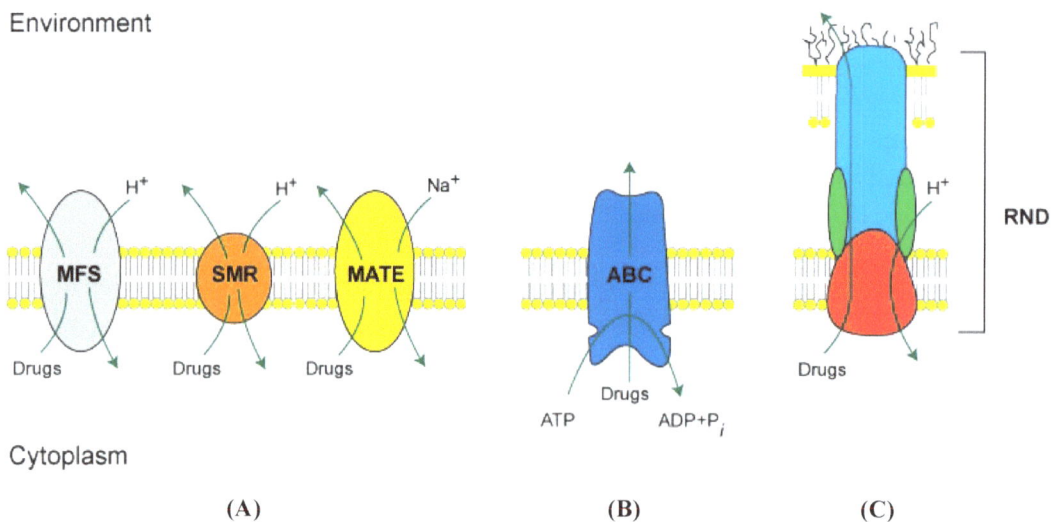

Figure 3: Different bacterial efflux pumps-indicating efflux of drugs (substrates) and energy sources as one of the antimicrobial resistance mechanisms. A) The MFS, SMR, and MATE families are powered by chemiosmotic energy, pumping drugs out of the cell while pumping H^+ or Na^+ into the cell. B) The ABC family of pumps is powered by ATP. C) The RND family is a multisubunit complex spanning the inner and outer membranes in Gram-negative bacteria (Adopted from Tegos et al., 2013).

It has been demonstrated that RND transporters are present in both gram negative and positive bacteria and they are involved in resistance to numerous drugs (Figure 3). Most of the mechanisms associated with resistance to Macrolides and Nalidixic acid in gram negative bacteria are attributed to ABC and MFS superfamilies of transporters. MATE dominates in gram positive bacteria and they are associated with aminoglycosides, fluoroquinolones, and cationic drugs resistance. Likewise, SMR predominate in gram positive bacteria where they are attributed to resistance to Benzalkonium, Cetrimide and Acriflavine

(Piddock, 2006). The two former agents are usually used as either preservatives or disinfectants and found in most of the household consumer products such as cosmetics and toothpastes.

The impact of efflux mechanisms on antimicrobial resistance is enormous; this is usually attributed to the following:

- The genetic elements encoding efflux pumps may be encoded on chromosomes and/or plasmids, thus contributing to both intrinsic (natural) and acquired resistance respectively. As an intrinsic mechanism of resistance, efflux pump genes can survive a hostile environment, which allows for the selection of mutants that over-express these genes. Because of its location on plasmids or transposons that are transportable genetic materials, they easily spread between different bacterial species. The following genes are associated with antimicrobial resistance: *Norm*, *QacA*, *QacC* for MATE, MFS and SMR efflux pumps respectively. The*AcrA-B* and LmrA genes play major roles in RND and ABC efflux pumps respectively (Figure 3).

- Antimicrobial agents, disinfectants inclusive may act as triggers and regulators of the expression of some efflux pumps.

- Broad spectrum of antimicrobial resistance is presumed to be one of the result of expression of several efflux pumps in a given bacterial species because of some shared substrates for MDR efflux pumps, thus one efflux pump may confer resistance to a wide range of antimicrobials (Li & Nikaido, 2009).

As previously described that MDR efflux pumps have many substrates, these include not only antibiotics but also agents like TCS that is increasingly used in the home as soap and hand-washing lotions, on farms and in food-processing plants. Similarly, the nonoxynol-9 widely used as a spermicide and can select mutants that overexpress *mtrCDE* in gonococcal isolates (Elkins & Mullis, 2006). Such widespread use of non-antimicrobial substrates of efflux pumps such as TCS and nonoxynol-9, could accidentally lead to the selection of mutants overexpressing MDR efflux pumps.

3.2.1.1 Experimental-based Evidences on Cross-resistance Development

Past laboratory studies have demonstrated that bacteria resistant to TCS, including strains of *Salmonella* and *E. coli*, habitually are resistant to common antibiotics as well, which doesn't come as a miracle for entities that can swap their genetic materials. The main mechanism for resistance: proteins on cell membranes called efflux pumps that shuttle harmful substances like TCS and antibiotics out of bacteria, leaving bacterial cells functioning normally (Figures 2& 3). These pumps might be specific to particular substances, or be more general and work with various kinds of substances/substrates. Although other processes can also confer resistance, but efflux pumps are predominantly powerful; genes that code for the pumps can freely be shared among bacteria (Hernández *et al.*, 2011).

Drury *et al* (2013) measured TCS concentrations in river sediment at six sites outside of Chicago, they found a clear pattern: Urban sites had greater concentrations than suburban sites, which in turn had greater concentrations than woodland sites. The urban sites were located downstream from sewers that overflow during heavy rains and thus feed soapy wastewater from sinks and showers, these included raw sewage from toilets that drained directly into the river. Examiningthe proportion of TCS-resistant bacteria at each site they found a similar pattern that is high concentrations of TCS meant a greater percentage of TCS-resistant bacteria in the microbial mix. Tosupport their field findings, a controlled laboratory experiment was set up: TCS was added to artificial streams, and TCS-resistant bacteria were generated (Drury *et al.*, 2013).

When a bacterial population is placed under a stressorsuch as an antimicrobial agent, a small sub-population armed with special defence mechanisms can develop. These lineages survive and reproduce as their weaker relatives perish. "What doesn't kill you makes you stronger" is the governing maxim here, as antibiotics or other antimicrobial agents select for bacteria that tolerate their presence.

As bacteria develop a tolerance for these medicated soaps/biocides there is also potential for developing a tolerance for certain antibiotics (Shatalin *et al.*, 2011). This phenomenon, called cross-resistance, has already been demonstrated in experimental studies using TCS, one of the most common antimicrobials in biocides used for various domestic and hospital decontamination and/or disinfection purposes. "TCS has a specific inhibitory target in bacteria similar to some antibiotics," says epidemiologist Allison Aiello at the University of Michigan.When bacteria are exposed to TCS for long periods of time, genetic mutations can arise. Some of these mutations bestow the bacteria with resistance to important antibiotics such as isoniazid (antituberculosis); whereas other microorganisms can boost their efflux pumps-protein machines in the cell membrane that can spit out several types of antibiotics (Aiello & Larson, 2003). These effects have been demonstrated only in the laboratory, not in households and other real world environments; thus Aiello& Larson believe that the few household studies may not have been sufficiently lengthy to depict a real image. "It's very possible that the emergence of resistant species takes quite some time to occur; the potential is there," they say.

Gusarov*et al.*(2009) &Heath& Rock (2000) provided details on how bacteria protect themselves from stressful condition such as "oxidative stress." Bacteria produce hydrogen sulfide, which, in combination with nitric oxide seems to protect them from antibiotic assaults. Researchers found three enzymes that are responsible for triggering the production of this gas in *S. aureus*, *E.coli* and other bacteria. When bacteria were treated with antibiotics, they spontaneously started producing more H_2S gas. Nguyen *et al.* (2011) investigating the biochemical characteristics of clinical isolates of *Pseudomonas aeruginosa;* they found that when the bacteria were deprived of nutrients, they showed signs of a stringent response. "As the bacteria sense starvation, they tend to produce an alarm signal called guanosine 5′-(tri) diphosphate, 3′-diphosphate [(p) ppGpp], "Nguyen explained."And this allows the cells to regulateenormous number of genes, which then allows it to better adapt and survive in response to starvation and stress."

To test whether stringent response could also be protecting the bacteria from antibiotics, the researchers created a mutant strain that lacked such an alarm. Definitely, antibiotics were much more effective against those bacterial strains that could not turn on their stringent response. On the other hand, when mice infected with bacteria lacking the response and were given antibiotics, their infections cleared up and the mice survived. "With normal, wild type bacteria, the mice would die even if you treated them with the antibiotics," Nguyen said.

In one of the largest phenotype studies ever performed on biocide and antibiotic reduced susceptibility, a total of 1632 world-wide clinical strains of*Staphylococcus aureus*strains were analyzed.Justifying the wide range of sensitivity(variability of susceptibility) observed on the antimicrobial action of antibiotics and biocides; Coelho *et al.*(2013) say this is because some microorganisms, by virtue of the absence of critical target sites or an inability of the agents to accumulate at those targets, are intrinsically resistant to particular groups of agents under all growth conditions. Other groups of microorganisms may undergo changes in susceptibility that reflect either the conditions under which they were cultivated or exposed (phenotypic change), the temporary expression of efflux pumps or synthesis and export of protective enzymes (inductive change), or mutations in the genes encoding or regulating a sensitive target site (chromosomal change). The acquisition of extrinsic genetic elements that encode such resistance (plasmid-mediated change) can be responsible for the rapid development and horizontal spread of resistance within populations, principally where this involves the expression of efflux pumps and drug-inactivating enzymes.

Phenotypic Changes in Biocide Susceptibility: The intrinsic susceptibility of a microorganism to a biocide, documented from the MIC or MBC determination by standard methods is not a fixed value. Somewhat, the susceptibility phenotype expressed by the microorganism can differ significantly according to the prevailing physicochemical conditions (Nett *et al.*, 2008; Harvey & Lund, 2007; Fux *et al.*, 2005). Changes in susceptibility are partly due to changes in the microbial outer membranes that increase barrier properties and prevent access of biocides to their site of action.The fact is, determination of antimicrobial effect used for antibiotics such as MICs are unsuitable for biocides (Fraise, 1999), because in real life, microorganismsusually exist in nutrient-depleted, slow-growing or non-growing states as adherent biofilms (Widmer*et al.*, 1991). Whereas, in clinical situations microorganisms may proliferate as biofilms, similarly they survive under nutrient-depleted conditions, on epithelial surfaces, or intracellularly in susceptible organisms or cells (Turner*et al.*, 2000). Navarro-Llorens*et al.* (2010) suggest that a general stress response to nutrient depletion and onset of stationary phase initiates the adoption of resting or dormant stages, similar to endospores, which are microbial phenotypes resistant to numerous physical and chemical agents (McBain *et al.*, 2012; Dixon, 2000).

Although phenotypic resistance to biocides and antibiotics is frequently overlooked as a cause of therapeutic catastrophe, its influence to the *in situ*microbial susceptibility is immense. Phenotypic resistance is not acquiescent to quantification with MIC or MBC determinations by conventional microbiological techniques or methods. Phenotypic change can cause alteration of microbial susceptibility to antimicrobial agents even 10 times, simply because the observed changes in the MIC areirrelevant. However, significant reductions in the susceptibility of clinical microorganisms (pathogens) over the reference strains increase the possibility of situations in which the concentration of biocide will be sub-inhibitory for some pathogenic microorganisms and thereby impose a selection pressure towards the less susceptible clones (Fraise, 2002). Such selection pressures will not occur when the mechanisms associated with decreased susceptibility relate to the adoption of a resting state. Rather, repeated treatments will cause a post-treatment clonal expansion of more resistant microorganisms (Skalet *et al.*, 2010).

Bacterial vomit response: Several studies have shown that efflux pumps, sometimes with extraordinarily specificity to certain kind of molecules viz. lipophilic or amphipathic, can also contribute to the intrinsic resistance of gram-negative bacteria to a variety of agents such as dyes, detergents, and antibiotics (Nishihara *et al.*, 2000). The efflux pumps are chromosomally encoded in gram-negative bacteria, and their expression is induced by exposure to sub-lethal antimicrobial concentrations (Levy, 2002).

The genes for multidrug efflux pumps *qacA* to *qacG* (Figure 3) have been shown to significantlycontribute to biocide tolerance in *Staphylococcus aureus* (Hegstad *et al.*, 2010; Smith *et al.*, 2008; Poole, 2005). These genes can become located on integrons and transferred between gram-positive organisms such as staphylococci and enterococci and also to gram-negative bacteria such as *P. aeruginosa* and the vibrios (Kazama *et al.*, 1999). If these efflux pumps indeed evolved as a defense against antimicrobial agents occurring in the environment (González-Lamothe *et al.*, 2009; Lewis & Ausubel, 2006), then "natural" antimicrobial agents would also contribute to this problem.

Previous studies had shown that low concentrations of antibiotics such as chloramphenicol and tetracycline and biocides such as pine oil act as weak inducers of the *mar* operon, just like what have been observed with a number of food supplements such as chili, mustard, and some herbs (Friedman & Juneja, 2010; Whyte *et al.*, 2001). Likewise, Meyer (2006) noted that a novel disinfectant based on extracts of grapefruit seeds also served to select for decreased susceptibility to itself and some quaternary ammonium-based agents. Sulavick *et al.* (1995) noted that the *marR*repressor of *marA* is inactivated by a variety of phenolic derivatives, of which majority are naturally occurring and of plant origin.

Efflux pumps significantly contribute to the resistance of microorganisms to antibiotics and biocides (Gilbert & McBain, 2003). Current knowledge suggests that efflux pumps are part of the natural defense mechanisms against natural environmental toxicants (Anselmo *et al.*, 2012; Epel *et al.*, 2008; Kingtong*et al.*, 2007). In such a fashion, efflux per se of biocides that are both inducers and substrates should be a transitory event. That kind of biocides will only impact the pattern of antibiotic resistance in the environment when their use leads to a selection of clones that hyper-express when induced.

In this regard, the level of expression of constitutive *mar* mutants could greatly be affected by the interactive binding of several transcriptional activators such as *marA*, Rob, SoxS, and Fis (Rosner & Martin, 2009; Martin *et al.*, 2008). With the appropriate selection pressures, this may result into selection of a microbial populations that inducibly hyperexpress efflux. For that matter, exposure of *mexAB*-deleted mutants of *P. aeruginosa*to sublethal concentration of many antimicrobials can select for microorganisms that hyperexpress an alternative efflux pump, MexCD and/or MexJK (Gilbert & McBain, 2003).MexJK is also part of the RND family of efflux systems, though it is not associated with the outer membrane porin (OprM) that may efflux TCS (Chuanchuen, *et al.*, 2002). Consequently, exposure to inhibitory molecules, such as TCS and fluoroquinolones, which are substrates for efflux pump but not inducers, will dictate towards constitutive efflux pump expression, provided that the selection pressure is maintained.

Destruction of biocide: Some microorganisms are able to demonstrate intrinsic resistance through inactivation of biocides and other antimicrobial agents. Biocides are comparatively less likely to be inactivated by bacteria as compared to antibiotics, but examples include the inactivation of phenols and some aldehydes in species of *Pseudomonas* (Gilbert & McBain, 2003) and of TCS (Hay*et al.*, 2001). Enzymatic degradation of formaldehyde by *Pseudomonas putida,* for instance, yields some agents of nutritive values for other bacterial species (secondary colonizers) resulting into further degradation of preservatives, which finally leads to product spoilage. Microbial inactivation of QACs, CHG, and phenylethanol has also been reported, but only at lower concentrations than those used in practice (Tumah, 2009; Beumer *et al.*, 2000).

Destruction of biocides/antimicrobial agents seems not to be a mechanism of resistance to these compounds, but will assist in the removal of such agents from the environment. Nishihara *et al.* (2000) described the inactivation of didecyldimethylammoniun chloride by a strain of *Pseudomonas fluorescens,* whiletwo more recent studies reported the detoxification of TCS (Murugesan *et al.* 2010; Bailey*et al.*, 2009). In both cases, it is probable that chronic exposure of populations to sub-inhibitory concentrations of such agents will lead to an induced expression of antimicrobial-degrading enzymes and a selection pressure towards those clones that can hyperexpress them. It is improbable that such enzymes would confer cross-resistance to third-party antibiotics; rather they seem to be very useful for biocide biodegradation and thus conserving the ecosystem.

Target modification: Since antibiotics usually act at specific sites within the bacteria, chromosomal mutations that change those targets are likely to modify not only the functionality of that target but also its susceptibility to the antibiotic. Chromosomal gene mutations that confer resistance to antibiotics have been relatively well studied (Alekshun & Levy, 2007; Cirz *et al.*, 2005; Chopra & Roberts, 2001).Mechanisms include evasion of delicate metabolic steps, modificationson the common antimicrobial target molecules such as a change in the bacterial ribosome affecting protein/enzyme synthesis, and hyper expression of target enzyme or the efflux pumps (Figure 3). Some biocides that also have specific singular target sites at growth-inhibitory concentrations have been identified), though only a few studies on the effects of mutations at those sites have been conducted (Ortega Morente*et al.*, 2013; Williams, 2006). The question iswhy the lessons learnt for chromosomal mutation and resistance to antibiotics should not apply to the inhibitory action of biocides when the biological effects are governed by action at a single target.

Such a view has been validated by the identification of *ENR* enzyme as growth-inhibitory targets for TCS in *E. coli* and *Mycobacterium smegmatis* (Kinjo *et al.*, 2013; Russell, 2004; Maillard, 2002).Exposure of *E. coli* to sub-lethal concentrations of TCS have been demonstrated that select, at quite high frequency, clonal mutations that are either altered in the *fabI* gene, which encodes the enzyme, or where the gene has been suppressed or deleted. Consequently, this leads to attenuated susceptibility to antimicrobial agents/antibiotics, ultimately producing a series of mutants with increased levels of antimicrobial resistance. Such mutant microorganisms have been characterized and found to relate to a single-amino-acid change in *fabI* at that codon for glycine 93 in *E. coli* and at the codon for glycine 95 in *P. aeruginosa* (Heath *et al.*, 1998).

The *S. aureus* mutants, like the *E. coli* mutants, show hyper-expression of a modified *fabI* gene product. In all cases, the mutant cells were no less sensitive to the bactericidal effects of TCS than were the parent wild-type isolates. This is in concordant with the view that the TCS has multiple antimicrobial targets that include the *ENR* as the most sensitive and responsible for growth inhibition (McDonnell & Pretzer, 1998).

The identification of specific, highly sensitive targets responsible for the growth-inhibitory action of TCS offers the possibility that exposure of populations of bacteria to sub-lethal levels of the agent might coincidentally select mutant populations with reduced susceptibility to third-party therapeutic agents which possess this as their sole target (Gilbert & McBain, 2003). The fact that the *ENR* enzyme in *M. smegmatis* (Kini*et al.*, 2009; McMurry& Levy,1998) is the target not only for TCS but also for the chemotherapeutic agent isoniazid is of major concern from pharmacological point of view. Demonstrating this association, it was revealed that deletion of the *inhI* gene, the *fabI* homologue, led to 1.2- to 8.5-timesupsurges in the MIC of isoniazid and 4- to 6.3-fold increases in the MIC of TCS. Fortunately, further studies have shown that isoniazid-resistant *ENR* enzyme in *Mycobacterium tuberculosis* retains its susceptibility to TCS, indicating that while the two agents have a common target enzyme; their interactions with that target are distinct. If adequately exploited, this may lead to discovery of novel antituberculosis molecules (Heath*et al.*, 2002).

As a biocide, TCS is probably not exclusive in having a singular critical process associated with its activity that is shared with other therapeutic agents. This could be related to the efflux pumps via the processes of uptake and/or interactive target. Other antimicrobial agents such as the aminoglycosides are well known to gain access to gram-negative bacteria through a self-promoted mechanism (Murtough *et al.*, 2000). In self-promoted uptake, the antimicrobial agent destabilizes microbial envelope-associated cations to cause a reorganization of the lipopolysaccharide and thus facilitate antibiotic uptake. A number of biocides, principally polymeric biguanides (Zhou *et al.*, 2010); share this mechanism of cellular uptake in order to access their target sites at the cytoplasmic membrane. Changes in the microbial envelope, such as those negatively affect the extent of cation binding to the outer membrane; coincidentally affect aminoglycoside and polymyxin susceptibility. Isolates of *P. aeruginosa* cultured by passage to demonstrate resistance against increasing concentrations of polymyxin show decreases in their susceptibility to QACs (Moore *et al.*, 2008).

Reduction in susceptibility to benzalkonium chloride among *Saccharomyces cerevisiae* isolates had been reported, which waslinked with loss of a cytoplasmic membrane and active-transport leucine pump (Perlstein *et al.*, 2007). The possibility arises that the quaternary ammonium biocides may also utilize such transport processes to gain access to bacterial cells, thus antimicrobial resistance will be obvious once deletion/repression of such proteins occurs. Mutants of *S. aureus* with simultaneous reductions in susceptibility to disinfectant/antimicrobial–containing pine oil and the antibiotics vancomycin and oxacillin have been reported (McMahon*et al.*, 2008; Price *et al.*, 2002).

Chromosomal efflux mutants: Multidrug efflux mechanisms are generally chromosome-encoded, with their expression normally resulting from mutations in regulatory genes, whereas drug-specific efflux mechanisms are encoded by mobile genetic elements whose acquisition is sufficient for resistance(Poole, 2007).Transposons and integrons significantly enhance the development of transferrable resistance due to their ability to move from plasmid to chromosome and subsequently pass resistance on to daughter cells (Alekshun & Levy, 2007). Transposons and integrons have also been found to possess a number of genetic determinants encoding resistance to QACs and heavy metals. Selective pressure, which is exerted by one antimicrobial agent, is likely to maintain co-resistance phenotypes arbitrated by adjacent genes. Therefore, it is possible that exposing integron-carrying bacteria to residual concentrations of biocides may encourage antibiotic resistance (Woods*et al.*, 2009; Percival *et al.*, 2005).

Chromosomal mutations to antibiotics are not uncommon. Nonetheless, only a few studies have demonstrated that such mutations confer resistance to biocides (Levy, 2002; White & McDermott,2001). A silver resistance determinant in enteric bacteria has recently been cloned and sequenced, but none has yet been identified in Gram-positive bacteria despite staphylococci and other Gram-positive bacteria being exposed to silver compounds in clinical use. In the hospital environment, it has been suggested that rather than plasmid-mediated resistance, continual exposure to sub-inhibitory antibiotic concentrations may cause subtle changes to the bacterial outer structure stimulating cell-to-cell contact.

Under extreme conditions or nutrient deprivation, microorganisms cannot survive unless evolve and adapt those conditions. The (p)ppGpp is a DNA fragment that assists bacteria to survive such harsh conditions or environments; this is a transcription-regulator gene associated with bacterial metabolic processes (Wu & Xie, 2009). Gilbert & McBain (2003) had previously reported the potential of various antimicrobial treatments to induce the expression of efflux pump either directly or indirectly through expression of pppGppp and *rpoS* genes. Under persistent exposure to antibacterial agents, it is undoubtedlybeneficial for microorganisms to maintain such efflux as an inducible function, which may select clones that can inducibly hyper-express this phenotype. Nevertheless, some antimicrobial agents, such as the antibiotic ciprofloxacin and the biocide TCS, that are substrates for efflux pumps but not inducers of their expression (Poole, 2007; Levy, 2002). Prolonged exposure to sub-lethal concentrations of such agents would select mutant microbial clones that express the efflux pumps constitutively. Further studies (Lister *et al.*, 2009; Linares *et al.*, 2005; Chuanchuen*et al.* 2001) have shown that exposure to TCS selected a multidrug-resistant strain that hyperexpressed the *mexCD* efflux system genes from a susceptible isolates of *P. aeruginosa* mutants in which *mexAB* was deleted.

Reduced Susceptibility to antimicrobial soaps/agentsassociated with plasmids: Horizontal transmission of resistance determinantsis possible and such genetic elements can fuse to produce large multi-resistance plasmids, the fusions are intrinsically unstable. The persistence of large multiple resistance plasmids therefore reflects the joint selection pressures to which the cells encompassing them are exposed. Henceforth, the plasmid-associated antimicrobial resistance in health facilities and community environments reflects the antimicrobial /antibiotic usage patterns, inclusive use of medicated soaps.

Plasmids have been implicated in encoding reduced susceptibility to biocidal agents as well as to antibiotics specifically related to heavy metals such as mercury, zinc, silver and copper resistance (Chopra, 2007; Perron *et al.*, 2004). Silver salts are used as antiseptics or disinfectants, and resistance to these has been observed in the clinic (Gupta*et al.*, 1999). Therefore most of the silver compounds are currently not widely used. Likewise, plasmid-carrying MRSA strains have changed susceptibilities to a variety of biocides that includingCHG, QACs, halogens, TCS and hydrogen peroxides (Brooks *et al.*, 2002).

Widespread reductions in susceptibility to ethidium bromide, benzalkonium chloride, acriflavine, cetrimide and diamidines are mediated by a group of structurally related plasmids encoding QAC efflux pumps (Pagedar *et al.*, 2011). The qacA gene can be found on the pSK1 family of multi-resistance plasmids and codes for a multidrug efflux pump, whileqacB is found on many beta-lactamase and heavy metal resistance plasmids such as pSK23 (Russell, 1998). The qacB gene codes for a similar protein, though is more specific and relates only to intercalating dyes and QACs (Wang, 2013; Jansen, 2012).However, it has been shown that antibiotic-sensitive *Staphylococcus* species, for which the MICs of various antimicrobial agents/biocides were high, were nevertheless less sensitive to a wide variety of antibiotics. Increased MICs for MRSA isolates have been reported for certain biocides, including biguanides, QACs, halogens and phenolic derivatives (Gilbert & McBain, 2003). These data bear testimony to the multiplicity of target sites implicated in the bactericidal action of biocides.

4   Medicated Soaps Toxicity and Environmental Impacts

4.1   Impact of Medicated Soaps on Human Health

Not only the inclusion of many antimicrobial active ingredients used in medicated soaps, personal care and other consumer products, together with pharmaceuticals have direct effects on clinical practice but also an apparent increase in the environmental impact. The main reasons for these concerns are: firstly because of the similarity of target sites between antibiotics or antimicrobial agents and medicated soaps' active ingredients that could influence selection of mutants transformed in such targets by any of these agents and the emergence of cross-resistance. Secondly the restrained differences in these agents (in medicated soaps) and antimicrobial susceptibility of antibiotic-resistant strains may expedite their selection and maintenance in the environment by low, sub-effective concentrations of these antimicrobial agents and the primary antibiotic (Gilbert & Moore, 2005). Lastly, indiscriminate use of medicated soaps might cause the evolution and selection of multidrug-resistant strains through other mechanisms such as efflux pumps (Fan *et al.*, 2002).

TCC is extensively used in household and personal care products including bar soaps, body washes, cleansing lotions, wipes and detergents. TCC-containing products have been marketed broadly in the United States and Europe for more than 45 years. Researchers have found two key effects: In human cells in the laboratory, TCC increased gene expression that is normally regulated by testosterone. In addition, when male rats were fed TCC, testosterone-dependent organs such as the prostate gland grew abnormally large, which has been attributed to increased risk of infertility and early puberty. Moreover, there have been several reports of contact dermatitis, or skin irritation, from exposure to TCS (Wojcik *et al.*, 2006;

Veldhoen *et al.*, 2006; Wilson *et al.*, 2003). There is also evidence that TCS may cause photo-allergic contact dermatitis (PACD), which occurs when the part of the skin exposed to TCS is also exposed to sunlight (Neumanna *et al.*, 2000; Dogra& Dua, 2005). A Swedish study found high levels TCS in three out of five human milk samples, indicating that TCS does in fact get absorbed into the body, often in high quantities (Adolfsson-Erici *et al.*, 2002). Furthermore, TCS is lipophilic, thus it can bio-accumulates in adipose tissues. TCS has not yet clearly been demonstrated to have carcinogenic, mutagenic, or terato-genic effects (McMurry *et al.*, 1998).

TCS has the potential to accumulate in humans, other animals and plants as results of physico-chemical properties and presence in soil and water bodies. Occasionally, humans are exposed to TCS through ingestion and dermal absorption, principally when they use TCS-containing products (Calafat *et al.*, 2008). Moss *et al.* (2000) demonstrated that 6.3% of the TCS applied to human skin tend to penetrate the skin 24 hours post application. In this era of HIV/AIDS pandemic, TCS should be cautiously use if not left alone completely, simply because it has also been demonstrated to possess immunosuppressive effects on natural killer cells responsible for early recognition and elimination of viral infected cells and participate in humoral immunity (Udoji *et al.*, 2010).

Persons, particularly children, who are constantly exposure to CHG and TCS, are more likely to develop allergies, including nut allergies and hay fever (Clayton *et al.*, 2011; Liippo *et al.*, 2011). Over use of antimicrobial agents or over sanitization of a child's environment deprive them of naturally developing their immune system through exposures to decreased number of normal flora and lessened microbial diversity. Simply because the relationship between the microorganism and the host (human) is mostly of mutual benefit, and they shape the human immune system throughout life (Kelly *et al.*, 2007; Guarner *et al.*, 2006; Macpherson & Harris, 2004).The median lethal dose of TCS (>99% pure) has been reported as 1090 ± 20 mg/kg in mice (22 gram body weight) following intraperitoneal injection in an ethanol/olive oil mixture (Kanetoshi *et al.* 1992).

On the other hand, p-chloro-m-cresol (PCMC) and PCMX are attributed to allergic contact dermatitis, inflammatory reactions/swelling of face or hands and difficulty in breathing. Skin rashes, redness, burning, itching, or swelling in the area where the agents have been applied are a few more of the side effects (Ogunshe *et al.*, 2011). However, TCS has also been shown to block the metabolism of thyroid hormones (Veldhoen *et al.*, 2006). This is due to its inhibitory effect on estrogen sulfotransferase, an enzyme which helps to metabolize the hormone and transport it to the developing fetus. Consequently the compound could be hazardous to pregnant women once enough of TCS get to the placenta (James *et al.*, 2010). Likewise, because of poor sanitary conditions in many of the developing countries, about 95% of TCS from of consumer products may get their way into rivers and thus affecting the ecosystem (Wilson *et al.*, 2003).

Dettol is one of the medicated soaps commonly used in households, especially to bath newborns. The soap contains PCMX (4.8%), Pine oil (9%) and Isopropyl alcohol (12%). PCMX is a phenol and is chemically related to the other phenolic disinfectants such as carbolic acid and cresols. Pine oil is made of secondary and tertiary terpene alcohols which cause central nervous system depression (CNS). The action is probably an additive to the depressant action of PCMX (Kumar, 2005). Iso-propyl alcohol is also associated with CNS depression (Kumar, 2008). The risk of serious complications and mortality following ingestion of Dettol has been reported to be around 8% and 1.8% respectively (Kumar, 2005). Monosulfiram has been associated with systemic adverse events such as dermal oedema, flushing, tachycardia, excessive sweating especially following ingestion of alcohol within 24 hours after treatment. This is due to the fact that monosulfiram is chemically related to disulfiram used for treatment of alcoholism (Fuller &

Gordis, 2004). Some of the nervous system side effects include cases of sensor neural deafness following direct instillation of CHG into the middle ear (Lai *et al.*, 2011).

Mercury poisoning (also known as hydrargyria or mercurialism) is a disease caused by exposure to mercury or its compounds. Because of differences in tissue distributions, mercury poisoning's effects will differ depending on whether it has been caused by exposure to elemental mercury, inorganic mercury compounds (as salts), or organomercury compounds (Clarkson & Magos, 2006; Ibrahim*et al.*, 2006). Studies have shown that almost all forms of mercury cause toxic effects in a number of tissues and organs, depending on the chemical form of mercury, the level of exposure, the duration of exposure, and the route of exposure (Jensen *et al.*, 2005). However, kidneys are the primary target organs where inorganic mercury is taken up, accumulated, and expresses toxicity. The main part of the kidney that is affected by mercury is the pars recta of the proximal tubule. The adverse effect of mercury in the body is through alterations in intracellular thiol metabolism, mercury can promote oxidative stress, lipid peroxidation, mitochondrial dysfunction, and changes in heme metabolism (Zalups, 2000).

In spite of its lethal effect, mercury iodide is used as a constituent of skin bleaching/lightening creams, soaps, an antiseptic in creams and ointments (Oyelakin *et al.*, 2010). Many of the mercury-containing products don't bear labels indicating that they contain it. Worldwide, lactating mothers are encouraged to breastfeed their babies; because breastfeeding has been associated with an advantage to infant neuro-behavioral development, possibly in part due to essential nutrients in breast milk. However, breast milk may be contaminated by environmental neurotoxicants, such as methylmercury (MeHg)-(Jansen *et al.*, 2005).

In several developing countries, Tanzania inclusive, even though mercury-containing products have been prohibited, they are clandestinely sold (Glahder *et al.*, 1999). The mercuric compounds' half-lives are long, thus over a long period of time; there would be accumulation in the body of consumers. Mercury exposure at high levels can harm the brain, kidneys, lungs, heart, and the immune system of people of all ages. Studies have shown that low levels of mercury do not cause a health concern (Holmes *et al.*, 2009; Mozaffarian & Rimm, 2006; Zalups, 2000). However, it has been demonstrated that high levels of methyl mercury, which is the microbial transformed bioactive form of mercury, in the bloodstream of unborn babies and young children may harm the developing nervous system, making the child less able to reason and teach (Wojcik *et al.*, 2006).

4.2   Environmental Impacts of Medicated Soaps

Mercury is present in the environment in a number of forms including elemental mercury (Hg^0), inorganic mercurous (Hg^+) and mercuric (Hg^{2+}) salts and as organic compounds such as MeHg, ethyl- and phenyl-mercury; each form possesses different physicochemical properties and toxicity profiles (Goldman &Shannon, 2001). Mercury has many harmful effects on health and environment. One of the important impacts of mercury to the environment is its ability to build up in the organisms and along the food chain. Almost all forms of mercury can accumulate to some degree; nonetheless MeHg is absorbed and accumulates to a greater extent than other forms. The bio-magnification of MeHg has the most substantial influence on the impact on animals and humans.

Bourdineaud *et al.* (2008) fed mice a diet containing as little as 0.1% of mercury-contaminated fish for a period of one month, and this resulted into a typical disorders of mercurial contamination.Fish appear to bind MeHgstrongly, nearly 100% of mercury that bio-accumulates in predator fish is MeHg. Once MeHg is absorbed in fish tissue, only half of it can be eliminated in 2 years, because it covalent binds to protein sulfhydryl groups (Wiener & Spry, 1996). Controlling for other factors, mercury contaminated fish are relatively found in larger quantity in small lakes as compared to large ones. The fact that small lakes are relatively warmer; the methylation of mercury is also higher. Consequently, perpetual mercury methylation and its accumulation in lakes and other aquatic organisms may negatively impact on climate change leading to further increase of levels of mercury in the environment (Jacob & Winner, 2009).

In microorganisms, effects of both inorganic and organic mercury compounds have been reported at concentrations of 5 mg/liter and 50mg/liter of culture medium (IPCS, 1991). Evidence suggests that mercury is responsible for a reduction of microbiological activity important to the ecosystem in soils over large parts of Europe and many other places worldwide with similar soil characteristics. In order to prevent ecological effects of mercury in organic soils, the acceptable content is from 0.07 to 0.3 mg/kg for the total mercury content in soil (Pirrone *et al.*, 2001). The Arctic Monitoring and Assessment Program(AMAP, 1998) had reported that when mercury concentrations exceed 25 mg/kg wet weight in kidneys and liver of marine and terrestrial mammals, tends to be very toxic and occasionally causes death.

Eggshell thinning in poultry and wild birdsis one of the first environmental consequences of the mercury contamination spreading (and other environmental toxins) as well as severe poisoning of wildlife has been witnessed in Scandinavia, North America and Greenland. Evidence of increasing mercury concentrations in some organisms found in these areas, is of concern with respect to ecosystem health (Dietz *et al.*, 2013). Such findingsnot only are attributable to medicated soaps-containing mercury compounds, but also household consumer products and other human activities such as mining, industrial and agricultural activities (Rugh *et al.*, 1996).

Researchers discovered that one of the most popular antimicrobials, TCC defies water treatment methods after has been used for various purposes, such as washing, in medicated soaps. Once it is flushed down drains, about 75% of TCC remain unaltered by sewages treatment and goes directly to surface water and in community sludge. The sludge is regularly applied as manure, which means TCC mighthypothetically accumulate in our food as well. Besides, TCC is known to cause cancer and reproductive problems in mammals, and blue-baby syndrome or methemoglobinemia in human infants. The use of nitrate-contaminated drinking water to prepare infant formula is a renowned risk factor for infant blue baby syndrome, which iscaused by decreased ability of blood to transport oxygen, causing oxygen deficiency in different body parts. Newborns are more prone than adults. The disease can be caused by in- take of water and vegetables high in nitrate (Knobeloch *et al.*, 2000).

Most of the medicated soaps contain antimicrobial agents (TCS, CHG and hexachlorophene) that are lipophilic, which stay in the body and accumulate over time. Some of these biocides are commonly detected in aquatic ecosystems, because they cannot be completely removed during the wastewater treatment process. For instance, biodegradation and photolytic degradation of TCS mitigate its availability to aquatic biota; yet the by-products such as methyltriclosan and other chlorinated phenols may be more resistant to degradation and have higher toxicity than the parent compounds. The incessant exposures of aquatic organisms to TCS and its bio-accumulation potential, have led to detectable levels of the antimicrobial in a number of aquatic species, in breast milk, urine and plasma, and these TCS levels correlate with consumer use patterns of the antimicrobial agents. The potential for endocrine disruption and antibiotic cross-resistance highlights the importance of the judicious use of such biocides (Dann & Hontela, 2011).

Assessing the presence of pollutant biocides of interest including volatile organic compounds (VOC) in child care facilities, the United States Environmental Protection Agency (EPA) for respiratory and irritant effects, revealed high levels of VOC such as aldehydes, chloroform, benzene, and ethyl benzene that surpassed child-specific "safe harbour levels" (Seltenrich, 2013). Some of these agents are common antimicrobials that are incorporated into medicated soaps and other biocide-containing house-hold consumer products.

Furthermore, there are growing concerns about the emergence and accumulation of numerous harmful chemicals resulting from biocides usage and other pharmaceutical products in the environment and their potential negative effects on human and animal health (Oyelakin *et al.*, 2010; James *et al.*, 2010). Wilson *et al* (2003) demonstrated that even treated wastewaters in the United States contain detectable quantities of surfactants (foaming agents, emulsifiers, and dispersants)-incorporated in medicated soaps, antibiotics, and other types of antimicrobial substances contained in pharmaceutical and personal-care products, which are released into stream ecosystems. Unfortunately the degradation characteristics of many of these chemicals are not yet known, nor are the chemical properties of their by-products. Kolpin *et al.* (2002) reported a consistent reduction of algal genus diversity as the concentrations of ciprofloxacin (an antibiotic), TCS and a common surfactant (Tergitol RNP) were increased. This suggests that direct and indirect effects of such chemicals on aquatic food-webs are also possible, both for parent compounds and for their degradation products (Drury *et al.*, 20013; Barber *et al.*, 2013).A dramatic loss of algal taxa even at low concentrations of these compounds was noticeable, which lead to cumulative, adverse impacts that might be incorrectly attributed to processes of natural change or ecological succession. Probably, the most crucial effects of biocides and pharmaceutical byproductswere those on inhibitors/inducers of multi-drug transport (efflux) systems and the cytochrome P450 monooxygenase isoforms in aquatic biota (Crofton *et al.*, 2007;Tsai *et al.*, 2001).

Wong & Pessah (1996) have been working on polychlorinated biphenyls (PCBs) and polybrominated diphenyl ethers (PBDEs) that are considered as environmental risk factors. PCBs have similar structure to TCS; the later interferes with the muscular contraction once stimulated, a response known as excitation-contraction coupling-(ECC). "Excitation-contraction coupling is essential for muscle contraction," "If you interfere with that process, it can be lethal and certainly debilitating''. TCS essentially impairs ECC in both cardiac muscle cells and skeletal muscle cells. This can happen at relatively low concentrations and relatively quickly. Although usage of TCS will not lead to immediate heart failure, since most people are able to metabolize TCS quickly so that it is readily excreted through urine. However, some people do not metabolize the compound quickly, thus TCS remains active in the circulatory system for a longer period of time. Therefore, the main concern the scientists have is the potential for TCS exposure to contribute to already debilitating heart conditions (Cherednichenko *et al.*, 2012).

5   Offsetting Antimicrobial Resistance Development

5.1   Rational use of medicated soaps

The issue of resistance to antimicrobial agents (including medicated soaps) is worrying, particularly in developing countries. The fundamental problems are largely economic and societal, and no ready solutions are available (Laxminarayan, *et al.*, 2013). Therefore, control of the emergence and spread of antimicrobial resistance requires a concerted effort on the part of all social and scientific agencies involved in health care (Baquero, 1996). One of the approaches is the rational use of medicated soaps, which mayinclude but not limited to theuse of right biocides for the intended purpose, using correct dose/concentration for a specified period of time on the appropriate object or body part. In order to comply with these conditions, consumers require professional advices or instructions. For that matter, an accurate diagnosis or environmental health analysis may also determine their use (Holloway, 2000).As medicated soaps contain antimicrobial agents; these need to be regulated by enforcing a policy for restricting their use and easy availability as consumer products (Tunger *et al.*, 2009).Similarly, medicated soaps should be used more judiciously in hospitals by intensive teaching of the principles of the use of antimicrobial agents and to establish better control measures for health care facility acquired infections for which medicated soaps and biocides are intended (Sharma *et al.*, 2005).

Showering or bathing with 2% TCS has been shown to be an effective regimen for the decolonization of patients whose skin is carrying MRSA as previously showed by Moran *et al.* (2006). This implies that it can also affect the protective human normal flora. Some recent studies have revealed that *Candida* strains exhibits intrinsic resistance to the medicated soaps; and some of the soaps had inappropriate active ingredients or concentrations and /or were adulterated (Ekanola *et al.*, 2012; Ogunshe *et al.*, 2011). Uses of lower concentrations of anti-infective agents (antimicrobials) always result into undesired effects such as development of drug-tolerance and ultimately resistance. Since all these biocides have several important medical uses, therefore in order to retain these applications we must eliminate the unnecessary ones. It is therefore advised that TCS usage need to be restricted to applications for which has proved to be still effective and most necessary. Alternatively, either isopropanol (60-80%) or n-propanol (60-80%) can be used instead of TCS, since they have demonstrated to be equally effective against viral particles and other microorganisms (Ansari *et al.*, 1989). The combination of the two may have synergistic effect. Likewise, hand hygiene that aims to reduce pathogenic microorganisms by the application of alcohol-based hand rubs (ABHR) without the addition of water, or by hand washing with plain soap or medicated soap and water has shown to be effective. ABHR has microbiologically demonstrated that is more effective than medicated or plain soap even in presence of blood (Larson & Bobo, 1992). To enhance the antimicrobial effect of ABHR, low concentration of CHG can be added and this has proved to be very effective (Zaragoza *et al.*, 1999).

5.2   Control of Easy Availability of Medicated Soaps

Undoubtedly, medicated soaps are drugs (antimicrobial agents) like any other currently known and used anti-infective agent. Several antimicrobial substances are found in medicated soaps and they have various mechanisms of action on microorganisms of which some resemble those of antibiotics (Ikpoh *et al.*, 2012). Investigating the antimicrobial effects of medicated soaps (1.0, 4.0 and 8.0 mg/ml) on strains of reference microorganisms namely*Candida albicans* (ATCC90028), *Staphylococcus aureus* (ATCC25923), *Pseudomonas aureginosa* (ATCC27853) and *Escherichia coli* (ATCC25922), using the disk diffusion technique; Mwambete & Lyombe, (2011) found apositive correlation (r =0.318; p<0.01) between zones of inhibition and soaps' concentrations. This buttresses their potential role as antimicrobial agents and usefulness in fighting topical microbial infections (Paulson, 2003).

Another study has showed thatthe use of medicated soaps containing CHG can provide persistent protection from infectious MRSA while soap products without CHG may not (Ferrara *et al.*, 2011). Presumably this explains why over 50% of soaps, or washing liquids easily available in Nigeria and other countries contain antimicrobial agents (Ekanola *et al.*, 2012). Many of the soaps even carry seals or endorsement from specific health bodies; though the Centre for Disease Control and Prevention claims there is so far no scientific proof that medicated soaps are better at preventing infections than regular soaps or even ordinary water (Ekanola *et al.*, 2012; Fulls *et al.*, 2008).

Study conducted by Mwambete and Lyombe (2011) revealed that regardless of a wide-spread availability of the so-called medicated soaps; a number of communicable infectious and food-borne diseases as well as poor-hygienic conditions-related health problems are rampant in communities. One of the very possible reasons was poor quality of these antimicrobial consumer products that could have lower concentration of antimicrobial active ingredients or adulterated (Ekanola *et al.*, 2012). In several resources-limited countries, this seems to be more of a marketing phenomenon. Long-term usage of such products has detrimental impacts such as emergence of antimicrobial-resistant microorganisms (Chuanchen *et al.*, 2001; White *et al.*, 2001; Russell, 1998). Mwambete & Lyombe, (2011) remonstrated that the tested medicated soaps, of which some are claimed to remove or kill over 99.99% of pathogenic microorganisms, were unable to neither eliminate fungi (*C. albicans*) nor demonstrate comparable antimicrobial effects at even higher concentrations of the medicated soaps (8mg/ml) as compared to that of ketaconazole (15μg) and ciprofloxacin (5μg) that as served positive control antibiotics (Figure 4).

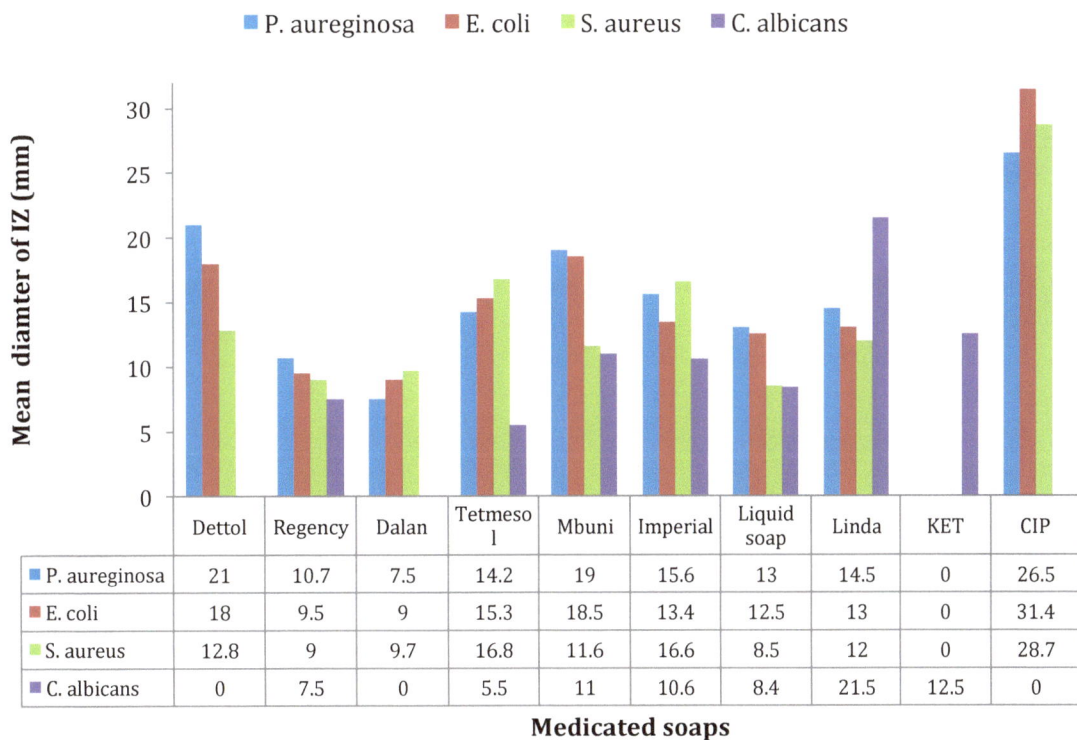

Legend: ■ P. aureginosa　■ E. coli　■ S. aureus　■ C. albicans

	Dettol	Regency	Dalan	Tetmesol	Mbuni	Imperial	Liquid soap	Linda	KET	CIP
■ P. aureginosa	21	10.7	7.5	14.2	19	15.6	13	14.5	0	26.5
■ E. coli	18	9.5	9	15.3	18.5	13.4	12.5	13	0	31.4
■ S. aureus	12.8	9	9.7	16.8	11.6	16.6	8.5	12	0	28.7
■ C. albicans	0	7.5	0	5.5	11	10.6	8.4	21.5	12.5	0

Medicated soaps

Key: KET-ketoconazole; CIP-ciprofloxacin; IZ-inhibition zone

Figure 4: Antimicrobial effects of different brands of soaps medicated on reference strains of microorganisms.

A survey conducted in the United States on national chains, regional grocery and internet consumer markets revealed that over 76% of liquid soaps and 29% bar soaps contained antibacterial additives. Overall, 45% of all surveyed soaps had antibacterial agents (Perencevich *et al.*, 2002).

Ekanola *et al.* (2012) determined the antimycotic effects of 18 different brands of soaps available in Ibadan, Nigeria. The active ingredients of the industrial soaps were respectively listed as-GIV soap [Cocos necitera oil, Elacsis guineensis oil, sodium hydroxide, perfume, glycerin, rode oil, titariumdioxide, tetrasodium EDTA, water, Cl 15880, Cl 45100], Halo soap [sodium tallowate, sodium palm kernelate, water (Aqua), fragrance (Parfum), glycerin, sodium chloride, tetrasodium EDTA, tetrasodium etidronate, titanium dioxide Cl 77891, menthol, trichlocarbon 1% w/w, Cl 12490, limonene, butylphynyl, methylpropional, linalool, geraniol], Imperial Leather soap [soap base, water, glycerin, fragrance, stabiliser and colour], London soap [1.2% w/w mercuric iodide included as 3% potassium mercuric solution], Lux soap [sodium tallowate, sodium palmate, aqua, sodium palm kernelate, glycerin, paraffin, sodium sulphate, titanium dioxide, phosphoric acid, tetra sodium EDTA, etidronic acid, tocophenol acetate, disodium distyrylbiphenyl disulfonate, hexyl cinnamol, Geraniol, benzyl salicylate, butylphenyl, methylpropionol, coumarin, Limonene, Cl 74160, Min TFM= 68%], Meriko soap [sodium tallowate, sodium cocoate, aqua, perfume, Cl 74160, Cl 12490, Cl 77266], Tetmosol soap [5% monosulfiram B.P., sodium tallowate, Citronella], Tura soap [TCS, allantoin, vitamin E, sodium tallowate, sodium palm kernelate, aqua, perfume, Cl 12940 (Pigment Red 5), Cl 77266 (Carbon Black), Cl 74160 (Pigment Blue 15)] and Zee soap [native black soap base, palm kernel oil, Shea butter (rich in natural vitamins), cocoa pod and palm bunch ash solution, camwood extract (osun), native honey, aloe vera, aqua, fragrance]. None of the soaps had *in vitro* inhibitory effects on any of the test Candida species viz. *C. albicans*, *C. glabrata*, C. *pseudotropicalis* and *C. tropicalis*.

Not all medicated soaps or antimicrobial products on the consumer market place contain toxic agents as active ingredients such as TCS, PCMC or TCC and the like. There is a myriad of other antimicrobial substances (chemicals) that are used; some of these agents are much effective at killing or inhibiting growth of the pathogenic microorganisms while others are not. Conversely, non-antimicrobial agent-containing soaps (plain soaps) have proved to be quite effective at cleansing microorganism from the body's surface (Aiello *et al.*, 2007).

6   Concluding Remarks

6.1   Conclusions

The fact that biocides/medicated soaps and antibiotics have similarities in mechanisms of action and the former have broader spectra of antimicrobial activity; hence biocides may also create a diversity of antimicrobial resistance spectra, which can result into expression of several efflux pumps that serve similar role for antibiotics. Therefore, it seems that medicated soaps usage may be doing more harm than good by significantly attributing to developing antimicrobial-resistant pathogens and thus rendering the existing and currently effective antimicrobial agents obsolete. The above elucidated experimental-based evidences and literature reviews, both indicate that extensive overuse of antimicrobial products in the consumer market place may significantlycontribute to the on-going problem of antimicrobial resistance. Not only better understanding of relationship between antimicrobial use and resistance but also earlier intervention on the easy availability of biocides and medicated soaps usage may decelerate the development and spread of antimicrobial resistance, particularly, if medicated soaps, just like other clinically used antibiotics, will also be controlled or regulated by responsible authorities.

The general public should recognize that antimicrobial product residues accumulate and pollute our environment; therefore we should minimize the use of antimicrobial agents-containing products such as medicated soaps for extra assurance. Besides, the use of medicated soaps may also deliver a false sense of security, resulting into abandonment or inadequate hand-washing practice as described by the alliance for prudent use of antibiotics (APUA, 2011). Active ingredients in medicated soaps and other household commonly used cleaning and antimicrobial agents have been associated with both mild and serious adverse effects, of those some are life threatening (Kumar, 2008; Kumar, 2005;Kolpin *et al.*, 2002).

6.2   Recommendations on Appropriate use of Medicated Soaps

Because of the above described effects of antimicrobial-containing soaps, it is recommended that irrational and long-time usage of these products should be discouraged. It is also important that during development of topical antimicrobial products, a multidimensional approach be adopted. This will ensure that the resultant product is designed for the specific needs of the market and that those needs are met. Drugs regulatory authorities should focus on the issues of easy availability of medicated soaps, particularly in developing countries in order to curtail the rapid spread of antimicrobial-resistance. The guidelines on medicated soaps and other biocides usage in household or for industrial purpose should be established, and its implementation closely monitored and regulated whenever necessary to avoid the emergence of any MDR strains. Modern and sophisticated methods (genetic and molecular)need to be employed for monitoringfurther spread and development ofantimicrobial resistance by effectively utilizing them during all stages of preclinical and clinical pharmacological studies (Gnanadhas *et al.*,2013).

The information to guide consumers on appropriate domestic use of biocides and other antimicrobial-containing products as well as recommendations as alternatives to TCSand other potentially toxic products have been published (APUA, 2011) as depicted in Table 3.

How to avoid irrational use of medicated soaps
• Wash hands frequently and thoroughly. Regular soaps lower the surface tension of water, and thus wash away unwanted bacteria.
• Lather hands for at least 10-15 seconds and then rinse off in warm water.
• Dry hands with a clean towel to help brush off any microorganisms that did not get washed down the drain.
• Complement with alcohol-containing hand sanitizer.
• Wash surfaces that come in contact with food with a detergent and water, or with bleach.
• Wash children's hands and toys regularly to prevent possible infections
• When selecting product such as hand soap, toothpastes, and deodorants, it is recommended to read the label. If the product states ''antibacterial'' one should locate the active ingredients list to see if the product contains TCS or other antibacterial agents. Consumers may opt to purchase products that either are not labelled ''antibacterial'' or contain alcohol or hydrogen peroxide as the antibacterial agent. In addition, non-organic antibiotics and organic biocides are effective alternatives to TCS.

Table 3: APUA guidelines on TCS usage to consumers

Lastly, it is obvious that the fight against emergence of resistant microbial strains and their worldwide spread requires concerted timely measures of all countries for better planning to slow down and possibly to prevent the eminent global health crisis.

Acknowledgements

I convey my heartedly felt gratitude to my resourceful wife Martha and daughters Erica and Careen for their offeredsupports during the confection of this chapter.

References

Adolfsson-Erici, M., Pettersson, M., Parkkonen, J., & Sturve, J. (2002). Triclosan, a commonly used bactericide found in human milk and in the aquatic environment in Sweden. Chemosphere,46(9):1485-1489.

Ahn, K. C., Zhao, B., Chen, J., Cherednichenko, G., Sanmarti, E., Denison, M. S., Hammock, B. D. (2008). In vitro biologic activities of the antimicrobials triclocarban, its analogs, and triclosan in bioassay screens: receptor-based bioassay screens. Environmental Health Perspectives, 116(9):1203.

Aiello, A.E., E.L. Larson, Levy, S.B. (2007). Consumer antibacterial soaps: effective or just risky? Clinical Infectious Disease, 45: S137-47.

Aiello, A.E., Larson, E. (2003). Antibacterial cleaning and hygiene products as an emerging risk factor for antibiotic resistance in the community.The Lancet Infectious Diseases,3(8):501-506.

Alekshun, M. N., & Levy, S. B. (2007). Molecular mechanisms of antibacterial multidrug resistance.Cell,128(6), 1037-1050.

AMAP (1998). AMAP Assessment Report: Arctic Pollution Issues. Oslo: Arctic Monitoring and Assessment Programme (AMAP).

Ansari, J., Hussain, S.A., Zarkar, A., Bliss, J., Tanguay, J.S. &Glaholm, J. (1989). In vivo protocol for testing efficacy of hand-washing agents against viruses and bacteria: experiments with rotavirus and Escherichia coli. Applied Environmental Microbiology, 55:3113–3118

Anselmo, H. M., van den Berg, J. H., Rietjens, I. M., & Murk, A. J. (2012). Inhibition of cellular efflux pumps involved in multi xenobiotic resistance (MXR) in echinoid larvae as a possible mode of action for increased ecotoxicological risk of mixtures.Ecotoxicology,21(8): 2276-2287.

APUA -The alliance for prudent use of antibiotics. Triclosan. White paper prepared by the alliance for prudent use of antibiotics: January 2011.

Bailey, A.M., Constantinidou, C., Ivens, A., Garvey, M.I., Webber, M.A., Coldham, N., Piddock, L.J. (2009). Exposure of Escherichia coli and Salmonella enterica serovar Typhimurium to triclosan induces a species-specific response, including drug detoxification. Journal of antimicrobial chemotherapy, 64(5): 973-985.

Baquero, F. (1996). Antibiotic resistance in Spain: What can be done?Clinical Infectious Diseases,23(4): 819-823.

Barber, L. B., Keefe, S. H., Brown, G. K., Furlong, E. T., Gray, J. L., Kolpin, D. W., Zaugg, S. D. (2013). Persistence and Potential Effects of Complex Organic Contaminant Mixtures in Wastewater-Impacted Streams.Environmental Science & Technology,47(5):2177-2188.

Beumer, R., Bloomfield, S.F., Exner, M., Fara, G.M., Nath, K.J., Scott, E. (2000).Microbial resistance and biocides.In A review by the International Scientific Forum on Home Hygiene (IFH).

Bourdineaud, J.P., Bellance, N., Bénard, G., Brèthes, D., Fujimura, M., Gonzalez, P., Laclau, M. (2008). Feeding mice with diets containing mercury-contaminated fish flesh from French Guiana: a model for the mercurial intoxication of the Wayana Amerindians.Environmental Health,7(1): 53.

Brooks, S.E., Walczak, M.A., Hameed, R., Coonan, P. (2002). Chlorhexidine resistance in antibiotic-resistant bacteria isolated from the surfaces of dispensers of soap containing chlorhexidine. Infection Control and Hospital Epidemiology, 23(11): 692-695.

Calafat, A.M., Ye, X., Wong, L.Y., Reidy, J.A., Needham, L.L. (2008). Urinary concentrations of triclosan in the U.S. population: 2003-2004. Environmental Health Perspectives, 116(3):303-307.

Cherednichenko, G., Zhang, R., Bannister, R.A., Timofeyev, V., Li, N., Fritsch, E. B., Pessah, I.N. (2012). Triclosan impairs excitation–contraction coupling and Ca2+ dynamics in striated muscle. Proceedings of the National Academy of Sciences, 109(35):14158-14163.

Chopra, I. (2007). The increasing use of silver-based products as antimicrobial agents: a useful development or a cause for concern? Journal of antimicrobial Chemotherapy,59(4): 587-590.

Chopra, I., Roberts, M. (2001). Tetracycline antibiotics: mode of action, applications, molecular biology, and epidemiology of bacterial resistance. Microbiology and Molecular Biology Reviews, 65(2): 232-260.

Chuanchuen, R., Beinlich, K., Hoang, T.T., Becher, A., Karkhoff-Schweitzer, R. R., Schweizer, H.P. (2001). Cross-resistance between Triclosan and antibiotics in Pseudomonas aeruginosa is mediated by multidrug efflux pumps: exposure of a susceptible mutant strain to triclosan selects for nfxB mutants overexpressing MexCD-OprJ. Antimicrobial Agents and Chemotherapy, 45:428–432.

Chuanchuen, R.K., Narasaki, C.T., Schweizer, H. P. (2002). The MexJK efflux pump of Pseudomonas aeruginosa requires OprM for antibiotic efflux but not for efflux of triclosan. Journal of Bacteriology, 184:5036-5044.

Cirz, R.T., Chin, J.K., Andes, D.R., de Crécy-Lagard, V., Craig, W.A., Romesberg, F.E. (2005). Inhibition of mutation and combating the evolution of antibiotic resistance.PLoS biology, 3(6): e176.

Clarkson, T.W., Magos, L. (2006). "The toxicology of mercury and its chemical compounds".Critical Reviews in Toxicology,36 (8): 609-662.

Clayton, E. M. R., Todd, M., Dowd, J. B., Aiello, A. E. (2011).The impact of bisphenol A and triclosan on immune parameters in the US population, NHANES 2003–2006.Environmental health perspectives,119(3), 390.

Coelho, J.R., Carriço, J.A., Knight, D., Martínez, J.L., Morrissey, I., Oggioni, M.R., Freitas, A.T. (2013). The use of machine learning methodologies to analyse antibiotic and biocide susceptibility in Staphylococcus aureus.PLoS one, 8(2): e55582.

Crofton, K. M., Paul, K. B., DeVito, M. J., Hedge, J. M. (2007). Short-term in vivo exposure to the water contaminant triclosan: Evidence for disruption of thyroxine.Environmental Toxicology and Pharmacology,24(2), 194-197.

Dann, A. B., Hontela, A. (2011). Triclosan: environmental exposure, toxicity and mechanisms of action. Journal of Applied Toxicology, 31(4): 285.

Davies, J., Davies, D. (2010). Origins and evolution of antibiotic resistance.Microbiology and Molecular Biology Reviews,74(3): 417-433.

Dietz, R., Sonne, C., Basu, N., Braune, B., O'Hara, T., Letcher, R. J., ... & Aars, J. (2013). What are the toxicological effects of mercury in Arctic biota?Science of the Total Environment, 443, 775-790. Evidence of increasing concentrations in mercury in some biota in Arctic Canada and Greenland is therefore a concern with respect to ecosystem health.

Dixon, B. (2000). Antibiotics as growth promoters: risks and alternatives. American Society for Microbiology News, 66:264–265.

Dogra, A., Dua, A. (2005). Cosmetic dermatitis.Indian Journal of Dermatology,50(4):191.

Drury, B., Scott, J., Rosi-Marshall, E. J., Kelly, J. J. (2013). TCS Exposure Increases TCS Resistance and Influences Taxonomic Composition of Benthic Bacterial Communities.Environmental science & technology,47(15): 8923-8930.

Ekanola, Y.A., Ogunshe, A.A.O., Azeez, D.L., Opasol, O. (2012) Studies on in vitro antimycotic potentials of local and industrial soaps on vuvlovaginal candfida species. International Journal of Plant, Animal and Environmental Sciences, 2(3): 69-74.

Elkins, C.A., Mullis, L.B. (2006). Mammalian steroid hormones are substrates for the major RND- and MFS-type tripartite multidrug efflux pumps of Escherichia coli. Journal of Bacteriology, 188:1191-1195.

Epel, D., Luckenbach, T., Stevenson, C. N., MacManus-Spencer, L. A., Hamdoun, A., Smital, A. T. (2008). *Efflux transporters: newly appreciated roles in protection against pollutants.Environmental Science & Technology,42(11): 3914-3920.*

Fan, F., Yan, K., Wallis, N.G., Reed, S., Moore, T.D., Rittenhouse, S.F., DeWolf, W.E. Jr. Huang, J., McDevitt, D., Miller, W.H., Seefeld, M.A., Newlander, K.A., Jakas, D.R., Head, M.S., Payne, D.J. (2002). *Defining and combating the mechanisms of triclosan resistance in clinical isolates of Staphylococcus aureus.Antimicrobial agents and chemotherapy,46(11): 3343-3347.*

Fangea, D., Nilssona, K., Tensonb, T., Ehrenberga, M. (2012).*Functional and Genetic Characterization of the Tap Efflux Pump in Mycobacterium bovis BCG.Antimicrobial Agents and Chemotherapy, 56 (4):2074-2083.*

FDA. (2013). *Triclosan: What Consumers Should Know Accessible at: Accessed on 8th December, 2013at: http://www.fda.gov/forconsumers/consumerupdates/ucm205999.htmPage Last Updated: 11/25/2013.*

Ferrara, M.S., Courson, R., Paulson, D.S. (2011). *Evaluation of persistent antimicrobial effects of an antimicrobial formulation. Journal of Athletic Training, 46(6): 629-633.*

Fraise, A.P. (1999). *Choosing disinfectants. Journal of Hospital Infection, 43(4):255-264.*

Fraise, A.P. (2002). *''Susceptibility of antibiotic resistant cocci to biocides'' Journal of Appplied Microbiology, 92; Suppl. 158S-62S.*

Friedman, M., Juneja, V.K. (2010).*Review of antimicrobial and antioxidative activities of chitosans in food.Journal of Food Protection, 73(9):1737-1761.*

Fuller, R.K., Gordis, E. (2004). *Does disulfiram have a role in alcoholism treatment today?Addiction99 21-24*

Fulls, J.L., Rodgers, N.D., Fischler, G.E., Howard, J.M., Patel, M., Weidner, P.L., Duran M.H. (2008). *Alternative hand contamination technique to compare the activities of antimicrobial and non-anytimicrobial soaps under different conditions Journal of Applied Environmental Microbiology, 74(12): 3739-44.*

Fux, C.A., Costerton, J.W., Stewart, P.S., Stoodley, P. (2005). *Survival strategies of infectious biofilms.Trends in microbiology, 13(1): 34-40.*

Gilbert, P., McBain AJ. (2003). *Potential impact of increased use of biocides in consumer products on prevalence of antibiotic resistance.Clinical Microbiology Reviews, 189-208.*

Gilbert, P., Moore, L. E. (2005). *Cationic antiseptics: diversity of action under a common epithet.Journal of applied microbiology,99(4), 703-715.*

Glahder, C.M., Appel, P. W. U., Asmund, G. (1999). *Mercury in Soap in Tanzania.National Environmental Research Institute.*

Gnanadhas, D. P., Marathe, S. A., Chakravortty, D. (2013).*Biocides-resistance, cross-resistance mechanisms and assessment.Expert opinion on investigational drugs, 22(2): 191-206.*

Goldman, L.R., Shannon, M.W. (2001). *The Committee on Environmental Health. Technical Report: mercury in the environment: implications for paediatricians. Pediatrics, 108 pp. 197–205.*

González-Lamothe, R., Mitchell, G., Gattuso, M., Diarra, M. S., Malouin, F., Bouarab, K. (2009).*Plant antimicrobial agents and their effects on plant and human pathogens.International Journal of Molecular Sciences, 10(8): 3400-3419.*

Guarner, F., Bourdet-Sicard, R., Brandtzaeg, P., Gill, H.S., McGuirk, P., Van Eden, W., Rook, G.A. (2006). *Mechanisms of disease: the hygiene hypothesis revisited.Nature Clinical Practice Gastroenterology & Hepatology,3(5):275-284.*

Gupta, A., Matsui, K., Lo, J. F., Silver, S. (1999). *Molecular basis for resistance to silver cations in Salmonella. Nature Medicine, 5:183–188*

Gusarov, I., Shatalin, K., Starodubtseva, M., & Nudler, E. (2009). *Endogenous nitric oxide protects bacteria against a wide spectrum of antibiotics. Science, 325(5946):1380-1384.*

Halden, R.U., Paull, D.H. (2005). Co-occurrence of triclocarban and TCS in US water resources.Environmental science & technology,39(6):1420-1426.

Harbarth, S., Dharan, S., Liassine, N., Herrault, P., Auckenthaler, R., Pittet, D. (1999). Randomized, placebo-controlled, double-blind trial to evaluate the efficacy of mupirocin for eradicating carriage of methicillin-resistant Staphylococcus aureus. Antimicrobial Agents and Chemotherapy, 43:1412-1416.

Harbarth, S., Samore, M.H. (2005).Antimicrobial resistance determinants and future control.Emerging Infectious Diseases,11(6), 794.

Harvey, R.J., Lund, V.J. (2007). Biofilms and chronic rhinosinusitis: systematic review of evidence, current concepts and directions for research. Rhinology, 45(1): 3.

Hassan, M., Kubmarawa, D., Modibbo, U.U. & Tunde, A. D. (2010).Production of medicated soap from butyrospermum paradoxum plant. Journal of Physical Sciences and Innovation, 2: 90-96.

Hay, A.G., Dees, P.M. Sayler, G.S. (2001). Growth of a bacterial consortium on triclosan.Federation of European Microbiologists Society- Microbiology Letter, 36:105–112.

Heath, J.H., Rubin, J.R., Holland, D.R., Zhang, E., Snow, M.E., Rock, C.O. (1999).Mechanism of triclosan inhibition of bacterial fatty acid synthesis.Journal of Biological Chemistry, 274:1110-114.

Heath, R., Yu, Y., Shapiro, M., Olson, E.,Rock, C.O. (1998).Broad spectrum antimicrobial biocides target the FabI component of fatty acid synthesis.Journal of Biological Chemistry,273(46), 30316-30320.

Heath, R. J., Rock, C.O. (2000). Microbiology: a Triclosan-resistant bacterial enzyme. Nature, 406(6792): 145-146.

Heath, R. J., White, S. W., Rock, C.O. (2002).Inhibitors of fatty acid synthesis as antimicrobial chemotherapeutics. Applied Microbiology and Biotechnology, 58:695–70.

Heath, R.J., g Li, J., Roland, G.E., Rock, C.O. (2000). Inhibition of the Staphylococcus aureus NADPH-dependent Enoyl-Acyl Carrier Protein Reductase by Triclosan and Hexachlorophene.The Journal of Biological Chemistry, 275(7): 4654 –4659.

Hegstad, K., Langsrud, S., Lunestad, B.T., Scheie, A.A., Sunde, M., Yazdankhah, S.P. (2010). Does the wide use of quaternary ammonium compounds enhance the selection and spread of antimicrobial resistance and thus threaten our health? Microbial Drug Resistance, 16(2): 91-104.

Hernández, A., Ruiz, F.M., Romero, A., Martínez, J.L. (2011). The Binding of Triclosan to SmeT, the Repressor of the Multidrug Efflux Pump SmeDEF, Induces Antibiotic Resistance in Stenotrophomonas maltophilia. PLoS Pathog, 7(6): e1002103

Holloway, K. (2000). Antimicrobial resistance: the facts. Essential Drug Monitor, WHO, 28&29:7-8.

Holmes, P., James, K. A. F., & Levy, L. S. (2009). Is low-level environmental mercury exposure of concern to human health?Science of the Total Environment,408(2):171-182.

Ibrahim, D., Froberg, B., Wolf, A., Rusyniak, D.E. (2006). "Heavy metal poisoning: clinical presentations and pathophysiology". Clinical Laboratory Medicine,26 (1): 67–97.

Ikpoh, I.S., Lennox, J.A., Agbo, B.E., Udoekong, N.S., Ekpo, I.A. Iyam, S.O. (2002). Comparative studies on the effect of locally made black soap and conventional medicated soaps on isolated human skin microflora. Journal of Mircobiology and Biotechnology Research, 2(4): 533-537.

IPCS (1991) Inorganic mercury.Geneva, World Health Organization, International Programme on Chemical Safety (Environmental Health Criteria 118).

Jack, D.L., Yang, N.M., Saier, M.H., Jr. (2001).The drug/metabolite transporter superfamily. European Journal of Biochemistry, 268(13):3620–39.

Jacob, D. J., & Winner, D. A. (2009). Effect of climate change on air quality.Atmospheric Environment,43(1), 51-63.

James, M.O., Li, W., Summerrlot, D.P., Rowland-Faux, L., Wood, C.E., (2010). Triclosan is a potent inhibitor of stradiol and estrone sulfonation in sheep placenta. Environmental International, Nov 36(8): 942-949.

Jawetz, A.M., Melnick, K.A., Adelberg, R.J. (2010). Normal human microbiota in: medical microbiology 25th ed. McGraw –Hill companies inc. USA. Pp159-164.

Jansen, A.C (2012). An Investigation of Resistance to Quaternary Ammonium Compound Disinfectants in Bacteria(Doctoral dissertation, University of the Free State).

Jensen, T.K., Grandjean, P., Jorgensen, E.B., White, R.F., Debes, F, Weihe, P. (2005). Effects of breast feeding on nueropsychologyical development in a community with methymerucury exposure from seafood. Journal of Exposure Analysis and Environmental Epidemiology, 15(5):423-30.

Kagan, L. J., Aiello, A. E., Larson, E. (2002). The role of the home environment in the transmission of infectious diseases.Journal of community health,27(4): 247-267.

Kaiser, N.E., Newman, J.L. (2006).Formulation technology as a key component in improving hand hygiene practices, American Journal of Infection Control,34(10):S81.

Kanetoshi, A., E. Katsura, H. Ogawa, T. Ohyama, H. Kaneshima, Miura, T. (1992). Acute Toxicity, Percutaneous Absorption and Effects on Hepatic Mixed Function Oxidase Activities of 2,4,4'-Tricholor-2'-hydroxydiphenyl Ether (Irgasan® DP300) and Its Chlorinated Derivatives. Archives of Environmental Contamination and Toxicology, 23: 91-98.

Kazama, H., Hamashima, H., Sasatsu, M., Arai, T. (1999).Characterization of the antiseptic-resistance gene qacE delta 1 isolated from clinical and environmental isolates of Vibrio parahaemolyticus and Vibrio cholera non-O1. Federation of European Microbiologists Society- Microbiology Letter, 74:379-384.

Kelly, D., King, T., Aminov, R. (2007).Importance of microbial colonization of the gut in early life to the development of immunity.Mutation Research/Fundamental and Molecular Mechanisms of Mutagenesis,622(1): 58-69.

Kingtong, S., Chitramvong, Y., Janvilisri, T. (2007). ATP-binding cassette multidrug transporters in Indian-rock oyster Saccostrea forskali and their role in the export of an environmental organic pollutant tributyltin.Aquatic Toxicology,85(2):124-132.

Kini, S.G., Bhat, A.R., Bryant, B., Williamson, J.S., & Dayan, F.E. (2009). Synthesis, antitubercular activity and docking study of novel cyclic azole substituted diphenyl ether derivatives.European journal of medicinal chemistry,44(2): 492-500.

Kinjo, T., Koseki, Y., Kobayashi, M., Yamada, A., Morita, K., Yamaguchi, K., Aoki, S. (2013). Identification of Compounds with Potential Antibacterial Activity against Mycobacterium through Structure-Based Drug Screening.Journal of chemical information and modeling, 53(5):1200-1212.

Knobeloch, L., Salna, B., Hogan, A., Postle, J., Anderson, H. (2000). Blue babies and nitrate-contaminated well water.Environmental Health Perspectives,108(7): 675.

Kolpin, D.W., Furlong, E.T., Meyer, M.T., Thurman, E.M., Zaugg, S.D., Barber, L.B., Buxton, H.T. (2002). Pharmaceuticals,Hormones, and Other Organic Wastewater Contaminants in U.S. Streams, 1999-2000: A National Reconnaissance. Environmental Science & Technology, 36:1202-1211.

Kumar, S. (2005). Dettol poisoning: Clinical features and management. Indian Journal of Forensic Medicine and Toxicol

Kumar, S. (2008). Dettol poisoning: Clinical features and management. Indian Journal of Forensic Medicine&Toxicology, 2(2): 29-31.

Kuroda, T., Tsuchiya, T. (2009).Multidrug efflux transporters in the MATE family. Biochimica et Biophysica Acta, 1794(5):763–8.

Lai, P., Coulson, C., Pothier, D.D., Rutka, J. (2011). Chlorhexidine ototoxicity in ear surgery, part 1: review of the literature. Journal of Otolaryngology Head Neck Surgery, Dec; 40(6):437-40.

Landrigan, P. J., Goldman, L. R. (2011). Children's vulnerability to toxic chemicals: a challenge and opportunity to strengthen health and environmental policy.Health Affairs,30(5): 842-850.

Larson, E. (1988). APIC guidelines for infection control practice. Guideline for use of topical antimicrobial agents. American Journal of Infections Control, 16(6):253-66.

Larson, E. (1999). Skin hygiene and infection prevention: more of the same or different approaches? Clinical Infectious Diseases, 29(5):1287-1294.

Larson, E., Bobo, L. (1992). Effective hand degerming in the presence of blood. Journal of Emergency Medicine, 10(1): 327-231.

Laxminarayan, R., Duse, A., Wattal, C., Zaidi, A.K., Wertheim, H.F., Sumpradit, N., Cars, O. (2013). Antibiotic resistance-the need for global solutions.The Lancet Infectious Diseases,13(12):1057-1098.

Levy, C.W., Roujeinikova, A., Sedelnikova, S., Baker, P.J., Stuitje, A.R., Slabas, A.R., Rice, D.W., Rafferty, J.B. (1999). Molecular basis of triclosan activity. Nature, 398: 383-384.

Levy, S. B. (2002). Active efflux, a common mechanism for biocide and antibiotic resistance. Journal of Applied Microbiology (Suppl.) 92:65s-71s.

Levy, S.B. (2001).Antibacterial household products: cause for concern.Emerging Infectious Diseases, 7(3):512-5.

Lewis, K., Ausubel, F.M. (2006). Prospects for plant-derived antibacterials.Nature Biotechnology, 24(12): 1504-1507.

Li, X., Nikaido, H. (2009). Efflux-Mediated Drug Resistance in Bacteria: an Update. Drugs, 69(12):1555-1623.

Liippo, J., Kousa, P., Lammintausta, K. (2011). The relevance of chlorhexidine contact allergy.Contact dermatitis,64(4): 229-234.

Linares, J.F., López, J.A., Camafeita, E., Albar, J.P., Rojo, F., Martínez, J.L. (2005). Overexpression of the multidrug efflux pumps MexCD-OprJ and MexEF-OprN is associated with a reduction of type III secretion in Pseudomonas aeruginosa.Journal of bacteriology,187(4): 1384-1391.

Lister, P. D., Wolter, D. J., Hanson, N. D. (2009). Antibacterial-resistant Pseudomonas aeruginosa: clinical impact and complex regulation of chromosomally encoded resistance mechanisms.Clinical Microbiology Reviews,22(4): 582-610

Macpherson, A.J., & Harris, N.L. (2004). Interactions between commensal intestinal bacteria and the immune system.Nature Reviews Immunology,4(6): 478-485.

Mahara, B., van Halteren, J., Verzijl, J.M., Wintermans, R.G., Buiting, A.G. (2002). Decolonization of methicillin-resistant Staphylococcus aureus using oral vancomycin and topical mupirocin.Clinical Microbiology and Infection, 8:671-675.

Maillard, J. Y. (2002). Bacterial target sites for biocide action.Journal of applied microbiology, 92(s1):16S-27S.

Martin, R.G., Bartlett, E.S., Rosner, J.L., Wall, M. E. (2008). Activation of the Escherichia coli marA/soxS/rob Regulon in Response to Transcriptional Activator Concentration.Journal of Molecular Biology, 380(2): 278-284.

McBain, A.J., Ledder, R.G., Sreenivasan, P., Gilbert, P.(2004). Selection for high-level resistance by chronic triclosan exposure is not universal.Journal of Antimicrobial Chemotherapy,53(5): 772-777.

McBain, A.J., Sufyaz, N., Rickard, A.H. (2012). Biofilm Recalcitrance: Theories and Mechanisms. Russell, Hugo and Ayliffe's Principles and Practice of Disinfection, Preservation and Sterilization, 87.

McDonnell, G., Pretzer, D. (1998). Action and targets of triclosan. American Society for Microbiology News, 64:670-671.

McMahon, M. A. S., Tunney, M. M., Moore, J. E., Blair, I. S., Gilpin, D. F., & McDowell, D. A. (2008). Changes in antibiotic susceptibility in staphylococci habituated to sub-lethal concentrations of tea tree oil (Melaleuca alternifolia).Letters in applied microbiology,47(4): 263-268.

McMurry, L. M., Levy S.B. (1998). Triclosan blocks lipid synthesis. Nature 394:621-622

McMurry, L.M., Oethinger, M., Levy, S.B. (1998).Triclosan targets lipid synthesis.Nature,394:531-32.

Meyer, B. (2006). Does microbial resistance to biocides create a hazard to food hygiene? International journal of food microbiology, 112(3): 275-279.

Miller, T.R., Heidler, J., Chillrud, S.N., DeLaquil, A., Ritchie, J.C., Mihalic, J.N., Halden, R.U. (2008). *Fate of triclosan and evidence for reductive dechlorination of triclocarban in estuarine sediments.Environmental science & technology, 42(12):4570-4576.*

Moore, L. E., Ledder, R. G., Gilbert, P., & McBain, A. J. (2008). *In vitro study of the effect of cationic biocides on bacterial population dynamics and susceptibility.Applied and environmental microbiology,74(15): 4825-4834.*

Moran, G.J., Krishnadasan, A., Gorwitz, R.J. (2006).*Methicillin-resistant S. aureus infection among patients in the emergency department. New England Journal of Medicine, 193(2):172-179.*

Moss, T., Howes, D., Williams, F.M. (2000).*Percutaneous penetration and dermal metabolism of triclosan (2, 4, 4'-trichloro-2'-hydroxydiphenyl ether). Food and Chemical Toxicology, 38(4): 361-370.*

Mozaffarian, D., & Rimm, E. B. (2006). *Fish intake, contaminants, and human health.JAMA: the journal of the American Medical Association,296(15):1885-1899.*

Murtough, S., Hiom, S.J., Palmer, M., Russell, A.D. (2000).*A survey of disinfectant use in hospital pharmacy aseptic preparation areas. Pharmaceutical Journal, 264:446–448*

Murugesan, K., Chang, Y.Y., Kim, Y.M., Jeon, J.R., Kim, E.J., Chang, Y.S. (2010). *Enhanced transformation of triclosan by laccase in the presence of redox mediators. Water research, 44(1): 298-308.*

Mwambete, K.D., Lyombe, F. (2011).*Antimicrobial Activity of Medicated Soaps commonly used by Dar es Salaam Residents in Tanzania. Indian Journal of Pharmaceutical Sciences, 73:92-98.*

Navarro Llorens, J.M., Tormo, A., Martínez-García, E. (2010). *Stationary phase in gram-negative bacteria.Federation of European Microbiologists-Microbiology Reviews, 34(4):476-495.*

Nester, M.T., Anderson, D.G., Roberts, Jr C.E., Pearsall, N.N. and Nester, M.T. Microbiology-A human perspective. Host-microorganism interactions. 3rd ed. Madrid: McGraw Hill; 2002.p451-72.

Nett, J.E., Guite, K.M., Ringeisen, A., Holoyda, K.A., Andes, D.R. (2008). *Reduced biocide susceptibility in Candida albicans biofilms. Antimicrobial agents and chemotherapy, 52(9): 3411-3413.*

Neumanna, N. J., Hölzleb, E., Plewigc, G., Schwarzd, T., Panizzone, R. G., Breitf, R., Lehmanna, P. (2000). *Photopatch testing: the 12-year experience of the German, Austrian, and Swiss photopatch test group.Journal of the American Academy of Dermatology,42(2): 183-192.*

Nguyen, D., Joshi-Datar, A., Lepine, F., Bauerle, E., Olakanmi, O., Beer, K., Singh, P.K. (2011). *Active starvation responses mediate antibiotic tolerance in biofilms and nutrient-limited bacteria.Science,334(6058): 982-986.*

Nishihara, T., Okamoto, T., Nishiyama, N. (2000). *Biodegradation of didecyldimethyl ammonium chloride by a strain of Pseudomonas fluorescens TN4 isolated from activated sludge. Journal of Applied Microbiology, 88:641–647*

Ogunshe, A. A.O., Omotoso, A.O., Akindele, T.M. (2011). *Soaps and disinfectants/germicides as adjunct antimycotic cleaning –agents in cases of vulvovigina candidiasis. Advances in Biological Research, 5(6): 282-290.*

Ortega Morente, E., Fernández-Fuentes, M. A., Grande Burgos, M. J., Abriouel, H., Pérez Pulido, R., Gálvez, A. (2013). *Biocide tolerance in bacteria. International Journal of Food Microbiology, 162(1):13-25.*

Oyelakin, O., Saidykhan, J., Secka, P., Adjivon, A. Acquaye, H.B. (2010).*Assessment of level of mercury present in soaps by the use of cold vapour atomic fluorescence spectrometric analysis-A Gambian case study.Ethiopian Journal of Environmental Studies and Management, 3(1): 8-12.*

Pagedar, A., Singh, J., Batish, V.K. (2011). *Efflux mediated adaptive and cross resistance to ciprofloxacin and benzalkonium chloride in Pseudomonas aeruginosa of dairy origin. Journal of Basic Microbiology, 51(3): 289-295.*

Paulson, D.S. (2003). *Handbook of topical antimicrobial: industry applications in consumers' products and pharmaceuticals. New York: Marcel Dekker, Inc. USA.*

Percival, S.L., Bowler, P.G., & Russell, D. (2005). *Bacterial resistance to silver in wound care.Journal of hospital infection,60(1), 1-7.*

Perencevich, E.N., Wong, M.T., Harris, A.D. (2002). National and regional assessment of the antibacterial soap market: A step toward determining the impact of prevalent antibacterial soaps. American Journal of Infection Control, 29(5): 281-283.

Perlstein, E. O., Ruderfer, D. M., Roberts, D. C., Schreiber, S. L., & Kruglyak, L. (2007). Genetic basis of individual differences in the response to small-molecule drugs in yeast.Nature genetics, 39(4):496-502.

Perron, K., Caille, O., Rossier, C., van Delden, C., Dumas, J. L., Köhler, T. (2004). CzcR-CzcS, a two-component system involved in heavy metal and carbapenem resistance in Pseudomonas aeruginosa.Journal of Biological Chemistry,279(10): 8761-8768.

Piddock L.J.V. (2006). Multidrug-resistance efflux pumps -not just for resistance. .Nature Reviews, 4: 626-636.

Pirrone, P., Costa, J.M., Pacyna, Ferrara, R. (2001). Mercury emissions to the atmosphere from natural and anthropogenic sources in the Mediterranean region. Atmospheric Environment, 35: 2997–3006.

Poole, K. (2002). Mechanisms of bacterial biocide and antibiotic resistance.Journal of Applied Microbiology, 92:55S-64S.

Poole, K. (2005). Efflux-mediated antimicrobial resistance.Journal of Antimicrobial Chemotherapy, 56(1): 20-51.

Poole, K. (2007). Efflux pumps as antimicrobial resistance mechanisms. Annals of medicine, 39(3):162-176.

Prescott, M.L., Harley, J.P., Klein, D.A. Microbiology, 6thed. New York: The McGraw Hill Companies. 2005, 35:p780-798.

Price, C.T., Singh, V.K., Jayaswal, R.K., Wilkinson, B.J., Gustafson, J.E. (2002). Pine oil cleaner-resistant Staphylococcus aureus: reduced susceptibility to vancomycin and oxacillin and involvement of SigB. Applied and Environmental Microbiology, 68(11):5417-5421.

Reiss, R., Lewis, G., Griffin, J. (2009). An ecological risk assessment for triclosan in the terrestrial environment.Environmental Toxicology and Chemistry,28(7): 1546-1556.

Richter, S.S., Galask, R.P., Messer, S.A., Hollis, R.J., Diekema, D.J., Pfaller, M.A. (2005). Antifungal susceptibilities of Candida species causing vulvovaginitis and epidemiology of recurrent cases.Journal of clinical microbiology, 43(5): 2155-2162.

Rolain, J.M., Parola, P.,Cornaglia,G. (2010). New Delhi metallo-beta-lactamase (NDM-1): towards a new pandemia?Clinical Microbiology and Infection,16(12):1699-1701.

Rosner, J.L., Martin, R.G. (2009). An excretory function for the Escherichia coli outer membrane pore TolC: upregulation of marA and soxS transcription and Rob activity due to metabolites accumulated in tolC mutants. Journal of bacteriology, 191(16):5283-5292.

Rugh, C. L., Wilde, H. D., Stack, N. M., Thompson, D. M., Summers, A. O., Meagher, R. B. (1996). Mercuric ion reduction and resistance in transgenic Arabidopsis thaliana plants expressing a modified bacterial merA gene.Proceedings of the National Academy of Sciences,93(8): 3182-3187.

Russell, A.D. (1998). Mechanisms of bacterial resistance to antibiotics and biocides.Progress in Medicinal Chemistry, 35:134–197.

Russell, A.D. (2003). Biocide use and antibiotic resistance: the relevance of laboratory findings to clinical and environmental situations.The Lancet infectious diseases,3(12): 794-803.

Russell, A.D. (2004). Whither triclosan? Journal of Antimicrobial Chemotherapy, 53(5): 693-695.

Russell, A.D., McDonnell, G. (2000). Concentration: a major factor in studying biocidal action. Journal of Hospital Infections, 44:1-3.

Seltenrich, N. (2013).Environmental Exposures in the Context of Child Care.Environmental health perspectives,121(5): 160.

Sharma, B.K. (2006). Industrial Chemistry, 5th Edition.pp. 1243-1245, 1249.

Sharma, R., Sharma, C., Kapoor, B. (2005). Antibacterial resistance: current problems and possible solutions. Indian journal of medical sciences, 59(3):120.

Shatalin, K., Shatalina, E., Mironov, A., Nudler, E. (2011). H$_2$S: a universal defense against antibiotics in bacteria. Science, 334(6058):986-990.

Silbergeld, E. K., Graham, J., Price, L. B. (2008). Industrial food animal production, antimicrobial resistance, and human health.Annu. Rev. Public Health,29:151-169.

Skalet, A. H., Cevallos, V., Ayele, B., Gebre, T., Zhou, Z., Jorgensen, J. H., Keenan, J. D. (2010). Antibiotic selection pressure and macrolide resistance in nasopharyngeal Streptococcus pneumoniae: a cluster-randomized clinical trial.PLoS medicine,7(12), e1000377.

Smith, K., Gemmell, C.G., Hunter, I. (2008). The association between biocide tolerances and the presence or absence of qac genes among hospital-acquired and community-acquired MRSA isolates. Journal of antimicrobial chemotherapy, 61(1): 78-84.

Sulavik, M.C., Gambino, L.F., Miller P.F. (1995). The MarR repressor of the multiple antibiotic resistance (mar) operons in Escherichia coli: pro-totypic member of a family of bacterial regulatory proteins involved in sensing phenolic compounds. Molecular Medicine, 1:436-446.

Tegos, G. P., Haynes, M., Strouse, J. J., Khan, M. T., Bologa, C. G., Oprea, T. I., & Sklar, L. A. (2013).Current Pharmaceutical Design,17, 1291–1302.

Tsai, C. H., Lin, P. H., Waidyanatha, S., Rappaport, S. M. (2001). Characterization of metabolic activation of pentachlorophenol to quinones and semiquinones in rodent liver.Chemico-biological interactions,134(1): 55-71.

Tumah, H.N. (2009). Bacterial biocide resistance.Journal of Chemotherapy, 21(1):5-15.

Tunger, O., Karakaya, Y., Cetin, C. B., Dinc, G., Borand, H. (2009).Rational antibiotic use.The Journal of Infection in Developing Countries,3(02): 088-093.

Turner, N. A., A. D. Russell, J. R. Furr, Lloyd, D. (2000). Emergence of resistance to biocides during differentiation of Acanthamoeba castellanii. Journal of Antimicrobial and Chemotherapy, 46:27-34

Udoji, F., Martin, T., Etherton, R., Whalen, M.M. (2010).Immunosuppressive effects of Triclosan, nonylphenol, and DDT on human natural killer cells in vitrol. Journal of Immunotoxicology, 7(3): 205-212.

Veldhoen, N., Skirrow, R.C., Osahoff, H., Wigmore, H., Clapson, D.J., Gunderson, M.P., Van, A.G., Helbing, C.C. (2006).The bacterial agent Triclosan modulate thyroid hormone-associate gene expression and disrupts postembryonic anuran development. Aquatic toxicology, 80(3): 217-227.

Walsh, C. (2000). Molecular mechanisms that confer antibacterial drug resistance.Nature,406(6797): 775-781.

Wang, J. (2013).Transmembrane Helix-Helix Interactions in a Bacterial Small Multidrug Transport Protein(Doctoral dissertation).

White, D.G., McDermott, P.F. (2001). Biocides, drug resistance and microbial evolution. Current Opinion on Microbiology, 4 (1):313–317.

Whyte, F.W., Allison, D.G., Jones, M.V., Gilbert, P. (2001). Abstract-101st Annual Meeting on American Society of Microbiology, Abstr. A99) and weak acids like salicylate.

Widmer, A. F., Wiestner, A., Frei, R., Zimmerli, W. (1991). Killing of non-growing and adherent Escherichia coli determines drug efficacy in de-vice-related infections. Antimicrobial Agents and Chemotherapy, 35:714-746.

Wiener, J. G., & Spry, D. J. (1996). Toxicological significance of mercury in freshwater fish. Environmental contaminants in wildlife: Interpreting tissue concentrations, 297-339.

Wilkinson, D. E., Gilbert, P. (1987).Permeation of the gram-negative cell envelope by some polymeric biguanides. Journal of Applied Bacteriology, 63:25

Williams, T.M. (2006). The mechanism of action of isothiazolone biocide.Corrosion, 2006.

Wilson, B.A., Smith, V.H., deNoyelles, Jr. F., Larive, C.K. (2003). *Effects of three pharmaceuticals and personal care products on natural freshwater algal assemblage. Environmental Science and Technology, 37(9):162A-164A.*

Wojcik, D.P., Godfrey, M.E., Christie, D., Haley, B.E. (2006). *Mercury toxicity presenting as chronic fatigue, memory impairment, and depression: Diagnosis, treatment, susceptibility, and outcomes in a New Zealand practice setting (1994-2006). 2006. Neuroendocrinology Letters. 27(4): 415-423.*

Wong, P.W., Pessah, I.N. (1996). *Ortho-substituted polychlorinated biphenyls alter calcium regulation by a ryanodine receptor-mediated mechanism: structural specificity toward skeletal-and cardiac-type microsomal calcium release channels.Molecular Pharmacology,49(4):740-751.*

Woods, E. J., Cochrane, C. A., & Percival, S. L. (2009). *Prevalence of silver resistance genes in bacteria isolated from human and horse wounds.Veterinary microbiology,138(3): 325-329.*

Wright, G.D. (2007). *The antibiotic resistome: the nexus of chemical and genetic diversity.Nature Reviews Microbiology,5(3): 175-186.*

Wu, J., Xie, J. (2009). *Magic spot:(p) ppGpp.Journal of cellular physiology,220(2): 297-302.*

Ying, G.G., Yu, X.Y., Kookana, R.S. (2007). *Biological degradation of triclocarban and triclosan in a soil under aerobic and anaerobic conditions and comparison with environmental fate modeling.Environmental Pollution, 150(3):300-305.*

Zalups, R.K. (2000). *Molecular Interactions with Mercury in the Kidney.Pharmacological Reviews, 52 (1):113-144.*

Zaragoza, M., Salles, M., Gomez, J., Bayas,J.M., Trilla, A.(1999). *Handwashing with soap or alcoholic solutions.A randomized clinical trial of its effectiveness. American Journal of Infections Control, 27(3):258-261.*

Zhou, Z. X., Wei, D. F., Guan, Y., Zheng, A. N., Zhong, J. J. (2010). *Damage of Escherichia coli membrane by bactericidal agent polyhexamethylene guanidine hydrochloride: micrographic evidences. Journal of applied Microbiology,108(3): 898-907.*

Melanoma and Immunosuppression: A Systematic Review

A. Bianca Stashak
Arizona College of Osteopathic Medicine
Midwestern University, Glendale, USA

Jerry D. Brewer
Division of Dermatologic Surgery, Department of Dermatology
Mayo Clinic/Mayo Clinic College of Medicine, Rochester, USA

1   Introduction

One of the deadliest forms of skin cancer, melanoma incidence has increased over the past three decades (Gray-Schopfer *et al.*, 2007) with metastatic melanoma carrying a 5 year survival rate of about 5% (Balch *et al.*, 2009; Rosenberg *et al.*, 2011). In the United States, melanoma incidence rates in 2010 were 27.4 and 16.7 per 100,000 for males and females, respectively (Ji *et al.*, 2013). Globally, the incidence of melanoma in Caucasians appears to increase with relative proximity to the equator, (de Vries and Coebergh, 2004; Little and Eide, 2012) with Australia exhibiting the greatest incidence worldwide (Little and Eide, 2012). This review focuses on the mechanisms by which melanoma induces immunosuppression, the behavior of melanoma in the setting of immunosuppression, and possible therapeutic targets in the treatment of malignant melanoma.

2   Melanoma-Induced Immunosuppression: 5 General Mechanisms

There are essentially five mechanisms by which melanoma appear to manipulate the host immune system. Often referenced in the literature as the "melanoma microenvironment," this malignancy-favorable medium develops due to induction of tolerance, mutations, secretion of immunosuppressive agents, surface antigen down-regulation and altered costimulatory function (McCarter *et al.*, 2007). The ability of melanoma to dampen immune function creates a unique barrier to the development of reliable therapies that target immune modulation.

2.1   Induction of Immune Tolerance

The capacity of melanoma cells to induce immune tolerance and immunosuppression is central to this malignancy's ability to thrive and progress within its host. Melanoma cells cause immunosuppression via multiple different mechanisms, including increased expression of genes that promote regulatory T cell function, inhibition of cytotoxic T lymphocyte (CTL) activity against malignant cells and altered secretion of cytokines (McCarter *et al.*, 2007). Under normal circumstances, T regulatory cells play a critical role in the suppression of autoimmune reactions by inducing tolerance of self-antigens. Without T regulatory cell activity, autoimmune disease would be rampant. However, in excessive numbers, these cells dampen the antitumor immune response, contributing to the progression of melanoma and other malignancies (Baumgartner *et al.*, 2007). In their analysis of cell populations in healthy patients versus patients with stage I and stage IV melanoma, McCarter *et al.* (2007) demonstrated that the number of T regulatory cells was greater in the latter two groups, and that the CD4+CD25+ cell frequency was found to be twice as high in metastatic melanoma than in either the healthy subjects or the subjects with stage I melanoma. These findings reinforce the notion that forced immune tolerance is an important mechanism in establishing and maintaining the melanoma microenvironment.

Although clearly more abundant in the setting of melanoma, the precise role of T regulatory cells in promoting a pro-malignant environment is not entirely clear. However, a transcription factor called FOXP3 that is found in greater numbers in the setting of melanoma, is expressed most abundantly by CD4+CD25+ cells (a phenotype of T regulatory cells) (Baumgartner *et al.*, 2007). Multiple studies have shown that greater expression of this transcription factor is correlated with various different malignancies, including melanoma. Not only does this transcription factor favor melanoma progression; it also has implications for the efficacy of melanoma therapy. Melanoma patients exhibiting greater expression of

CD4+CD25+FOXP3+ cells are particularly resistant to treatment with immunologic therapies (Baumgartner *et al.*, 2007; Polak *et al.*, 2007; Viguier *et al.*, 2004).

At this time, the mechanism by which melanoma induces T regulatory cell activity has not yet been explained. It is important to note that the finding of elevated numbers of T regulatory cells and FOXP3 expression is not exclusive to melanoma, or even to malignancy for that matter, as these cell populations are also upregulated in the setting of various inflammatory and disease states (Baumgartner *et al.*, 2007; Levings *et al.*, 2006).

The activity of dendritic cells (DCs), whose roles include the T cell activation and promotion of T lymphocyte tolerance of self-antigens, is also important in the understanding of melanoma. Studies of murine models have shown that samples exhibiting greater numbers of DCs also have greater numbers of T regulatory cells (Choi *et al.*, 2012). Although an underlying relationship between DC populations and melanoma progression is likely, investigators at this point have failed to demonstrate a direct influence of melanoma on DC induction and activity (Baumgartner *et al.*, 2012).

2.2   Mutations

An association between malignancy and production of myeloid derived suppressor cells (MDSCs) has also been identified. MDSCs, which stimulate T regulatory cell activity *in vivo* and antagonize cytotoxic T cell activity *in vitro* accumulate under the influence of factors produced by the tumor. The action of MDSCs results in depression of innate and adaptive immunity and diminished antitumor immunogenicity (Lindenberg *et al.*, 2013). The FDA-approved BRAF inhibitor, vemurafenib, has recently been shown to exhibit anti-MDSC tendencies, indicating a possible dual mechanism of action for this therapy in the treatment of melanoma in patients with the BRAF^{V600E} mutation (Schilling *et al.*, 2013). Furthermore, in their analysis of human metastatic melanoma samples treated with vemurafenib, Khalili *et al.* (2012) demonstrated that BRAF inhibition can be used to retransform the melanoma microenvironment via the suppression of IL-1 cytokine expression. The role of BRAF mutations in melanoma and resistance to treatment is further discussed later in this chapter.

2.3   Secretion of Immunosuppressive Agents

The signaling factors most implicated in clinical research on melanoma and immunosuppression include IL-10, TGF-β and indoleamine 2,3 dioxygenase. Previous studies have demonstrated that IL-10 has a suppressive effect on both DCs and T lymphocytes (Lindenberg *et al.*, 2013). During their laboratory investigation of Wnt/β-catenin signaling in melanoma cells, Yaguchi *et al.* found that with increasing expression of IL-10 in melanoma cells, DCs' activity was suppressed via β-catenin expression by malignant cells. Furthermore, as cutaneous melanoma evolves from a radial to vertical growth phase, IL-10 expression is found to be greater as well (Itakura *et al.*, 2011).

A specific regulator of cytokine signaling, Socs-1 (suppressor of cytokine signaling-1), plays an important role in the inhibition of cytokines IL-10 and TGF-β (Fu *et al.*, 2009; Hong *et al.*, 2009) and has been shown to augment the immunogenicity of DCs. In their investigation of a possible therapeutic target in DC immune function, Song *et al.* (2012) used murine subjects injected with Socs-1 treated B-16 melanoma cells. The investigators found that Socs-1 silenced samples demonstrated improved antigen presentation by DCs.

An enzyme implicated in melanoma-induced immunosuppression is indoleamine 2,3 dioxygenase (IDO). In a study of CD4+ cells and IDO in patients with melanoma, breast cancer, or renal cell carcinoma, Danish investigators found that melanoma-expressed IDO inhibits antitumor activity by catalyzing the conversion of tryptophan to toxic metabolites that in turn suppress T cell effector function and promote conversion of naïve T cells to T regulatory cells (Munir *et al.*, 2012). In contrast, the presence of IDO-reactive CD8+ T cells, which target tumor cells and DCs expressing IDO, is associated with stronger anti-tumor activity (Munir *et al.*, 2012). In addition, melanoma cells expressing IDO portend a worse prognosis (Curti *et al.*, 2009; Munn *et al.*, 2004). This improved understanding of IDO-induced immunosuppression may provide a promising therapeutic target in the treatment of melanoma as well as other malignancies.

2.4   Antigen Down-Regulation

Evasion of host immune system surveillance is another important mechanism of melanoma-induced immunosuppression. Melanoma cells are capable of "masking" themselves from the immune system by down-regulating surface major histocompatibility complex class I (MHC I) tumor cell antigens. Integral to the preparation of antigenic peptides for display on these MHC I molecules are the transporter-associated antigen processing (TAP) heterodimers. A decrease in the activity of both TAP1 and TAP2 has been observed in the setting of melanoma (Kirkwood *et al.*, 2008; Zhang *et al.*, 2007). The result is a diminished host immune response to melanoma antigens. In fact, in a comparison of TAP1 and TAP2 expression in malignant melanoma (MM), Tao *et al.* (2008) found that malignancies with the lowest frequency of TAP1 and TAP2 exhibited more invasive growth, greater Clark level and more tumor infiltrating lymphocytes (TILs).

2.5   Altered Co-Stimulatory Function

A co-inhibitory molecule called B7-H1 (also known as PD-L1), has recently earned appreciation for its role in immunosuppression in the setting of melanoma. Under normal circumstances, the programmed death-1 receptor (PD-1) is activated by B7-H1 when CD4+ and CD8+ cells are chronically stimulated by T lymphocytes. By inhibiting T cell receptor (TCR) production and cytokine secretion, B7-H1 impairs antitumor immune function through induction of T cell anergy and apoptosis (Ahmadzadeh *et al.*, 2009; Dong *et al.*, 2002; Taube *et al.*, 2012). Although the exact mechanism by which melanoma manipulates this process has not yet been elucidated, a definite correlation between this malignancy and B7-H1/PD-1 activity exists. Interestingly, greater quantities of PD-1 have not only been observed in melanoma, but also in cases of heightened viral load in HIV and hepatitis C infections (Taube *et al.*, 2012). Conversely, PD-1 deficient mice have been found to exhibit a greater frequency of autoimmune diseases (Postow *et al.*, 2012). A number of antibodies to PD-1 (Postow *et al.*, 2012) are currently undergoing clinical testing for the treatment of melanoma and are discussed later in this review.

The inhibition of natural killer (NK) cells' stimulation and cytolytic activity is yet another mechanism through which melanoma cells evade immunosurveillance. These effects are mediated by the malignant cells' disruption of NK cell ligands such as NKG2D ligand, Fas ligand and APO2 ligand/tumor necrosis factor-related apoptosis-associated ligand. In fact, IDO, the melanoma-expressed enzyme found to antagonize T cell effector function, has also been identified as an important player in this process of NK cell inhibition in melanoma pathogenesis (Martínez-Lorenzo *et al.*, 2004; Pietra *et al.*, 2012).

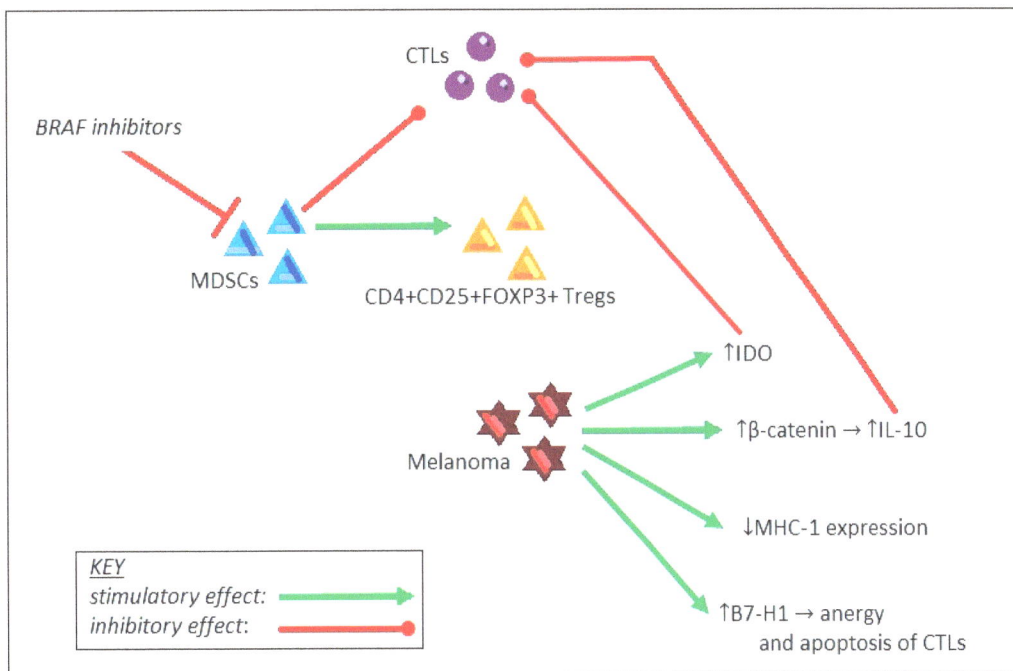

Figure 1: Mechanisms of Melanoma-Induced Immunosuppression. Illustration of immunosuppression in the melanoma microenvironment. Melanoma induces suppression of the human immune system through multiple different mechanisms, including induction of tolerance, mutations, secretion of immunosuppressive agents, surface antigen down-regulation and altered costimulatory function (Ahmadzadeh *et al*., 2009; Baumgartner *et al*., 2007; Baumgartner *et al*., 2012; Choi *et al*., 2012; Curti *et al*., 2009; Dong *et al*., 2002; Fu *et al*., 2009; Hong *et al*., 2009; Itakura *et al*., 2011; Khalili *et al*., 2012; Kirkwood *et al*., 2008; Levings *et al*., 2006; Lindenberg *et al*., 2013; Martínez-Lorenzo *et al*., 2004; McCarter *et al*., 2007; Munir *et al*., 2012; Munn *et al*., 2004; Pietra *et al*., 2012; Polak *et al*., 2007; Postow *et al*., 2012; Schilling *et al*., 2013; Song *et al*., 2012; Tao *et al*., 2008; Taube *et al*., 2012; Viguier *et al*., 2004; Zhang *et al*., 2007).

3   HLA and Melanoma Cell Antigenicity

Supporting the understanding of melanoma as a highly immunogenic malignancy is the research on peptide prediction algorithms and HLA binding by Bredenbeck *et al*. (2005) and Jarmalavicius *et al*. (2012). Cancer immunogenicity is in part determined by the interactions of T cells with HLA-bound peptides originating from malignant cells (Jarmalavicius *et al*., 2012). Although peptide prediction algorithms that determine the ability of peptides to bind HLA class 1 molecules have elucidated some tumor-associated epitopes, they sometimes fall short (Bredenbeck *et al*., 2005). Bredenbeck *at al.* sought to identify tumor antigens exhibiting poor HLA-binding capacity that would otherwise have been neglected by currently available peptide prediction algorithms. They suggested that the obstacles to the identification of tumor associated peptides with established algorithms are the assumption that such peptides are universally strong HLA-binders, as well as the focus on individual amino acids rather than on the sequences that they compose (Bredenbeck *et al*., 2005). Through their work with multiple melanoma cell lines, Bredenbeck *at al.* found that, although a number of the identified epitopes were suboptimal HLA-binders, they were equally efficient stimulators of T cells from both healthy donors and from cancer patients (Bredenbeck *et al.*, 2005). The investigators anticipate that these findings will have significant implications for the development of antitumor vaccines (Bredenbeck *et al.*, 2005).

Antigenic heterogeneity and cross-immunogenicity of tumor cells are important concepts for anti-melanoma therapy. By assessing the antigenicity of metastatic tumor cells extracted from 4 different human melanoma cell lines, Jarmalavicius *et al.* (2012) found that approximately only 10% of the HLA-bound peptides were shared across the strains, indicating a high degree of heterogeneity between the 4 cell lines extracted from four unrelated patients. Furthermore, the unique HLA sequences of each of the lines was found to be immunogenic not only for those peripheral blood mononuclear cells (PBMCs) of the patients from whom the samples originated, but also when introduced to healthy donor PBMCs (Jarmalavicius *et al.*, 2012). Perhaps not surprisingly, 43% of the HLA ligands identified had originated from nuclear proteins, where the processes of DNA replication, gene regulation, cell cycle control and tumor suppression occur (Jarmalavicius *et al.*, 2012). The authors expect that the HLA and origin of their associated proteins may guide future efforts in the modifications of HLA peptide prediction algorithms.

4   Melanoma and Solid Organ Transplantation

There are three different scenarios in which melanoma may emerge after organ transplantation. Subsequent to transplantation, a patient may develop melanoma as a consequence of immunosuppressive agents for the prevention of organ rejection, (Penn, 2000) may acquire malignant cells directly via donor tissue, or may experience recurrence of formerly dormant melanoma (Dreno, 2003).

4.1   Post-Transplantation De Novo Melanoma

Post-transplantation skin cancer is a very common phenomenon and follows a more aggressive course than in non-transplant patients (Kovach and Stasko, 2009). Compared to melanoma, the development of non-melanoma skin cancer (NMSC) in organ transplant recipients (OTRs) is difficult to refute, given the abundance of evidence in support of this relationship (Fekecs *et al.*, 2010; Lindelöf *et al.*, 2000; Stockfleth *et al.*, 2002; Wisgerhof *et al.*, 2010; Zavos *et al.*, 2011). The task of establishing a similar connection between organ transplantation and de novo melanoma has proven more challenging. From their analysis of a population-based cohort of 5,356 OTRs, Lindelöf *et al.* (2000) concluded that, while there was a greatly increased risk of NMSC in this population, there was no significant evidence of increased risk of melanoma. In contrast, a review of Medicare billing claims for de novo cancer in post-renal transplant recipients (RTRs) demonstrated that the incidence of melanoma in RTRs was approximately 5-fold higher than in the general population. However, the authors concede that given the use of Medicare claims in gathering information, a selection bias was inherently present (Kasiske et al., 2004). A more recent analysis supports the assertion that melanoma does indeed develop more frequently in OTRs: Chatrath and associates determined a standardized incidence ratio (SIR) of 5.8 for melanoma post-liver transplant (95% CI: 4.7 to 7.0) (Chatrath *et al.*, 2013).

4.2   Melanoma Transmitted from Donor Organs

The transmission rate of melanoma from graft to recipient is very low, particularly compared to the proportion of patients on immunosuppressive therapy who develop de novo skin cancer (Buell *et al.*, 2004).

Still, evidence for this phenomenon is available, mostly in individual case studies where PCR has been employed to prove donor origin of malignancy (Bilal *et al.*, 2013; Chen *et al.*, 2012). Further complicating the picture is the fact that melanoma can remain dormant for decades, possibly only being identified after death of the donor. In fact, postmortem investigation of cause of death of organ donors who were later determined to have transmitted melanoma, reveals that several had suffered cerebral hemorrhages, and that these were retrospectively attributed to occult melanoma metastases (Zwald *et al.*, 2010). In practice, it is prudent to carefully consider each patient's case independently, as the risk of not receiving a life-saving organ transplant may outweigh the future risk of donor-derived skin cancer.

4.3   Melanoma Recurrence Post-Transplantation

Data on the recurrence of melanoma post-transplantation is limited, with most research yielding little evidence for increased risk of melanoma recurrence in the OTR population. In a review of the Cincinnati Transplant Tumor Registry (CTTR) from 1968 to 1995, Penn observed that 19% of the 31 patients who had melanoma before receiving donor organs developed recurrences after transplantation (Penn, 1996 (Penn, 1996) as cited in Colegio *et al.* (2009). Of note, all 6 of these patients were RTRs. However, Breslow depth was not disclosed for any of these 6 patients, making interpretation of these findings difficult. Certainly, not all melanoma is created equal, as Breslow depth and time elapsed from original melanoma diagnosis to transplantation appear to be critical criteria in the evaluation of melanoma recurrence risk in the OTR population (Colegio *et al.*, 2009). Melanoma staging factors also considered for OTRs are the presence of ulceration, lactate dehydrogenase level and mitotic rate (Balch *et al.*, 2009). Colegio *et al.* (2009) also address the utility of sentinel lymph node biopsy to determine relative risk of melanoma recurrence after transplant. A sentinel lymph node biopsy negative for micrometastases coupled with a period of at least 2 years between melanoma diagnosis and transplant portends a better prognosis. The authors conclude that the risk of recurrence as estimated by these criteria ought to be carefully weighed against the implications of withholding transplantation.

4.4   Prognosis of Malignant Melanoma in the Setting of Organ Transplantation

Multiple studies have demonstrated a more aggressive course for malignant melanoma in OTRs than is expected for the general population. In the same analysis of the CTTR, Penn observed more rapid tumor growth and development of metastases due to MM in OTRs, with median survival of 10.5 months after surgery (Penn, 1996). In their comparison of 95 patients from SCOPE (Skin Care in Organ Transplant Patients, Europe) versus age, sex, tumor thickness and ulceration-status matched controls (Matin *et al.*, 2008) from AJCC (American Joint Committee on Cancer), Matin *et al.* (2008) demonstrated worse prognosis in the OTR group at melanoma stages T3 and T4, but no significant reduction in survival rates for T1 and T2. A more recent Mayo Clinic retrospective review of 638 patients with melanoma diagnosed post-transplant supports this trend: compared to expected survival according to the SEER (Surveillance, Epidemiology and End Results) Program, melanoma cause specific survival was significantly lower among immunosuppressed OTRs for lesions with Breslow thickness of 1.51 to 3.00 mm and Clark level III or IV. A similar trend was not observed in patients with more shallow Breslow measurements (≤ 1.50 mm), nor in Clark levels I and II, indicating that MM exhibits especially aggressive behavior in more advanced lesions in the setting of organ transplantation. However, overall survival rates were lower for the OTR group, regardless of lesion thickness (Brewer *et al.*, 2011).

5   Melanoma in Lymphoproliferative Disease

Similar to the iatrogenic immunosuppression for OTRs, the impediment of immune function inherent in lymphoproliferative diseases, combined with iatrogenic immunomodulation, increases patients' susceptibility to malignancies, including skin cancer. The most commonly addressed diseases in the literature are non-Hodgkin lymphoma (NHL) and chronic lymphocytic leukemia (CLL), a particular form of NHL. Several studies have highlighted this potential link between melanoma and non-cutaneous malignancies like lymphoma. A recent review of a melanoma registry in Rome revealed that 14.8% of patients with melanoma developed lymphoma, the majority of which (72.7%) were non-Hodgkin lymphoma (NHL) (Bottoni *et al.*, 2013).

5.1   Lymphoma and Melanoma: Molecular and Genetic Associations

Characterized by a monoclonal proliferation of B cells, CLL is associated with a greater risk of melanoma according to multiple studies. This augmented risk is attributed to a number of different mechanisms through which CLL causes immunosuppression. Through the down-regulation of CD154 (a CD40 ligand on T cells), malignant B cells interfere with T cell-APC interactions (Aslakson *et al.*, 1999, as cited in Brewer *at al.*) (Aslakson *et al.*, 1999; Brewer *et al.*, 2011; Cantwell *et al.*, 1997). Expressed on B cells and other potential APCs, the purpose of CD40 is to engage CD154 to induce costimulatory interactions between cells. Inhibition of CD154 expression by the B cells of CLL results in a failure to solicit antigen presentation by the malignant cells (Wierda *et al.*, 2000). As a risk factor for the development of melanoma, immune dysfunction resulting from lymphoproliferative disease results from suboptimal antigen presentation by monoclonal B cells, disruption of MHC I and II expression, altered expression of TCR variable genes and lower levels of immunoglobulins and complement (Kipps, 2000; Wierda *et al.*, 2000).

Childhood survivors of cancer are at increased risk of developing melanoma in adulthood. According to the Childhood Cancer Survivor Study (CCSS) composed of 14,358 patients, a 2.5-fold risk of melanoma was seen in patients diagnosed in childhood with various cancers, including soft tissue and bone sarcoma, leukemia and lymphoma (subsequent invasive melanoma SIR: 2.42, 95% CI 1.77-3.23; AER: 0.10, 95% CI 0.05-0.15) (Meadows *et al.*, 2009; Pappo *et al.*, 2013).

Overexpression of antiapoptotic proteins such as BCL-2, a proto-oncogene, inappropriately permits survival of cells that normally should be eliminated through programmed cell death. Consequently, overexpression of BCL-2 by malignant cells provides a survival advantage that is particularly apparent in melanoma and lymphoproliferative diseases (Anvekar *et al.*, 2011). In fact, 95% of CLL and 90% of melanoma exhibit BCL-2 overexpression (Mikhail *et al.*, 2005; Thomadaki and Scorilas, 2006). Also often disrupted in CLL is the chromosomal domain of TP53, the "guardian of the genome." In CLL, deletions of 17p, within which TP53 is located, are associated with a worse prognosis and greater resistance to treatment. Although TP53 is rarely mutated in melanoma, disruption of apoptotic pathways is often present. Researchers have recently identified a TP53 relative, TP63, that is often mutated in melanoma, contributing to apoptotic evasion by malignant cells (Matin *et al.*, 2013). Interestingly, p63 deficiency in mice results in immature, non-stratified skin without expression of differentiation markers as well as severe developmental anomalies of the limbs (Mills *et al.*, 1999).

Similar to the correlation between melanoma and lymphoproliferative diseases, breast cancer and melanoma appear to be related in the context of certain genetic predispositions. Mutations in CDKN2A are known to contribute to the development of melanoma, (Goldstein *et al.*, 2006; Hansson, 2010) while BRCA2 mutations are correlated with female breast cancer (Nasir *et al.*, 2009). Evidence suggests that a mutual relationship exists: patients with CDKN2A mutations are predisposed to developing breast cancer and those with BRCA2 mutations are at greater than average risk of developing melanoma (Goggins *et al.*, 2004). In a review of 1,884 patients from the SEER database, investigators found a statistically significant (p = 0.0002) elevated risk of cutaneous melanoma among survivors of female breast cancer treated with surgery and irradiation, and that survivors of melanoma were similarly more susceptible to developing breast cancer. A history of radiation for breast cancer likely also contributed to the elevated the risk of melanoma in this population, although the melanomas did not necessarily develop in the previously irradiated field (Galper *et al.*, 2002). Notwithstanding, these findings raise the question of a relationship between the pathogenesis of melanoma and breast cancer (Goggins *et al.*, 2004).

5.2   Lymphoma and Melanoma Epidemiology

First noted in 1973, the connection between lymphoma and melanoma has been a topic of considerable interest over the past three decades and yet, a distinct explanation for this correlation has not been described. However, it is clear that with melanoma, there is an increased risk of lymphoma, and vice versa. Studies demonstrate a greater melanoma risk in NHL patients ranging from 1.8 to 2.4 fold, (Adami *et al.*, 1995; Brennan *et al.*, 2005; Dong and Hemminki, 2001; Goggins *et al.*, 2001; Hisada *et al.*, 2001; McKenna *et al.*, 2003; Travis *et al.*, 1991; Travis *et al.*, 1992; Tsimberidou *et al.*, 2009) while others show an increased risk of NHL in melanoma patients ranging from 1.3 to 2.7,(Adami *et al.*, 1995; Brennan *et al.*, 2005; Crocetti and Carli, 2004; Goggins *et al.*, 2001; McKenna *et al.*, 2003; Riou *et al.*, 1995; Spanogle *et al.*, 2010) suggesting a mutual relationship between these two malignancies. In their analysis of 109,000 cases of NHL, Brennan *et al.* determined a SIR of 1.92 for melanoma as a second primary cancer developing within 10 years of the first primary NHL (Brennan *et al.*, 2005). In a retrospective review (1995 to 2009) of 52 patients with both CLL and melanoma who were treated at the Mofitt Cancer Center, subjects with melanoma were at greater risk of CLL compared to other malignancies. In the context of melanoma, CLL was 10-fold more common than colorectal cancer, 8-fold more common than prostate cancer and 4-fold more common than breast cancer (Farma *et al.*, 2013). A review of patients treated for CLL at MD Anderson also supports this correlation, demonstrating an 8% incidence of melanoma in this CLL population, with a ratio of observed to expected cases of 6.17 (Farma *et al.*, 2013; Tsimberidou *et al.*, 2009).

5.3   Clinical Course of Melanoma in Lymphoma Patients

Most research on the survival rates of patients with both melanoma and lymphoproliferative diseases are based on small sample populations. However, a recent relatively large SEER population-based study of 212,245 patients conducted by Brewer *et al.* demonstrated that the overall survival of patients with MM and a preceding history of either CLL or NHL was in fact worse than expected, as evidenced by standardized mortality ratios (SMR for CLL, 2.6; 95% CI 2.3 to 3.0; SMR for NHL 2.3; 95% CI, 2.1 to 2.6). Malignant melanoma cause-specific survival was also worse than expected for both CLL (SMR, 2.8; 95% CI, 2.2 to 3.4) and NHL (SMR, 1.9; 95% CI, 1.3 to 2.8) (Brewer *et al.*, 2012). This supports the earlier finding by Brewer *et al.* that patients with a diagnosis of CLL before the development of melanoma had worse overall survival (60.9%) compared to those whose melanoma preceded their CLL (96.2%) (Brewer *et al.*, 2010).

6   Melanoma and Iatrogenic Immunosuppression

The very medications used in the treatment of malignancy and prevention of organ rejection may have pro-malignant effects via their suppression of the immune system. The offenders most referenced in the literature include: cyclosporine A (CsA), tacrolimus, azathioprine, corticosteroids, methotrexate, myco-phenolate mofetil, 5-fluorouracil, the biologic response modifiers ("biologics") and various chemothera-pies (Kubica and Brewer, 2012). For example, cyclophosphamide has been employed as a tumor-suppressing agent because of its ability to reduce T regulatory cell numbers. However, recent evidence suggests that this medication also promotes the production of MDSCs, which in turn stimulate T regulato-ry cell production and suppress CTL activity (Becker and Schrama, 2013; Lindenberg *et al.*, 2013; Sevko *et al.*, 2013).

The use of azathioprine for immune system attenuation in OTRs has been correlated with the de-velopment of dysplastic keratosis, BCC and SCC. However, these findings appear to be attributable to mechanisms independent of the immunosuppressive action of this medication. Conjecture for this phe-nomenon addresses the UV-sensitizing effects of azathioprine's imidazole degradation product and the carcinogenic behavior of its active metabolite, 6-thioguanine (Hemmens & Moore 1986, Taylor & Shus-ter 1992, Lennard *et al.*, 1985, as cited in Penn, 1996 (Penn, 1996)). A similar relationship between the use of azathioprine and melanoma is uncertain (Penn, 1996).

As of yet, there lacks a clear consensus as to whether or not immunosuppressive modalities as a class permit malignant changes. A portion of the research on medications used in OTRs has suggested that the specific immunosuppressive agent is less important as a contributor to tumorigenesis than is the overall effect of immunosuppression (Baron and Krol, 2005; Bouwes Bavinck *et al.*, 1996). The chal-lenge of accurately attributing pro-oncogenic effects of immunosuppressive therapies is significant con-sidering the many other risk factors, comorbidities and polypharmacy in the OTR population. Of note, these studies addressed malignancy in general and were not specific to melanoma (Kubica and Brewer, 2012).

Conversely, numerous other studies have shown that specific classes of immunosuppressive agents are particularly tumorigenic. The class of calcineurin inhibitors, which includes cyclosporine A, exhibits pro-oncogenic properties through increased production of Bcl-2, fibronectin-guided migration of meta-static melanoma cells, (Juhász *et al.*, 2009) disruption of DNA repair, (Dapprich *et al.*, 2008; Kubica and Brewer, 2012) and promotion of angiogenesis via a TGF-β dependent mechanism (Koehl *et al.*, 2004). For these reasons, the mTOR (mammalian target of rapamycin) inhibitors such as sirolimus and everoli-mus may be substituted for the calcineurin inhibitor class, as the latter family has even been associated with lower risk of malignancy (Kauffman *et al.*, 2005). In fact, rapamycin (sirolimus) has been shown to oppose the oncogenic mechanisms of UV radiation, including the UV-induced down-regulation of Akt1, a protein kinase with tumor suppressing function. Sully *et al.* describe the finding of selective up-regulation of Akt1 after treatment with rapamycin in the setting of non-melanoma skin cancers such as squamous cell carcinoma (Sully *et al.*, 2013). This observation is particularly intriguing, as it highlights a medication that appears to reverse a detrimental effect of UV radiation on the epidermis (Sully *et al.*, 2013).

As the application of TNF-α inhibitors increases, and as the indications for these therapies expand, the concern over heightened risk of infection and malignancy similarly grows. The relationship between TNF-α and cancer is quite complicated because this cytokine has both pro- and anti-malignant properties (Balkwill, 2009). Analysis of melanoma's association with TNF-α inhibitor therapy is limited, especially compared to the data available on the biologics' association with other malignancies including lymphoma. A review of 71 clinical trials to discuss the long-term safety of adalimumab (a TNF-α inhibitor) revealed an increased risk of melanoma in those treated for psoriasis (SIR 4.37, 95% CI, 1.89 to 8.61), but no greater incidence of the malignancy in the rheumatoid arthritis (RA) population (SIR 1.5, 95% CI, 0.84 to 2.47) (Burmester *et al.*, 2013). Factors associated with psoriasis itself are potential contributors to this trend. For example, this patient population is more likely to have a history of psoralin-UV-A (PUVA) treatment than the RA population (Paul *et al.*, 2003). Data for the relationship between TNF-α inhibitor treatment for RA and NMSC or melanoma risk is mixed, with the latter being more ambiguous (Askling *et al.*, 2009; Chakravarty *et al.*, 2005; Leombruno *et al.*, 2009; Raaschou *et al.*, 2013). With regard to outcomes in RA patients treated with TNF-α inhibitors, prognosis after melanoma diagnosis does not appear to be worse than compared to the TNF-α inhibitor-naïve population (Raaschou *et al.*, 2011).

7   Melanoma and Autoimmunity

Because melanoma is a highly immunogenic cancer, vigorous immune surveillance and execution are critical to suppressing this malignancy. To that end, one might imagine that diseases in which immune activity is especially robust may provide protection against malignant melanoma. In fact, the epitome of super-vigilant immune function, autoimmunity, has been associated with better prognosis for melanoma (Satzger *et al.*, 2007). In a randomized trial of 200 melanoma patients treated with high dose interferon-α, Gogas *et al.* compared the relapse free survival and overall survival in those who developed signs of autoimmunity compared to those who did not (Gogas *et al.*, 2006). While relapse occurred in 73% (108 of 148) of patients without evidence of autoimmunity, only 13% (7 of 52) of patients with either autoantibodies or clinical signs of autoimmune disease experienced relapse of melanoma (Gogas *et al.*, 2006). Supported by their univariate analysis of relapse-free survival demonstrating a positive relationship between autoimmunity and lack of melanoma recurrence (p<0.001), the investigators concluded that autoimmunity itself was a prognostic marker for greater relapse-free survival and overall survival (Gogas *et al.*, 2006). A subsequent study by Satzger *et al.* provided the same conclusions for melanoma patients treated with low dose interferon alpha (Satzger *et al.*, 2007).

8   Melanoma in Patients with HIV Infection and AIDS

The introduction of highly active antiretroviral therapy (HAART) in the 1990s represented a major turning point in the treatment of HIV infection and AIDS. Typically comprised of 3 medications with independent mechanisms of action, HAART has significantly decreased the number of AIDS-defining illnesses (Kubica and Brewer, 2012). As a result of its effect on the natural course of HIV/AIDS, HAART has allowed for greater survival with this chronic infection. However, with increased longevity emerged increased incidence of associated maladies such as lipodystrophy, osteopenia, metabolic syndrome, and non-AIDS defining cancers (NADCs) (Patel *et al.*, 2008). Melanoma is among these various malignancies.

Patients with HIV infection are at 1.5 to 2-fold increased risk of developing malignancies compared to the general population (Burgi *et al.*, 2005; Patel *et al.*, 2008; Wilkins *et al.*, 2006). In their 1996 to 2008 comparison of demographically matched HIV infected versus HIV non-infected patients from

California, Silverberg and coworkers determined a relative risk of 1.8 (95% CI, 1.3 to 2.6) for melanoma in the HIV+ population (p = 0.001) (Silverberg *et al.*, 2011). Although they also correlated the increased melanoma incidence with CD4 count < 500 cells/μL, this finding was not statistically significant (p = 0.092) (Silverberg *et al.*, 2011).

In an earlier study, melanoma was associated with a standardized rate ratio of 2.6 (95% CI, 1.9 to 3.6) in HIV+ patients (p value not provided) (Patel *et al.*, 2008). In their prospective cohort analysis of 54,780 HIV+ patients from 1992 to 2003, Patel *et al.* (2008) found that melanoma was more prevalent in HIV+ patients and that the incidence of melanoma increased over time. In contrast, melanoma incidence remained unchanged for the same time periods in the general population. Although an attribute of this study was its large patient population, the inability to account for numerous confounding factors, including tobacco use, alcohol abuse, and infection with oncogenic viruses (Silverberg *et al.*, 2011) presents a challenge in assessing the contribution of HIV-induced immunosuppression to the development of melanoma in this patient population (Kubica and Brewer, 2012; Patel *et al.*, 2008).

8.1   Clinical Course in Patients with Melanoma and HIV Infection/AIDS

Considering the role of the immune system in suppressing malignant transformation, it stands to reason that the probability of developing cancer in the immunosuppressed state of HIV/AIDS is greater than that of the general population. One small study demonstrated that HIV+ patients' disease-free and overall survival were lower than for patients in an HIV-negative control population (median OS: 2.8 years for HIV+, 6.4 years for HIV-; p = 0.045). This study illustrated that HIV+ patients experienced a more aggressive course of melanoma, highlighting the need for closer cancer surveillance in this patient population. Although not statistically significant, the same study also indicated shorter survival time for HIV+ melanoma patients as CD4 count declined (Rodrigues *et al.*, 2002).

In the previously referenced study, Silverberg *et al.* (2011) also noticed a possible trend in the development of melanoma in HIV+ patients as CD4 counts declined. Once again, this relationship between HIV-induced immunosuppression and the appearance of melanoma was not statistically significant. Beyond these two studies, others have failed to illustrate a similar relationship between CD4 count and melanoma. With regard to the evolution of melanoma, the role of HIV-induced immunosuppression as well as the level of immune system compromise (indicated by CD4 count and HIV RNA viral load) is still unclear.

8.2   Immune Dysregulation in HIV Infection

Increased risk of melanoma in patients with HIV/AIDS results from the distortion of relative cytokine ratios, causing an imbalance of immune cell populations. Reuter *et al*'s analysis of two HIV+ patient populations, the "elite controllers (EC)" and the "chronic progressors (CP)," has provided valuable insight into HIV-induced immune dysfunction. The elevated levels of IL-4 found in HIV infection lead to a shift of CD4 specialization away from Th1 and toward Th2 phenotype, resulting in greater levels of cytokines associated with the latter, including IL-4, IL-5, IL-6, IL-10 and IL-13 (Reuter *et al.*, 2012; Wang *et al.*, 1994). In turn, IL-4 induces B cells to produce immunoglobulins and provides positive feedback for further Th2 expansion. Conversely, IL-4 and IL-10 inhibit Th1 production (Reuter *et al.*, 2012). This trend is consistent with the earlier findings by Clerici and Shearer, who recognized an HIV-associated Th1 to Th2 shift as levels of IL-4 and IL-10 rose and that HIV infection progressed to AIDS as IL-2 and IFN-γ declined. Effective immune control over HIV infection was correlated with more robust Th1 responses to HIV antigens, further supporting the understanding that Th1 responses are critical in preventing HIV progression to AIDS (Clerici and Shearer, 1993).

9   Surgical Management of Melanoma

Although extensive research efforts have focused on pharmacologic strategies for malignant melanoma, wide surgical resection of the primary tumor remains the standard of care, with medical management serving an adjuvant role in MM (Dzwierzynski, 2013). Surgical excision that achieves deep margins down to the fascia and a specified safety margin is currently the only intervention that may offer a cure in malignant melanoma (Sladden *et al.*, 2009). The factors considered during surgical planning of melanoma excision include anatomic location and size of the primary tumor, Breslow depth and histologic features. The National Comprehensive Cancer Network (NCCN) has established guidelines for adequate resection margins according to the size of the primary lesion (Wasif *et al.*, 2013). For example, the recommended margin for lesions ≤ 1.0 mm is 1.0 cm, while a clinical margin of 1-2 cm is recommended for lesions measuring 1.01 to 2 mm (Wasif *et al.*, 2013).

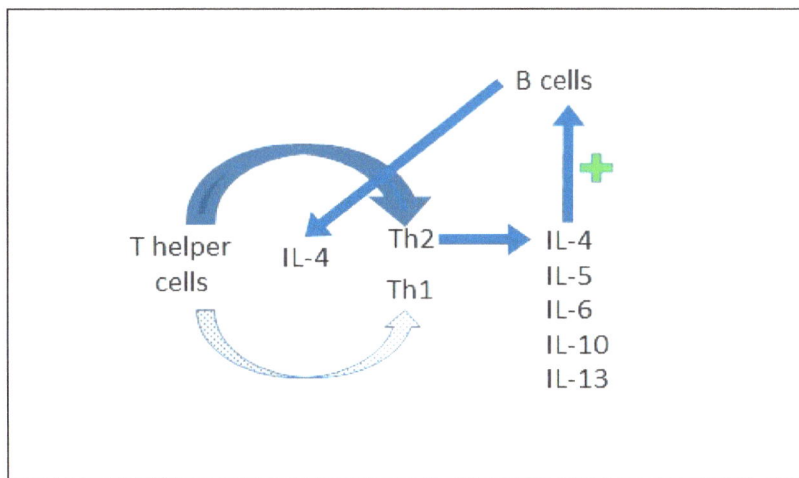

Figure 2: The Th1 to Th2 Shift in HIV Infection. Immune dysregulation in HIV infection. HIV-induced immune dysfunction is characterized by elevated IL-4, which preferentially stimulates helper T cells to differentiate into Th2 cells in greater ratios than into Th1 cells. Greater numbers of Th2 cells results in elevations of cytokines such as IL-4 and IL-10, which are responsible for further inhibiting the production of Th1 cells. This dampening of the Th1 response contributes to progression of HIV to AIDS (Clerici and Shearer, 1993; Reuter *et al.*, 2012; Wang *et al.*, 1994).

Interestingly, in their assessment of nation-wide observance of the guidelines for resection margins and sentinel lymph node biopsies, Wasif *et al.* show that there is significant room for improvement in the surgical care of melanoma patients in terms of compliance with these established protocols. In their review of 60,194 patients with MM from the SEER database from 2004 to 2008, Wasif *et al.* demonstrated that 66.2% of patients with T1 stage melanoma received clinical margins measuring < 1 cm (CI: 1.36 to 1.63, p < 0.001). They also found that only 53% of patients eligible for sentinel lymph node biopsy (stages Ib and II melanoma) received this intervention. However, interpretation of this latter finding is difficult due to the possibility that some sentinel lymph node biopsy candidates may have declined the procedure (Wasif et al., 2013).

The application of Mohs micrographic surgery to the treatment of melanoma remains a controversial subject. While Zitelli et al. argue that a benefit of Mohs surgery compared to traditional excision for melanoma is the ability to examine complete margins rather than simply representative sections, (Zitelli et al., 1997) artifact resulting from frozen specimen preparation may prevent accurate assessment for malignant cells (Dzwierzynski, 2013). Although Mohs for MM may be employed in investigational endeavors, there is not enough evidence to support its use for the general population at this time (Dzwierzynski, 2013). Dzwierzynski offers a detailed discussion of the surgical management of melanoma, addressing functionally and aesthetically sensitive anatomical concerns (Dzwierzynski, 2013).

10   Medical Management of Melanoma

Current Medical Therapy for Melanoma		
Category	**Specific therapy**	**Actions**
Chemotherapy (Middleton et al., 2000)	Temozolomide (TMZ) Dacarbazine (DTIC)	Alkylating agents → DNA methylation, double stranded breaks (Middleton et al., 2000)
Kinase inhibitors (Mackiewicz and Mackiewicz, 2012; Ngiow et al., 2013)	BRAF inhibitors: Vemurafenib Dabrafenib MEK 1/2 inhibitor: Trametinib	Mutations in components of the MAPK pathway, such as BRAF and MEK, favor melanoma cell expansion and survival (Mackiewicz and Mackiewicz, 2012; Ngiow et al., 2013) BRAF inhibitors target the most common location for BRAF mutations ($BRAF^{V600E}$) (Ngiow et al., 2013)
Immunotherapy (Den Otter et al., 2008; Rosenberg et al., 1985)	IL-2	Promotes proliferation and antitumor activity of CTLs Most promising for fast growing, highly vascularized tumors with pre-existing peritumoral leukocytic infiltrates (Den Otter et al., 2008; Rosenberg et al., 1985)
CTLA-4 inhibitors (Contardi et al., 2005; Ribas, 2007)	Ipilimumab Tremelimumab	CTLA-4 is a T cell regulator constitutively expressed on T regulatory cells (Ribas, 2007) and tumor cells (Contardi et al., 2005) CTLA-4 suppresses immune function by inhibiting production of IL-2 and IFN-γ and by inducing DC expression of IDO (Ribas, 2007)
Dendritic cell vaccines (Bocchia et al., 2000; Nestle et al., 1998; Schreibelt et al., 2013)	Nil	Mature monocyte-derived DCs loaded with laboratory-produced peptides → bind MHC class I molecules → tumor specific CTL responses (Schreibelt et al., 2013) May be especially useful in patients whose specific TAAs are unknown (Bocchia et al., 2000; Nestle et al., 1998)
ACT (Turcotte et al., 2013; Wu et al., 2012)	Nil	Antigen-specific T cells (usually TILs expanded by IL-2 ex vivo) are infused into the patient to augment the immune response to tumor cells (Turcotte et al., 2013; Wu et al., 2012)

Table 1: Current medical therapies for melanoma.

10.1   Chemotherapy

There are two first line chemotherapy agents for metastatic melanoma: temozolomide (TMZ) and dacarbazine (DTIC). Both of these alkylating agents are converted to the active form of 5-(3-methyltriazen-1-yl)imidazole-4-carboximide (MTIC) and therefore have the same ultimate mechanism of action: DNA methylation resulting in double stranded breaks (Middleton *et al.*, 2000). A significant difference between these two agents is TMZ's capacity to penetrate the blood brain barrier, making it a useful therapy for CNS malignances such as astrocytoma, glioblastoma and brain metastases from MM. Unfortunately, outcomes of these individual chemotherapies in the treatment of MM have been disappointing with objective response rates of < 20% for DTIC (Quirt *et al.*, 2007) and 21% for TMZ (Middleton *et al.*, 2000). In reaction to these findings, subsequent studies have sought to investigate the impact of one chemotherapy agent in conjunction with immunotherapy. A 2007 analysis of 526 patients that examined chemoimmunotherapy (TMZ plus IFN-α) versus TMZ alone in metastatic MM showed no significant difference in survival time between the two populations (Larkin and Gore, 2008; Sasse *et al.*, 2007). However, a smaller study of 73 patients conducted at the University of Pretoria, South Africa, demonstrated that DTIC combined with IFN-α compared to DTIC alone had a significantly greater overall response (20% for DTIC alone, 95% CI: 7 to 39; 50% for combination, 95% CI: 26 to 72; p = 0.007) (Falkson, 1995). Most studies currently in progress are investigating the combination of the main chemotherapy agents with other therapies in an effort to sensitize malignant cells to the chemotherapy regimens.

10.2   Kinase Inhibitors

The mitogen-activated protein kinase pathway (RAS/RAF/MAPK/ERK) favors melanoma cell expansion and survival. Mutations in one of this pathway's components, the oncogenic serine-threonine protein kinase BRAF, are present in approximately 50% of human melanomas. BRAF mutations result in heightened tumor cell expression of IL-1α and IL-1β, ultimately augmenting PD-L1 expression and suppressing T cell antitumor activity (Khalili *et al.*, 2012). Hence, therapies have been introduced to target the most common location for these mutations, occurring at V600 (BRAF^{V600E}). These therapies are vemurafenib and dabrafenib, the BRAF inhibitors (Ngiow *et al.*, 2013). Overall survival as demonstrated by the BRIM3 study (a phase III clinical trial) was greater with vemurafenib than with DTIC, with a median OS of 13.6 months versus 9.7 months (95% CI 0.57 to 0.87; p < 0.001). Similar findings were seen for progression free survival (PFS) in the BREAK-3 study comparing efficacies of dabrafenib and DTIC, although overall survival data is not yet available (Mackiewicz and Mackiewicz, 2012). Unfortunately, as with other anti-melanoma agents, resistance to these therapies has been observed, prompting consideration of other potential targets along the MAPK pathway, such as MEK. The METRIC study, a phase III trial comparing MEK1/2 inhibitor trametinib with paclitaxel/DTIC showed greater PFS in the trametinib arm (4.8 months) compared to the chemotherapy group (1.4 months) (95% CI: 0.31 to 0.64; p < 0.0001) (Mackiewicz and Mackiewicz, 2012). Investigators suspect that combination therapy to target multiple steps of this pathway simultaneously may help to circumvent melanoma's resistance to individual therapies (Ngiow *et al.*, 2013).

In their assessment of patients with BRAF^{V600E} positive metastatic melanoma treated with either a BRAF inhibitor alone or with a combination of a BRAF inhibitor and a MEK inhibitor, Frederick *et al.* found that BRAF inhibition in general caused lower levels of the inhibitory cytokines IL-6 and IL-8 and higher levels of perforin and granzyme, markers of T cell cytotoxic activity (Frederick *et al.*, 2013). Regarding the two comparison groups, melanoma treated solely with BRAF inhibitors yielded lower tumor antigen expression and suppressed levels of CD8 cells, coinciding with the progression of melanoma. Interestingly, when one patient from this group was secondarily treated with the BRAF/MEK inhibitor combination therapy, both melanoma antigen expression and CD8 levels were reestablished (Frederick *et al.*, 2013).

10.3   Immunotherapy

Interleukin-2 (IL-2), a cytokine responsible for the proliferation and antitumor activity of CTLs, has been the subject of extensive research for years. In 1985, after promising results with IL-2 administration in murine models, Rosenberg *et al.* demonstrated objective cancer regression in 11 of 25 patients with various types of malignancies. In fact, one of these patients experienced complete regression of metastatic melanoma (Rosenberg *et al.*, 1985). However, severe toxicity associated with systemic administration of recombinant IL-2 has limited its application in the treatment of human cancer. Den Otter *et al.* (2008) offer an extensive review of studies investigating local administration of IL-2 to avoid adverse events associated with systemic administration, such as vascular leak phenomenon. Although a comprehensive explanation of their findings is not included here, their work suggests that local IL-2 may be most appropriate for fast growing, highly vascularized tumors with pre-existing peritumoral leukocytic infiltrates.

10.4   The CTLA-4 Inhibitors

A therapeutic target of interest is the cytotoxic T lymphocyte-associated protein 4 (CTLA-4, also known as CD152), a key T cell regulator that is constitutively expressed on T regulatory cells (Ribas, 2007) and tumor cells. (Contardi *et al.*, 2005). The functional analog of CTLA-4, CD28, competes for the same ligands (B7-1, B7-2), but serves the opposing role of providing the secondary activation signal for T cells (Wolchok and Saenger, 2008). Whereas CTLA-4 induces tolerance, CD28 augments antitumor immunity (Wolchok and Saenger, 2008). Upon receiving a costimulatory signal, CTLA-4 inhibits the production of IL-2 and IFN-γ and induces DC expression of IDO, making this negative regulator integral to the prevention of autoimmunity and lymphoproliferative disease as has been demonstrated in knock-out murine models (Ribas, 2007). In turn, inhibition of CTLA-4 has attracted much research interest, leading to the introduction of the CTLA-4 inhibitors, which are fully human monoclonal antibodies (Hodi *et al.*, 2010).

In a clinical trial that ultimately led to the 2011 FDA approval of ipilimumab (a CTLA-4 inhibitor) for metastatic melanoma, greater overall survival was demonstrated with ipilimumab when compared to glycoprotein 100 (gp100), a melanosomal protein vaccine with immunogenic properties but questionable antitumor capabilities. All of the 676 subjects had unresectable stage III or IV melanoma and each was randomly assigned to one of 3 treatment arms: ipilimumab alone or in combination with a gp100 vaccine and the gp100 vaccine alone. Overall survival rates for the 3 groups were: 10.1 months, 10.0 months and 6.4 months respectively. The difference in OS between the ipilimumab treatment arm alone and the combination arm was not statistically significant (p = 0.76) (Hodi *et al.*, 2010). A phase III trial for CTLA-4 inhibitor tremelimumab failed to demonstrate statistically significant increased overall survival (OS) compared to the first line chemotherapy treatments TMZ and DTIC, with median OS for tremelimumab at 12.6 months (95% CI, 10.8 to 14.3) and for chemotherapy at 10.7 months (95% CI, 9.36 to 11.96) (Ribas *et al.*, 2013).

Small clinical trials involving the CTLA-4 inhibitors, ipilimumab and tremelimumab, with or without chemotherapy have shown mixed results. In a multicenter phase II trial of ipilimumab combined with DTIC versus ipilimumab alone, better response rates were observed in the combination arm (17% versus 5%), although also accompanied by greater toxicity (28% versus 18%) (Ribas, 2007). With overlapping confidence intervals, however, the significance of these findings is questionable. Further investigation in the form of a phase III trial of DTIC plus ipilimumab versus DTIC alone is currently ongoing (Fischkoff *et al.*, as cited in Ribas 2007).

As with numerous other therapeutic strategies for melanoma, resistance to the CTLA-4 inhibitors has been observed. One proposed offender in the resistance to anti-CTLA-4 therapy is host-derived IDO (Holmgaard *et al.*, 2013). Through the use of murine subjects, Holmgaard *et al.* (2013) sought to determine the inhibitory influence of tumor-derived and/or host-derived IDO on antitumor immune function in the setting of CTLA-4 inhibitor therapy. They found that IDO deficiency was associated with greater T cell infiltration of tumor after anti-CTLA-4 therapy, and that combination therapy of an IDO inhibitor called 1MT (1-methyl-tryptophan) with anti-CTLA-4 yielded greater ratios of T effector to T regulatory cells in the vicinity of the tumor.

Other investigators have examined the implications of certain CTLA-4 polymorphisms for treatment response to anti-CTLA-4 antibodies such as ipilimumab (Queirolo *et al.*, 2013). In an attempt to elucidate predictive markers for positive response to anti-CTLA-4 therapy, Queirolo *et al.* (2013) assessed responsiveness among patients with variable SNPs (single nucleotide polymorphisms) of the CTLA-4 gene. Their work yielded greater overall survival in patients with 2 particular heterozygous CTLA-4 genotypes ($p < 0.001$): -1577G/A and CT60G/A. Although a number of patients who succumbed to melanoma also exhibited these heterozygous mutations, all surviving patients carried the 2 CTLA-4 heterozygous genoptyes (Queirolo *et al.*, 2013). Because no therapy is devoid of risk, the availability of predictive markers for positive outcomes with anti-CTLA-4 therapy may guide clinicians to carefully select for the patients most likely to benefit from these medications (Queirolo *et al.*, 2013).

A particularly interesting study by Hodi *et al.* (2003) examined the antitumor effects of MDX-CTLA-4 (a CTLA-4 inhibitor) in melanoma patients who had previously received irradiated tumor vaccines. With the intention of increasing antitumor immunity, vaccination stimulates the secretion of granulocyte-macrophage colony-stimulating factor (GM-CSF), generating greater numbers of activated DCs that in turn phagocytose tumor cells and present their antigens to lymphocytes within the lymph nodes. To the investigators' surprise, pathologic analysis of MDX-CTLA-4 treated tissues demonstrated significant increases in neutrophils, possibly explaining the abundant tumor necrosis that was observed. Hodi *et al.* (2003) suggest that the substantial neutrophilic infiltrate may have been the result of T cell activation.

It has been demonstrated that CTLA-4 is also constitutively expressed in tumor cells and that, via recombinant CTLA-4 ligand stimulation, apoptosis of malignant cells can be induced. In their experimentation with various human tumor cell lines (including melanoma) expressing CTLA-4, Contardi *et al.* (2005) showed that recombinant CD80 and CD86, both ligands for CTLA-4, can be employed to induce apoptosis of the malignant cells expressing CTLA-4. Such findings suggest that, aside from CTLA-4 inhibition by monoclonal antibodies, CTLA-4 itself can be used as a target in the treatment of MM.

10.5 Dendritic Cell Vaccines

As antigen presenting cells intimately in tune with their surrounding environment by way of molecular signaling, DCs play an essential role in immunosurveillance and thus in anti-tumor immunity as well. Upon loading antigen, DCs degrade the proteins to peptides and display them in MHCs in order to present the antigens to B and T cells in lymphoid organs (Palucka and Banchereau, 2012). In a similar fashion, most clinically tested DC vaccines involve mature monocyte-derived DCs that are loaded with laboratory-produced peptides that bind MHC class I molecules, with the ultimate effect of producing tumor specific CTL responses (Schreibelt *et al.*, 2013). In a trial with 16 advanced melanoma patients, Nestle *et al.* (1998) examined the effects of DC vaccines pulsed with tumor lysate or with various different tumor associated antigens (TAAs) (depending on individual patients' specific HLA haplotypes). They observed regression of metastases (skin, soft tissue, lung and pancreas) in 5 of the patients, 2 of whom experienced complete responses. Notably, 2 of the responding patients received the tumor lysate-pulsed DC vaccine without previous exposure to TAAs, indicating that the DC vaccine alone may be effective in tumors whose specific antigens are not known (Bocchia *et al.*, 2000; Nestle *et al.*, 1998). Since then, numerous other studies have employed DC vaccines in combination with other therapies and continue to show promising results, warranting continued investigation.

10.6   Adoptive Cell Transfer Therapy (ACT)

Adoptive cell transfer therapy (ACT) is the process by which antigen-specific T cells are infused into a patient to augment the immune response to tumor cells. Although various different types of ACT have been developed, the use of tumor infiltrating lymphocytes (TILs) that have been expanded with IL-2 *ex vivo*, is the most extensively studied and clinically successful of the methods, with response rates > 50% (Turcotte *et al.*, 2013; Wu *et al.*, 2012). In their clinical analysis of ACT with TILs for the treatment of GI adenocarcinoma or melanoma metastases, Turcotte *et al.* (2013) demonstrated that 43% (105 out of 246) of the melanoma cultures exhibited MHC-I mediated CD8+ reactivity. This is in comparison to 9% (17 out of 188) MHC-I mediated CD8+ reactivity in the GI metastases group (p < 0.001). The investigators speculated that the discrepancy between melanoma and GI tumor sensitivity to ACT was likely related to the former malignancy's uniquely immunologic features compared to other cancers.

Thus far, the greatest limitation of ACT has been the failure to induce sustained antitumor activity via TILs. Possible explanations include persistence of T regulatory cells that dampen the antitumor activity of CTLs and an imbalance of T cell regulatory mechanisms (Rosenberg *et al.*, 2011; Wrzesinski *et al.*, 2010). As demonstrated by Wrzesinski *et al.* using murine models, lymphodepletion induced by total body irradiation (TBI) prior to the initiation of ACT improves the outcome of cell transfer therapy by abating T regulatory cell numbers and improving the T cell homeostatic regulation (Dudley *et al.*, 2002). Their work illustrated a direct correlation between levels of fractionated TBI administered and the efficacy of subsequent ACT treatment. Also noteworthy, was the augmentation of the ratio of tumor reactive CD8+ T cells to CD4+ T cells, which was proportional to TPI dose (Wrzesinski *et al.*, 2010). This data was supported by a subsequent clinical trial by Rosenberg *et al.* (2011) who studied 93 patients with metastatic melanoma, 95% of whose disease continued to progress despite intensive prior therapy. Objective response rates for the 3 trial groups with regimens of chemotherapy alone versus chemotherapy plus 2 or 12 Gy irradiation were 49%, 52% and 72%, respectively. As extensive exploration into the field continues, ACT offers hope in the search for therapies offering enduring metastatic melanoma regression. We refer the reader to more extensive reviews and research on the topic of ACT (Jensen *et al.*, 2012; Turcotte *et al.*, 2013; Wu *et al.*, 2012).

11   Potential for New Therapies

The following is a brief introduction to newly identified targets and potential therapies for the management of melanoma. This is not intended to be a comprehensive review. Perhaps one of the most studied treatments for metastatic melanoma, IL-2 therapy has demonstrated consistent antitumor response *in vitro* and *in vivo* (Chou *et al.*, 2013; Chu *et al.*, 2013; Den Otter *et al.*, 2008). However, the systemic toxicity of

IL-2, characterized by vascular leak syndrome and other phenomena, has limited the clinical utility of this immunotherapy (Chou *et al.*, 2013). Therefore, recent research has focused on producing a therapy with the same mechanism of action but milder toxicity. Researchers Chou *et al.* (2013) have produced palmitate-derivatized (Ribas, 2007) IL-2 (pIL-2), a form of recombinant human IL-2 (rhIL-2) whose properties allow for localization of the drug to the tumor site, minimizing its systemic effects. In their investigations with murine subjects, Chou *et al.* (2013) demonstrated that, compared to rhIL-2, pIL-2 stimulated more CD8+ cells, promoted survival of antitumor immune cells, decreased incidence of lung metastasis and increased overall survival. These findings were applicable to both pIL-2 adoptive T cell transfer with CTLs and to intra-tumorally injected pIL-2 models. Although further investigation into pIL-2's interactions with the immune system is necessary, the development of this modified form of IL-2 with theoretical lower toxicity is encouraging.

Potential Future Treatments for Melanoma		
Proposed therapy	**Description**	**Actions**
pIL-2 (Chou *et al.*, 2013)	Palmitate-derivatized form of rhIL-2 that localizes to tumor site, minimizing systemic toxicity	Stimulation of CD8+ cells Improved survival of antitumor immune cells Decreased incidence of lung metastasis Increased overall survival
Nanoparticles (Zheng *et al.*, 2013)	Liposomes conjugated with targeting molecules to a) label and b) expand ACT and endogenous T cells *in vivo*	Liposome-conjugated molecules: - Anti-Thy1.1-Lip: antibodies to ACT T cell antigens → successful labeling of transferred cells *in vivo* - IL-2-Fc-Lip: recombinant IL-2 → greater antitumor T cell expansion; more robust expansion of ACT T cells with each subsequent IL-2-Fc-Lip injection
LV-tSMAC (Emeagi *et al.*, 2012)	SMAC-encoding lentiviral vectors	Greater antitumor immunity ↓ *in vivo* T regulatory cells Greater CTL activation
Oblimersen (Jain, 2001, 2005; Semenza, 2003; Shang *et al.*, 2012; Stein *et al.*, 2009)	Bcl-2 antisense	Sensitizes MM cells to subsequent chemotherapy - ↓ Bcl-2 synthesis - Potentiates FBF-2 activity to promote tumor angiogenesis, preventing hypoxia-induced MM upregulation
Mebendazole (Doudican *et al.*, 2008; Doudican *et al.*, 2013)	Antihelminthic	Promotes MM cell apoptosis - Interferes with interaction between Bcl-2 and Bax - ↓XIAP, ↑proteosomal degradation Inhibition of tubulin polymerization during cellular proliferation

Table 2: New therapies for melanoma

The proposed use of nanoparticles as an adjunct to ACT may enable persistent *in vivo* T cell expansion without the systemic administration of highly toxic IL-2. Zheng *et al.* (2013) have shown that liposomes conjugated with targeting molecules can both specifically and nonspecifically augment ACT cells and endogenous T cell proliferation (respectively) to enhance antitumor activity. The liposome-conjugated targeting molecules used in these murine experiments were a) antibodies specific to ACT T cell antigens (anti-Thy1.1-Lip) and b) recombinant IL-2 (IL-2-Fc-Lip), a nonspecific T cell activator. Their work demonstrated successful *in vivo* labeling of transferred T cells via anti-Thy1.1-Lip and greater antitumor T cell expansion with liposome-bound IL-2 than with injection of equivalent free IL-2 doses, with each subsequent injection of IL-2-Fc-Lip inducing greater ACT cell expansion.

Considering its direct role in the interaction between CTLs and tumor cells, the programmed death (PD-1) receptor and its ligand (PD-L1) have garnered significant interest in the development of melanoma therapy. By suppressing the antitumor activity of CD4+ and CD8+ T cells, the PD-1/PD-L1 interaction may contribute to the progression of malignancy in PD-L1 expressing tumors (Brahmer *et al.*, 2012). There are currently 3 anti-PD-1 antibodies undergoing clinical trials for the treatment of melanoma and other malignancies including renal cell carcinoma, non-small cell lung cancer and colorectal cancer (Postow *et al.*, 2012). These PD-1 inhibitory antibodies are BMS-936558 (formerly MDX-1106), MK-3475 and CT-011 (Postow *et al.*, 2012). In a phase I study of 296 patients with various advanced solid tumors (104 of whom had melanoma), Topalian *et al.* (2012) assessed the antitumor activity of a fully human monoclonal anti-PD-1 antibody, BMS-936558, the most thoroughly studied anti-PD-1 antibody (Postow *et al.*, 2012). In this study, PD-L1 expression in tumors was assessed in 42 patients, 18 of whom had melanoma. Of those 42 patients, 25 demonstrated immunohistochemical positivity for PD-L1 expression and 9 of those 25 patients exhibited an objective response. The lack of objective response in all 17 patients who were negative for PD-L1 expression necessitates a thorough investigation into PD-L1 as a marker in the selection of patients for therapy with anti-PD-1 antibody (Topalian *et al.*, 2012). The investigators also found that all doses tested showed antitumor activity and that objective responses were particularly notable in melanoma, non-small cell lung cancer, renal cell carcinoma and various sites of metastasis (Topalian *et al.*, 2012). Phase II trials for the use of anti-PD-1 antibodies against PD-L1 expressing tumors are currently underway.

A particularly elegant cancer therapy is the oncolytic virus or OV. This therapeutic modality employs a live virus deprived of certain genes while enhanced with others in order to target cancer cells and disrupt the tumor microenvironment (Bartlett *et al.*, 2013; Donnelly *et al.*, 2013). Vulnerability to viral assault and replication is a feature inherently characteristic of malignant cells that distinguishes them from normal cells (Donnelly *et al.*, 2013). Rampant viral replication within malignant cells essentially labels them for the immune system, while protecting normal cells whose antiviral mechanisms remain intact (Donnelly *et al.*, 2013). T-VEC or Talimogene laherperevec (formerly OncoVex or JS1/ICP34.5-/ICP47-/CM-CSF) is an OV engineered from herpes simplex virus that does not express neurovirulent genes of the wild-type virus and instead, is equipped to express granulocyte-macrophage colony stimulating factor to enhance antitumor immunity (Bartlett *et al.*, 2013). Intratumoral T-VEC injections have recently demonstrated promise in phase II clinical trials in metastatic melanoma. In a study of 50 patients with IIIc or IV metastatic melanoma, 74% of whom had received previous nonsurgical treatment for their disease, Senzer *et al.* (2009) demonstrated an overall response rate of 26% with most responses (92%) enduring for 7 to 31 months after treatment. Both un-injected and injected lesions exhibited regression, leading the authors to speculate that the effects on distant, un-injected lesions is probably immune mediated.

Evasion of apoptosis is a survival mechanism common to many malignancies and is particularly important in melanoma. Although there are two general pathways for apoptosis to proceed, they ultimately converge to the same end. There are many participants in this mechanism, one of which is called second mitochondria-derived activator of caspase (SMAC) or direct inhibitor of apoptosis-binding protein with low pI (DIABLO), (Emeagi *et al.*, 2012) hereafter referred to as SMAC. SMAC functions to antagonize IAPs (inhibitors of apoptosis) whose role is regulation of capsases (Vucic *et al.*, 2002). More specifically, SMAC and SMAC-like peptides have been shown to inhibit the function of various types of IAPs, including XIAPs (X-linked IAPs) and ML-IAPs (melanoma IAPs), both of which are expressed in human malignancies (Vucic *et al.*, 2002). This interaction highlights a promising therapeutic target, one which has recently been further explored by Emeagi *at al.* In their investigation using murine melanoma models, Emeagi *et al.* (2012) were able to harness the pro-apoptotic effects of SMAC through transduction of SMAC-encoding lentiviral vectors (LV-tSMAC). Though requiring more extensive exploration, the results are encouraging: LV-tSMAC bearing mice exhibited greater antitumor immunity, more activated CTLs and decreased *in vivo* T regulatory cells.

Although DTIC is a first-line therapy for metastatic melanoma, overall improvement in prognosis is marginal due to the chemotherapy resistant features of melanoma (Avril *et al.*, 2004; Bedikian *et al.*, 2006; Chiarion Sileni *et al.*, 2001). Thus, a key component of anti-melanoma therapy is the administration of a sensitizing agent that combats the melanoma microenvironment of immune evasion. Recognizing that B-cell lymphoma 2 (Bcl-2) overexpression contributes to melanoma cells' capacity to avoid apoptosis, researchers introduced oblimersen (G2139), a relatively new therapy currently in clinical trials. Oblimersen, also known as Bcl-2 antisense, would be used as an adjunct or pretreatment for patients to be treated subsequently with a medication such as DTIC, TMZ or albumin-bound paclitaxel (Ott *et al.*, 2013). (Antisense refers to a factor that prohibits the translation of a certain protein's mRNA) (Bedikian *et al.*, 2006).

Oblimersen-induced sensitization of melanoma cells to chemotherapy may involve mechanisms beyond suppression of Bcl-2 synthesis. Stein *et al.* (2009) demonstrate that oblimersen promotes tumor angiogenesis in rat models by potentiating FGF-2 induced cellular mitogenesis. Although seemingly contradictory to tumor eradication principles, Jain *et al.* (2001, 2005) explain that antiangiogenic factors actually dampen chemotherapeutics' efficacy through hypoxia, diminishing the amount of medication that can reach the target site. Evidence also suggests that antiangiogenic-induced tumor hypoxia results in more aggressive and metastatic cancer (Shang *et al.*, 2012). As an example, in response to hypoxic conditions, Bcl-2 may promote angiogenesis by enhancing production of hypoxia-inducible factor-1α (HIF-1α) and ultimately vascular endothelial growth factor (VEGF) (Semenza, 2003).

In an experiment of drug repositioning, where a known therapy is implemented in a novel application, (Doudican *et al.*, 2013). The authors demonstrated the pro-apoptotic features of the antihelminthic mebendazole (MBZ) and its relationship to XIAP. Mebendazole's capacity to induce apoptosis *in vitro* and *in vivo* can be attributed to several mechanisms. Through phosphorylation, MBZ prevents Bcl-2 from interacting with pro-apoptotic factor Bcl-2 associated X protein (Bax), causing selectively higher rates of apoptosis of melanoma cells compared with melanocytes (Doudican *et al.*, 2008). Mebendazole also promotes melanoma cell apoptosis via the interaction between XIAP and SMAC, which results in abatement of XIAP levels and proteosomal degradation. In addition, as an inhibitor of tubulin polymerization, MBZ can suppress cellular proliferation from a structural standpoint (Doudican *et al.*, 2013). The investigators observed that the decline in XIAP levels was correlated with tumor cell susceptibility to MBZ's cell cycle suppressive effects. Although MBZ impeded melanoma xenograft growth *in vivo*, its application did not result in xenograft tumor regression.

12   Recommendations

Although the scientific community's understanding of melanoma continues to grow, establishing concrete protocols for the treatment of malignant melanoma in the immunosuppressed presents an ongoing challenge. Along with the modification of greater vigilance and a higher index of suspicion, it is recommended that melanoma screening and care of the immunosuppressed patient essentially parallel that of the immunocompetent population. Particularly in the settings of lymphoproliferative malignancy and organ transplantation, a multidisciplinary approach is growing more popular, integrating dermatologists, oncologists and surgeons, and offering transplant clinic dermatology visits for surveillance of these patients (Otley and Pittelkow, 2000). Considering both the increased incidence and more aggressive nature of MM in these patients, especially attentive regimented screening is prudent (Brewer *et al.*, 2011; Rodrigues *et al.*, 2002).

A significant challenge in the management of immunosuppressed OTR patients is balancing the prevention of donor organ rejection with the potential for de novo, recurrent, or (rarely) graft-transmitted melanoma. When appropriate, immunosuppressive therapy may be reduced to temporize this risk. Recommendations for adjusting immunosuppressive therapy dose according to melanoma stage and donor organ type are provided by SCOPE (Otley, 2006).

Lymph node assessment and evaluation for distant metastases are critical components in the determination of the appropriate level of immunomodulation. The multidisciplinary approach is especially key here, where cooperation between dermatologist, oncologist and surgeon provides expert input, consideration of adjuvant therapy and the option of lymphadenectomy if indicated (Berg and Otley, 2002). In the event of extensive regional or distant metastases, indefinite postponement of transplantation has been recommended (Dinh and Chong, 2007).

Recommendations regarding organ transplant candidates with a history of melanoma are limited, with Penn's analysis of the CTTR providing the most information for this patient population (Penn, 1996). As of yet, there does not appear to be evidence for contraindication to organ transplant and associated immunosuppression in patients with a history of thin melanomas, but careful consideration of risk of recurrence versus implications of withholding organ transplantation is crucial in cases of advanced melanoma, requiring the cooperation of the entire medical team involved.

Specific recommendations for the management of melanoma in HIV/AIDS patients are sparse. Optimal medical control of this chronic infection with HAART is crucial, as the immune dysfunction making these patients more susceptible to malignancy is the target of antiretroviral therapy. Some authors also recommend the implementation of cancer surveillance programs within HIV clinics, although with an emphasis on non-melanoma cancer such as prostatic and anal carcinoma (Burgi *et al.*, 2005). It is also wise to consider the potential for medication interactions between anti-neoplastic agents and members of the HAART regimen when managing this patient population (Spano *et al.*, 2008). As with other immunosuppressed patients, HIV/AIDS status warrants more frequent surveillance and compliance with preventative measures (sun protection).

13   Conclusion

A substantial amount of research exists regarding melanoma's immunogenic properties as well as its presence in various forms of immunosuppression. Yet, much is to be learned about the long-term implications of malignant melanoma in these settings, as well as the appropriate treatment modifications for the special patient populations of the iatrogenically and otherwise immunosuppressed. With continued advancements in our understanding of melanoma and identification of new therapeutic targets, treatment of this malignancy will likely become more personalized, as immunotherapies approach the forefront of our anti-melanoma arsenal. As we anticipate new developments and recommendations in the surveillance and treatment of melanoma in said populations, vigilant screening and early intervention remain the standard of care.

Appendix: Abbreviations and Acronyms

CCSS = Childhood Cancer Survivor Study; SCOPE = Skin Care in Organ Transplant Patients, Europe; SEER = Surveillance, Epidemiology and End Results; AJCC = American Joint Committee on Cancer; IDO = indoleamine 2,3-dioxygenase; TNF = tumor necrosis factor; TGF = transforming growth factor; CI = confidence interval; SIR = standardized incidence ratio; SMR = standardized mortality ratio; PAF = phospholipid platelet-activating factor; PAF-R = phospholipid platelet-activating factor receptor; Treg = regulatory T cell; APC = antigen presenting cell; DC = dendritic cell; MDSC = myeloid derived suppressor cell; CLL = chronic lymphocytic leukemia; PUVA = psoralin-UV-A; HAART = highly active antiretroviral therapy; HIV = human immunodeficiency virus; AIDS = acquired immunodeficiency syndrome; IL = interleukin; NHL = non-Hodgkin lymphoma; OTR = solid organ transplant recipient; PBMC = peripheral blood mononuclear cell; TAP = transporter-associated antigen processing; TMZ = temozolomide; DTIC = dacarbazine; MTIC = 5-(3-methyltriazen-1-yl)imidazole-4-carboximide; mTOR = mammalian target of rapamycin.

References

Adami, J., M. Frisch, J. Yuen, B. Glimelius, and M. Melbye, 1995, Evidence of an association between non-Hodgkin's lymphoma and skin cancer: BMJ, v. 310, p. 1491-5.

Ahmadzadeh, M., L. A. Johnson, B. Heemskerk, J. R. Wunderlich, M. E. Dudley, D. E. White, and S. A. Rosenberg, 2009, Tumor antigen-specific CD8 T cells infiltrating the tumor express high levels of PD-1 and are functionally impaired: Blood, v. 114, p. 1537-44.

Anvekar, R. A., J. J. Asciolla, D. J. Missert, and J. E. Chipuk, 2011, Born to be alive: a role for the BCL-2 family in melanoma tumor cell survival, apoptosis, and treatment: Front Oncol, v. 1.

Askling, J., E. Baecklund, F. Granath, P. Geborek, M. Fored, C. Backlin, L. Bertilsson, L. Cöster, L. T. Jacobsson, S. Lindblad, J. Lysholm, S. Rantapää-Dahlqvist, T. Saxne, R. van Vollenhoven, L. Klareskog, and N. Feltelius, 2009, Anti-tumour necrosis factor therapy in rheumatoid arthritis and risk of malignant lymphomas: relative risks and time trends in the Swedish Biologics Register: Ann Rheum Dis, v. 68, p. 648-53.

Aslakson, C. J., G. Lee, J. S. Boomer, A. Gilman-Sachs, O. Kucuk, and K. D. Beaman, 1999, Expression of regeneration and tolerance factor on B cell chronic lymphocytic leukemias: a possible mechanism for escaping immune surveillance: Am J Hematol, v. 61, p. 46-52.

Avril, M. F., S. Aamdal, J. J. Grob, A. Hauschild, P. Mohr, J. J. Bonerandi, M. Weichenthal, K. Neuber, T. Bieber, K. Gilde, V. Guillem Porta, J. Fra, J. Bonneterre, P. Saïag, D. Kamanabrou, H. Pehamberger, J. Sufliarsky, J. L. Gonzalez Larriba, A. Scherrer, and Y. Menu, 2004, Fotemustine compared with dacarbazine in patients with disseminated malignant melanoma: a phase III study: J Clin Oncol, v. 22, p. 1118-25.

Balch, C. M., J. E. Gershenwald, S. J. Soong, J. F. Thompson, M. B. Atkins, D. R. Byrd, A. C. Buzaid, A. J. Cochran, D. G. Coit, S. Ding, A. M. Eggermont, K. T. Flaherty, P. A. Gimotty, J. M. Kirkwood, K. M. McMasters, M. C. Mihm, D. L. Morton, M. I. Ross, A. J. Sober, and V. K. Sondak, 2009, Final version of 2009 AJCC melanoma staging and classification: J Clin Oncol, v. 27, p. 6199-206.

Balkwill, F., 2009, Tumour necrosis factor and cancer: Nat Rev Cancer, v. 9, p. 361-71.

Baron, J., and A. Krol, 2005, Management of nevi in transplant patients: Dermatol Ther, v. 18, p. 34-43.

Bartlett, D. L., Z. Liu, M. Sathaiah, R. Ravindranathan, Z. Guo, Y. He, and Z. S. Guo, 2013, Oncolytic viruses as therapeutic cancer vaccines: Mol Cancer, v. 12, p. 103.

Baumgartner, J., C. Wilson, B. Palmer, D. Richter, A. Banerjee, and M. McCarter, 2007, Melanoma induces immunosuppression by up-regulating FOXP3(+) regulatory T cells: J Surg Res, v. 141, p. 72-7.

Baumgartner, J. M., K. R. Jordan, L. J. Hu, C. C. Wilson, A. Banerjee, and M. D. McCarter, 2012, DC maturation and function are not altered by melanoma-derived immunosuppressive soluble factors: J Surg Res, v. 176, p. 301-8.

Becker, J. C., and D. Schrama, 2013, The dark side of cyclophosphamide: cyclophosphamide-mediated ablation of regulatory T cells: J Invest Dermatol, v. 133, p. 1462-5.

Bedikian, A. Y., M. Millward, H. Pehamberger, R. Conry, M. Gore, U. Trefzer, A. C. Pavlick, R. DeConti, E. M. Hersh, P. Hersey, J. M. Kirkwood, F. G. Haluska, and O. M. S. Group, 2006, Bcl-2 antisense (oblimersen sodium) plus dacarbazine in patients with advanced melanoma: the Oblimersen Melanoma Study Group: J Clin Oncol, v. 24, p. 4738-45.

Berg, D., and C. C. Otley, 2002, Skin cancer in organ transplant recipients: Epidemiology, pathogenesis, and management: J Am Acad Dermatol, v. 47, p. 1-17; quiz 18-20.

Bilal, M., J. D. Eason, K. Das, P. B. Sylvestre, A. G. Dean, and J. M. Vanatta, 2013, Donor-Derived Metastatic Melanoma in a Liver Transplant Recipient Established by DNA Fingerprinting: Exp Clin Transplant.

Bocchia, M., V. Bronte, M. P. Colombo, A. De Vincentiis, M. Di Nicola, G. Forni, L. Lanata, R. M. Lemoli, M. Massaia, D. Rondelli, P. Zanon, and S. Tura, 2000, Antitumor vaccination: where we stand: Haematologica, v. 85, p. 1172-206.

Bottoni, U., R. Clerico, G. Paolino, M. Ambrifi, C. Luci, P. Corsetti, and S. Calvieri, 2013, Appearance of malignant melanoma after a non-cutaneous cancer diagnosis: Ecancermedicalscience, v. 7, p. 315.

Bouwes Bavinck, J. N., D. R. Hardie, A. Green, S. Cutmore, A. MacNaught, B. O'Sullivan, V. Siskind, F. J. Van Der Woude, and I. R. Hardie, 1996, The risk of skin cancer in renal transplant recipients in Queensland, Australia. A follow-up study: Transplantation, v. 61, p. 715-21.

Brahmer, J. R., S. S. Tykodi, L. Q. Chow, W. J. Hwu, S. L. Topalian, P. Hwu, C. G. Drake, L. H. Camacho, J. Kauh, K. Odunsi, H. C. Pitot, O. Hamid, S. Bhatia, R. Martins, K. Eaton, S. Chen, T. M. Salay, S. Alaparthy, J. F. Grosso, A. J. Korman, S. M. Parker, S. Agrawal, S. M. Goldberg, D. M. Pardoll, A. Gupta, and J. M. Wigginton, 2012, Safety and activity of anti-PD-L1 antibody in patients with advanced cancer: N Engl J Med, v. 366, p. 2455-65.

Bredenbeck, A., F. O. Losch, T. Sharav, M. Eichler-Mertens, M. Filter, A. Givehchi, W. Sterry, P. Wrede, and P. Walden, 2005, Identification of noncanonical melanoma-associated T cell epitopes for cancer immunotherapy: J Immunol, v. 174, p. 6716-24.

Brennan, P., G. Scélo, K. Hemminki, L. Mellemkjaer, E. Tracey, A. Andersen, D. H. Brewster, E. Pukkala, M. L. McBride, E. V. Kliewer, J. M. Tonita, A. Seow, V. Pompe-Kirn, C. Martos, J. G. Jonasson, D. Colin, and P. Boffetta, 2005, Second primary cancers among 109 000 cases of non-Hodgkin's lymphoma: Br J Cancer, v. 93, p. 159-66.

Brewer, J. D., L. J. Christenson, A. L. Weaver, D. C. Dapprich, R. H. Weenig, K. K. Lim, J. S. Walsh, C. C. Otley, W. Cherikh, J. F. Buell, E. S. Woodle, C. Arpey, and P. R. Patton, 2011, Malignant melanoma in solid transplant recipients: collection of database cases and comparison with surveillance, epidemiology, and end results data for outcome analysis: Arch Dermatol, v. 147, p. 790-6.

Brewer, J. D., L. J. Christenson, R. H. Weenig, and A. L. Weaver, 2010, Effects of chronic lymphocytic leukemia on the development and progression of malignant melanoma: Dermatol Surg, v. 36, p. 368-76.

Brewer, J. D., T. D. Shanafelt, C. C. Otley, R. K. Roenigk, J. R. Cerhan, N. E. Kay, A. L. Weaver, and T. G. Call, 2012, Chronic lymphocytic leukemia is associated with decreased survival of patients with malignant melanoma and Merkel cell carcinoma in a SEER population-based study: J Clin Oncol, v. 30, p. 843-9.

Buell, J. F., T. M. Beebe, J. Trofe, T. G. Gross, R. R. Alloway, M. J. Hanaway, and E. S. Woodle, 2004, Donor transmitted malignancies: Ann Transplant, v. 9, p. 53-6.

Burgi, A., S. Brodine, S. Wegner, M. Milazzo, M. R. Wallace, K. Spooner, D. L. Blazes, B. K. Agan, A. Armstrong, S. Fraser, and N. F. Crum, 2005, Incidence and risk factors for the occurrence of non-AIDS-defining cancers among human immunodeficiency virus-infected individuals: Cancer, v. 104, p. 1505-11.

Burmester, G. R., R. Panaccione, K. B. Gordon, M. J. McIlraith, and A. P. Lacerda, 2013, Adalimumab: long-term safety in 23 458 patients from global clinical trials in rheumatoid arthritis, juvenile idiopathic arthritis, ankylosing spondylitis, psoriatic arthritis, psoriasis and Crohn's disease: Ann Rheum Dis, v. 72, p. 517-24.

Cantwell, M., T. Hua, J. Pappas, and T. J. Kipps, 1997, Acquired CD40-ligand deficiency in chronic lymphocytic leukemia: Nat Med, v. 3, p. 984-9.

Chakravarty, E. F., K. Michaud, and F. Wolfe, 2005, Skin cancer, rheumatoid arthritis, and tumor necrosis factor inhibitors: J Rheumatol, v. 32, p. 2130-5.

Chatrath, H., K. Berman, R. Vuppalanchi, J. Slaven, P. Kwo, A. J. Tector, N. Chalasani, and M. Ghabril, 2013, De novo malignancy post-liver transplantation: a single center, population controlled study: Clin Transplant.

Chen, K. T., A. Olszanski, and J. M. Farma, 2012, Donor transmission of melanoma following renal transplant: Case Rep Transplant, v. 2012, p. 764019.

Chiarion Sileni, V., R. Nortilli, S. M. Aversa, A. Paccagnella, M. Medici, L. Corti, A. G. Favaretto, G. L. Cetto, and S. Monfardini, 2001, Phase II randomized study of dacarbazine, carmustine, cisplatin and tamoxifen versus dacarbazine alone in advanced melanoma patients: Melanoma Res, v. 11, p. 189-96.

Choi, Y. S., J. A. Jeong, and D. S. Lim, 2012, Mesenchymal stem cell-mediated immature dendritic cells induce regulatory T cell-based immunosuppressive effect: Immunol Invest, v. 41, p. 214-29.

Chou, S. H., A. V. Shetty, Y. Geng, L. Xu, G. Munirathinam, A. Pipathsouk, I. Tan, T. Morris, B. Wang, A. Chen, and G. Zheng, 2013, Palmitate-derivatized human IL-2: a potential anticancer immunotherapeutic of low systemic toxicity: Cancer Immunol Immunother, v. 62, p. 597-603.

Chu, M. B., M. J. Fesler, E. S. Armbrecht, S. W. Fosko, E. Hsueh, and J. M. Richart, 2013, High-Dose Interleukin-2 (HD IL-2) Therapy Should Be Considered for Treatment of Patients with Melanoma Brain Metastases: Chemother Res Pract, v. 2013, p. 726925.

Clerici, M., and G. M. Shearer, 1993, A TH1-->TH2 switch is a critical step in the etiology of HIV infection: Immunol Today, v. 14, p. 107-11.

Colegio, O. R., C. M. Proby, J. S. Bordeaux, J. M. McGregor, and E. r. S. Melanoma Working Group of the International Transplant Skin Cancer Collaborative (ITSCC) & Skin Care in Organ Transplant Patients, 2009, Prognosis of pretransplant melanoma: Am J Transplant, v. 9, p. 862.

Contardi, E., G. L. Palmisano, P. L. Tazzari, A. M. Martelli, F. Falà, M. Fabbi, T. Kato, E. Lucarelli, D. Donati, L. Polito, A. Bolognesi, F. Ricci, S. Salvi, V. Gargaglione, S. Mantero, M. Alberghini, G. B. Ferrara, and M. P. Pistillo, 2005, CTLA-4 is constitutively expressed on tumor cells and can trigger apoptosis upon ligand interaction: Int J Cancer, v. 117, p. 538-50.

Crocetti, E., and P. Carli, 2004, Risk of second primary cancers, other than melanoma, in an Italian population-based cohort of cutaneous malignant melanoma patients: Eur J Cancer Prev, v. 13, p. 33-7.

Curti, A., S. Trabanelli, V. Salvestrini, M. Baccarani, and R. M. Lemoli, 2009, The role of indoleamine 2,3-dioxygenase in the induction of immune tolerance: focus on hematology: Blood, v. 113, p. 2394-401.

Dapprich, D. C., R. H. Weenig, A. L. Rohlinger, A. L. Weaver, K. K. Quan, J. H. Keeling, J. S. Walsh, C. C. Otley, and L. J. Christenson, 2008, Outcomes of melanoma in recipients of solid organ transplant: J Am Acad Dermatol, v. 59, p. 405-17.

de Vries, E., and J. W. Coebergh, 2004, Cutaneous malignant melanoma in Europe: Eur J Cancer, v. 40, p. 2355-66.

Den Otter, W., J. J. Jacobs, J. J. Battermann, G. J. Hordijk, Z. Krastev, E. V. Moiseeva, R. J. Stewart, P. G. Ziekman, and J. W. Koten, 2008, Local therapy of cancer with free IL-2: Cancer Immunol Immunother, v. 57, p. 931-50.

Dinh, Q. Q., and A. H. Chong, 2007, Melanoma in organ transplant recipients: the old enemy finds a new battleground: Australas J Dermatol, v. 48, p. 199-207.

Dong, C., and K. Hemminki, 2001, Second primary neoplasms among 53 159 haematolymphoproliferative malignancy patients in Sweden, 1958-1996: a search for common mechanisms: Br J Cancer, v. 85, p. 997-1005.

Dong, H., S. E. Strome, D. R. Salomao, H. Tamura, F. Hirano, D. B. Flies, P. C. Roche, J. Lu, G. Zhu, K. Tamada, V. A. Lennon, E. Celis, and L. Chen, 2002, Tumor-associated B7-H1 promotes T-cell apoptosis: a potential mechanism of immune evasion: Nat Med, v. 8, p. 793-800.

Donnelly, O., K. Harrington, A. Melcher, and H. Pandha, 2013, Live viruses to treat cancer: J R Soc Med, v. 106, p. 310-4.

Doudican, N., A. Rodriguez, I. Osman, and S. J. Orlow, 2008, Mebendazole induces apoptosis via Bcl-2 inactivation in chemoresistant melanoma cells: Mol Cancer Res, v. 6, p. 1308-15.

Doudican, N. A., S. A. Byron, P. M. Pollock, and S. J. Orlow, 2013, XIAP downregulation accompanies mebendazole growth inhibition in melanoma xenografts: Anticancer Drugs, v. 24, p. 181-8.

Dreno, B., 2003, Skin cancers after transplantation: Nephrol Dial Transplant, v. 18, p. 1052-8.

Dudley, M. E., J. R. Wunderlich, P. F. Robbins, J. C. Yang, P. Hwu, D. J. Schwartzentruber, S. L. Topalian, R. Sherry, N. P. Restifo, A. M. Hubicki, M. R. Robinson, M. Raffeld, P. Duray, C. A. Seipp, L. Rogers-Freezer, K. E. Morton, S. A. Mavroukakis, D. E. White, and S. A. Rosenberg, 2002, Cancer regression and autoimmunity in patients after clonal repopulation with antitumor lymphocytes: Science, v. 298, p. 850-4.

Dzwierzynski, W. W., 2013, Managing malignant melanoma: Plast Reconstr Surg, v. 132, p. 446e-60e.

Emeagi, P. U., S. Van Lint, C. Goyvaerts, S. Maenhout, A. Cauwels, I. A. McNeish, T. Bos, C. Heirman, K. Thielemans, J. L. Aerts, and K. Breckpot, 2012, Proinflammatory characteristics of SMAC/DIABLO-induced cell death in antitumor therapy: Cancer Res, v. 72, p. 1342-52.

Falkson, C. I., 1995, Experience with interferon alpha 2b combined with dacarbazine in the treatment of metastatic malignant melanoma: Med Oncol, v. 12, p. 35-40.

Farma, J. M., J. S. Zager, V. Barnica-Elvir, C. A. Puleo, S. S. Marzban, D. E. Rollison, J. L. Messina, and V. K. Sondak, 2013, A collision of diseases: chronic lymphocytic leukemia discovered during lymph node biopsy for melanoma: Ann Surg Oncol, v. 20, p. 1360-4.

Fekecs, T., Z. Kádár, Z. Battyáni, K. Kalmár-Nagy, P. Szakály, O. P. Horváth, G. Wéber, and A. Ferencz, 2010, Incidence of nonmelanoma skin cancer after human organ transplantation: single-center experience in Hungary: Transplant Proc, v. 42, p. 2333-5.

Frederick, D. T., A. Piris, A. P. Cogdill, Z. A. Cooper, C. Lezcano, C. R. Ferrone, D. Mitra, A. Boni, L. P. Newton, C. Liu, W. Peng, R. J. Sullivan, D. P. Lawrence, F. S. Hodi, W. W. Overwijk, G. Lizée, G. F. Murphy, P. Hwu, K. T. Flaherty, D. E. Fisher, and J. A. Wargo, 2013, BRAF inhibition is associated with enhanced melanoma antigen expression and a more favorable tumor microenvironment in patients with metastatic melanoma: Clin Cancer Res, v. 19, p. 1225-31.

Fu, H., S. Song, F. Liu, Z. Ni, Y. Tang, X. Shen, L. Xiao, G. Ding, and Q. Wang, 2009, Dendritic cells transduced with SOCS1 gene exhibit regulatory DC properties and prolong allograft survival: Cell Mol Immunol, v. 6, p. 87-95.

Galper, S., R. Gelman, A. Recht, B. Silver, A. Kohli, J. S. Wong, T. Van Buren, E. H. Baldini, and J. R. Harris, 2002, Second nonbreast malignancies after conservative surgery and radiation therapy for early-stage breast cancer: Int J Radiat Oncol Biol Phys, v. 52, p. 406-14.

Gogas, H., J. Ioannovich, U. Dafni, C. Stavropoulou-Giokas, K. Frangia, D. Tsoutsos, P. Panagiotou, A. Polyzos, O. Papadopoulos, A. Stratigos, C. Markopoulos, D. Bafaloukos, D. Pectasides, G. Fountzilas, and J. M. Kirkwood, 2006, Prognostic significance of autoimmunity during treatment of melanoma with interferon: N Engl J Med, v. 354, p. 709-18.

Goggins, W., W. Gao, and H. Tsao, 2004, Association between female breast cancer and cutaneous melanoma: Int J Cancer, v. 111, p. 792-4.

Goggins, W. B., D. M. Finkelstein, and H. Tsao, 2001, Evidence for an association between cutaneous melanoma and non-Hodgkin lymphoma: Cancer, v. 91, p. 874-80.

Goldstein, A. M., M. Chan, M. Harland, E. M. Gillanders, N. K. Hayward, M. F. Avril, E. Azizi, G. Bianchi-Scarra, D. T. Bishop, B. Bressac-de Paillerets, W. Bruno, D. Calista, L. A. Cannon Albright, F. Demenais, D. E. Elder, P. Ghiorzo, N. A. Gruis, J. Hansson, D. Hogg, E. A. Holland, P. A. Kanetsky, R. F. Kefford, M. T. Landi, J. Lang, S. A. Leachman, R. M. Mackie, V. Magnusson, G. J. Mann, K. Niendorf, J. Newton Bishop, J. M. Palmer, S. Puig, J. A. Puig-Butille, F. A. de Snoo, M. Stark, H. Tsao, M. A. Tucker, L. Whitaker, E. Yakobson, and M. G. C. (GenoMEL), 2006, High-risk melanoma susceptibility genes and pancreatic cancer, neural system tumors, and uveal melanoma across GenoMEL: Cancer Res, v. 66, p. 9818-28.

Gray-Schopfer, V., C. Wellbrock, and R. Marais, 2007, Melanoma biology and new targeted therapy: Nature, v. 445, p. 851-7.

Hansson, J., 2010, Familial cutaneous melanoma: Adv Exp Med Biol, v. 685, p. 134-45.

Hisada, M., R. J. Biggar, M. H. Greene, J. F. Fraumeni, and L. B. Travis, 2001, Solid tumors after chronic lymphocytic leukemia: Blood, v. 98, p. 1979-81.

Hodi, F. S., M. C. Mihm, R. J. Soiffer, F. G. Haluska, M. Butler, M. V. Seiden, T. Davis, R. Henry-Spires, S. MacRae, A. Willman, R. Padera, M. T. Jaklitsch, S. Shankar, T. C. Chen, A. Korman, J. P. Allison, and G. Dranoff, 2003, Biologic activity of cytotoxic T lymphocyte-associated antigen 4 antibody blockade in previously vaccinated metastatic melanoma and ovarian carcinoma patients: Proc Natl Acad Sci U S A, v. 100, p. 4712-7.

Hodi, F. S., S. J. O'Day, D. F. McDermott, R. W. Weber, J. A. Sosman, J. B. Haanen, R. Gonzalez, C. Robert, D. Schadendorf, J. C. Hassel, W. Akerley, A. J. van den Eertwegh, J. Lutzky, P. Lorigan, J. M. Vaubel, G. P. Linette, D. Hogg, C. H. Ottensmeier, C. Lebbé, C. Peschel, I. Quirt, J. I. Clark, J. D. Wolchok, J. S. Weber, J. Tian, M. J. Yellin, G. M. Nichol, A. Hoos, and W. J. Urba, 2010, Improved survival with ipilimumab in patients with metastatic melanoma: N Engl J Med, v. 363, p. 711-23.

Holmgaard, R. B., D. Zamarin, D. H. Munn, J. D. Wolchok, and J. P. Allison, 2013, Indoleamine 2,3-dioxygenase is a critical resistance mechanism in antitumor T cell immunotherapy targeting CTLA-4: J Exp Med, v. 210, p. 1389-402.

Hong, B., W. Ren, X. T. Song, K. Evel-Kabler, S. Y. Chen, and X. F. Huang, 2009, Human suppressor of cytokine signaling 1 controls immunostimulatory activity of monocyte-derived dendritic cells: Cancer Res, v. 69, p. 8076-84.

Itakura, E., R. R. Huang, D. R. Wen, E. Paul, P. H. Wünsch, and A. J. Cochran, 2011, IL-10 expression by primary tumor cells correlates with melanoma progression from radial to vertical growth phase and development of metastatic competence: Mod Pathol, v. 24, p. 801-9.

Jain, R. K., 2001, Normalizing tumor vasculature with anti-angiogenic therapy: a new paradigm for combination therapy: Nat Med, v. 7, p. 987-9.

Jain, R. K., 2005, Normalization of tumor vasculature: an emerging concept in antiangiogenic therapy: Science, v. 307, p. 58-62.

Jarmalavicius, S., Y. Welte, and P. Walden, 2012, High immunogenicity of the human leukocyte antigen peptidomes of melanoma tumor cells: J Biol Chem, v. 287, p. 33401-11.

Jensen, S. M., C. G. Twitty, L. D. Maston, P. A. Antony, M. Lim, H. M. Hu, U. Petrausch, N. P. Restifo, and B. A. Fox, 2012, Increased frequency of suppressive regulatory T cells and T cell-mediated antigen loss results in murine melanoma recurrence: J Immunol, v. 189, p. 767-76.

Ji, A. L., M. R. Baze, S. A. Davis, S. R. Feldman, and A. B. Fleischer, 2013, Ambulatory melanoma care patterns in the United States: J Skin Cancer, v. 2013, p. 689261.

Juhász, T., C. Matta, G. Veress, G. Nagy, Z. Szíjgyártó, Z. Molnár, J. Fodor, R. Zákány, and P. Gergely, 2009, Inhibition of calcineurin by cyclosporine A exerts multiple effects on human melanoma cell lines HT168 and WM35: Int J Oncol, v. 34, p. 995-1003.

Kasiske, B. L., J. J. Snyder, D. T. Gilbertson, and C. Wang, 2004, Cancer after kidney transplantation in the United States: Am J Transplant, v. 4, p. 905-13.

Kauffman, H. M., W. S. Cherikh, Y. Cheng, D. W. Hanto, and B. D. Kahan, 2005, Maintenance immunosuppression with target-of-rapamycin inhibitors is associated with a reduced incidence of de novo malignancies: Transplantation, v. 80, p. 883-9.

Khalili, J. S., S. Liu, T. G. Rodríguez-Cruz, M. Whittington, S. Wardell, C. Liu, M. Zhang, Z. A. Cooper, D. T. Frederick, Y. Li, R. W. Joseph, C. Bernatchez, S. Ekmekcioglu, E. Grimm, L. G. Radvanyi, R. E. Davis, M. A. Davies, J. A. Wargo, P. Hwu, and G. Lizée, 2012, Oncogenic BRAF(V600E) promotes stromal cell-mediated immunosuppression via induction of interleukin-1 in melanoma: Clin Cancer Res, v. 18, p. 5329-40.

Kipps, T. J., 2000, Chronic lymphocytic leukemia: Curr Opin Hematol, v. 7, p. 223-34.

Kirkwood, J. M., A. A. Tarhini, M. C. Panelli, S. J. Moschos, H. M. Zarour, L. H. Butterfield, and H. J. Gogas, 2008, Next generation of immunotherapy for melanoma: J Clin Oncol, v. 26, p. 3445-55.

Koehl, G. E., J. Andrassy, M. Guba, S. Richter, A. Kroemer, M. N. Scherer, M. Steinbauer, C. Graeb, H. J. Schlitt, K. W. Jauch, and E. K. Geissler, 2004, Rapamycin protects allografts from rejection while simultaneously attacking tumors in immunosuppressed mice: Transplantation, v. 77, p. 1319-26.

Kovach, B. T., and T. Stasko, 2009, Skin cancer after transplantation: Transplant Rev (Orlando), v. 23, p. 178-89.

Kubica, A. W., and J. D. Brewer, 2012, Melanoma in immunosuppressed patients: Mayo Clin Proc, v. 87, p. 991-1003.

Larkin, J., and M. Gore, 2008, Malignant melanoma (metastatic): Clin Evid (Online), v. 2008.

Leombruno, J. P., T. R. Einarson, and E. C. Keystone, 2009, The safety of anti-tumour necrosis factor treatments in rheumatoid arthritis: meta and exposure-adjusted pooled analyses of serious adverse events: Ann Rheum Dis, v. 68, p. 1136-45.

Levings, M. K., S. Allan, E. d'Hennezel, and C. A. Piccirillo, 2006, Functional dynamics of naturally occurring regulatory T cells in health and autoimmunity: Adv Immunol, v. 92, p. 119-55.

Lindelöf, B., B. Sigurgeirsson, H. Gäbel, and R. S. Stern, 2000, Incidence of skin cancer in 5356 patients following organ transplantation: Br J Dermatol, v. 143, p. 513-9.

Lindenberg, J. J., R. van de Ven, S. M. Lougheed, A. Zomer, S. J. Santegoets, A. W. Griffioen, E. Hooijberg, A. J. van den Eertwegh, V. L. Thijssen, R. J. Scheper, D. Oosterhoff, and T. D. de Gruijl, 2013, Functional characterization of a STAT3-dependent dendritic cell-derived CD14(+) cell population arising upon IL-10-driven maturation: Oncoimmunology, v. 2, p. e23837.

Little, E. G., and M. J. Eide, 2012, Update on the current state of melanoma incidence: Dermatol Clin, v. 30, p. 355-61.

Mackiewicz, J., and A. Mackiewicz, 2012, Recent advances in melanoma treatment - American Society of Clinical Oncology (ASCO) 2012 perspective: Contemp Oncol (Pozn), v. 16, p. 197-200.

Martínez-Lorenzo, M. J., A. Anel, M. A. Alava, A. Piñeiro, J. Naval, P. Lasierra, and L. Larrad, 2004, The human melanoma cell line MelJuSo secretes bioactive FasL and APO2L/TRAIL on the surface of microvesicles. Possible contribution to tumor counterattack: Exp Cell Res, v. 295, p. 315-29.

Matin, R. N., A. Chikh, S. L. Chong, D. Mesher, M. Graf, P. Sanza', V. Senatore, M. Scatolini, F. Moretti, I. M. Leigh, C. M. Proby, A. Costanzo, G. Chiorino, R. Cerio, C. A. Harwood, and D. Bergamaschi, 2013, p63 is an alternative p53 repressor in melanoma that confers chemoresistance and a poor prognosis: J Exp Med, v. 210, p. 581-603.

Matin, R. N., D. Mesher, C. M. Proby, J. M. McGregor, J. N. Bouwes Bavinck, V. del Marmol, S. Euvrard, C. Ferrandiz, A. Geusau, M. Hackethal, W. L. Ho, G. F. Hofbauer, B. Imko-Walczuk, J. Kanitakis, A. Lally, J. T. Lear, C. Lebbe, G. M. Murphy, S. Piaserico, D. Seckin, E. Stockfleth, C. Ulrich, F. T. Wojnarowska, H. Y. Lin, C. Balch, C. A. Harwood, and E. r. S. g. Skin Care in Organ Transplant Patients, 2008, Melanoma in organ transplant recipients: clinicopathological features and outcome in 100 cases: Am J Transplant, v. 8, p. 1891-900.

McCarter, M. D., J. Baumgartner, G. A. Escobar, D. Richter, K. Lewis, W. Robinson, C. Wilson, B. E. Palmer, and R. Gonzalez, 2007, Immunosuppressive dendritic and regulatory T cells are upregulated in melanoma patients: Ann Surg Oncol, v. 14, p. 2854-60.

McKenna, D. B., D. Stockton, D. H. Brewster, and V. R. Doherty, 2003, Evidence for an association between cutaneous malignant melanoma and lymphoid malignancy: a population-based retrospective cohort study in Scotland: Br J Cancer, v. 88, p. 74-8.

Meadows, A. T., D. L. Friedman, J. P. Neglia, A. C. Mertens, S. S. Donaldson, M. Stovall, S. Hammond, Y. Yasui, and P. D. Inskip, 2009, Second neoplasms in survivors of childhood cancer: findings from the Childhood Cancer Survivor Study cohort: J Clin Oncol, v. 27, p. 2356-62.

Middleton, M. R., J. J. Grob, N. Aaronson, G. Fierlbeck, W. Tilgen, S. Seiter, M. Gore, S. Aamdal, J. Cebon, A. Coates, B. Dreno, M. Henz, D. Schadendorf, A. Kapp, J. Weiss, U. Fraass, P. Statkevich, M. Muller, and N. Thatcher, 2000, Randomized phase III study of temozolomide versus dacarbazine in the treatment of patients with advanced metastatic malignant melanoma: J Clin Oncol, v. 18, p. 158-66.

Mikhail, M., E. Velazquez, R. Shapiro, R. Berman, A. Pavlick, L. Sorhaindo, J. Spira, C. Mir, K. S. Panageas, D. Polsky, and I. Osman, 2005, PTEN expression in melanoma: relationship with patient survival, Bcl-2 expression, and proliferation: Clin Cancer Res, v. 11, p. 5153-7.

Mills, A. A., B. Zheng, X. J. Wang, H. Vogel, D. R. Roop, and A. Bradley, 1999, p63 is a p53 homologue required for limb and epidermal morphogenesis: Nature, v. 398, p. 708-13.

Munir, S., S. K. Larsen, T. Z. Iversen, M. Donia, T. W. Klausen, I. M. Svane, P. T. Straten, and M. H. Andersen, 2012, Natural CD4+ T-cell responses against indoleamine 2,3-dioxygenase: PLoS One, v. 7, p. e34568.

Munn, D. H., M. D. Sharma, D. Hou, B. Baban, J. R. Lee, S. J. Antonia, J. L. Messina, P. Chandler, P. A. Koni, and A. L. Mellor, 2004, Expression of indoleamine 2,3-dioxygenase by plasmacytoid dendritic cells in tumor-draining lymph nodes: J Clin Invest, v. 114, p. 280-90.

Nasir, A., R. E. Shackelford, F. Anwar, and T. J. Yeatman, 2009, Genetic risk of breast cancer: Minerva Endocrinol, v. 34, p. 295-309.

Nestle, F. O., S. Alijagic, M. Gilliet, Y. Sun, S. Grabbe, R. Dummer, G. Burg, and D. Schadendorf, 1998, Vaccination of melanoma patients with peptide- or tumor lysate-pulsed dendritic cells: Nat Med, v. 4, p. 328-32.

Ngiow, S. F., D. A. Knight, A. Ribas, G. A. McArthur, and M. J. Smyth, 2013, BRAF-targeted therapy and immune responses to melanoma: Oncoimmunology, v. 2, p. e24462.

Otley, C. C., 2006, Non-Hodgkin lymphoma and skin cancer: A dangerous combination: Australas J Dermatol, v. 47, p. 231-6.

Otley, C. C., and M. R. Pittelkow, 2000, Skin cancer in liver transplant recipients: Liver Transpl, v. 6, p. 253-62.

Ott, P. A., J. Chang, K. Madden, R. Kannan, C. Muren, C. Escano, X. Cheng, Y. Shao, S. Mendoza, A. Gandhi, L. Liebes, and A. C. Pavlick, 2013, Oblimersen in combination with temozolomide and albumin-bound paclitaxel in patients with advanced melanoma: a phase I trial: Cancer Chemother Pharmacol, v. 71, p. 183-91.

Palucka, K., and J. Banchereau, 2012, Cancer immunotherapy via dendritic cells: Nat Rev Cancer, v. 12, p. 265-77.

Pappo, A. S., G. T. Armstrong, W. Liu, D. K. Srivastava, A. McDonald, W. M. Leisenring, S. Hammond, M. Stovall, J. P. Neglia, and L. L. Robison, 2013, Melanoma as a subsequent neoplasm in adult survivors of childhood cancer: a report from the childhood cancer survivor study: Pediatr Blood Cancer, v. 60, p. 461-6.

Patel, P., D. L. Hanson, P. S. Sullivan, R. M. Novak, A. C. Moorman, T. C. Tong, S. D. Holmberg, J. T. Brooks, and A. a. A. S. o. D. P. a. H. O. S. Investigators, 2008, Incidence of types of cancer among HIV-infected persons compared with the general population in the United States, 1992-2003: Ann Intern Med, v. 148, p. 728-36.

Paul, C. F., V. C. Ho, C. McGeown, E. Christophers, B. Schmidtmann, J. C. Guillaume, V. Lamarque, and L. Dubertret, 2003, Risk of malignancies in psoriasis patients treated with cyclosporine: a 5 y cohort study: J Invest Dermatol, v. 120, p. 211-6.

Penn, I., 1996, Malignant melanoma in organ allograft recipients: Transplantation, v. 61, p. 274-8.

Penn, I., 2000, Post-transplant malignancy: the role of immunosuppression: Drug Saf, v. 23, p. 101-13.

Pietra, G., C. Manzini, S. Rivara, M. Vitale, C. Cantoni, A. Petretto, M. Balsamo, R. Conte, R. Benelli, S. Minghelli, N. Solari, M. Gualco, P. Queirolo, L. Moretta, and M. C. Mingari, 2012, Melanoma cells inhibit natural killer cell function by modulating the expression of activating receptors and cytolytic activity: Cancer Res, v. 72, p. 1407-15.

Polak, M. E., N. J. Borthwick, F. G. Gabriel, P. Johnson, B. Higgins, J. Hurren, D. McCormick, M. J. Jager, and I. A. Cree, 2007, Mechanisms of local immunosuppression in cutaneous melanoma: Br J Cancer, v. 96, p. 1879-87.

Postow, M. A., J. Harding, and J. D. Wolchok, 2012, Targeting immune checkpoints: releasing the restraints on anti-tumor immunity for patients with melanoma: Cancer J, v. 18, p. 153-9.

Queirolo, P., A. Morabito, S. Laurent, S. Lastraioli, P. Piccioli, P. A. Ascierto, G. Gentilcore, M. Serra, A. Marasco, E. Tornari, B. Dozin, and M. P. Pistillo, 2013, Association of CTLA-4 polymorphisms with improved overall survival in melanoma patients treated with CTLA-4 blockade: a pilot study: Cancer Invest, v. 31, p. 336-45.

Quirt, I., S. Verma, T. Petrella, K. Bak, and M. Charette, 2007, Temozolomide for the treatment of metastatic melanoma: a systematic review: Oncologist, v. 12, p. 1114-23.

Raaschou, P., J. F. Simard, M. Holmqvist, J. Askling, and A. S. Group, 2013, Rheumatoid arthritis, anti-tumour necrosis factor therapy, and risk of malignant melanoma: nationwide population based prospective cohort study from Sweden: BMJ, v. 346, p. f1939.

Raaschou, P., J. F. Simard, M. Neovius, J. Askling, and A.-R. T. i. S. S. Group, 2011, Does cancer that occurs during or after anti-tumor necrosis factor therapy have a worse prognosis? A national assessment of overall and site-specific cancer survival in rheumatoid arthritis patients treated with biologic agents: Arthritis Rheum, v. 63, p. 1812-22.

Reuter, M. A., C. Pombo, and M. R. Betts, 2012, Cytokine production and dysregulation in HIV pathogenesis: lessons for development of therapeutics and vaccines: Cytokine Growth Factor Rev, v. 23, p. 181-91.

Ribas, A., 2007, Anti-CTLA4 Antibody Clinical Trials in Melanoma: Update Cancer Ther, v. 2, p. 133-139.

Ribas, A., R. Kefford, M. A. Marshall, C. J. Punt, J. B. Haanen, M. Marmol, C. Garbe, H. Gogas, J. Schachter, G. Linette, P. Lorigan, K. L. Kendra, M. Maio, U. Trefzer, M. Smylie, G. A. McArthur, B. Dreno, P. D. Nathan, J. Mackiewicz, J. M. Kirkwood, J. Gomez-Navarro, B. Huang, D. Pavlov, and A. Hauschild, 2013, Phase III randomized clinical trial comparing tremelimumab with standard-of-care chemotherapy in patients with advanced melanoma: J Clin Oncol, v. 31, p. 616-22.

Riou, J. P., S. Ariyan, K. R. Brandow, and L. P. Fielding, 1995, The association between melanoma, lymphoma, and other primary neoplasms: Arch Surg, v. 130, p. 1056-61.

Rodrigues, L. K., B. J. Klencke, K. Vin-Christian, T. G. Berger, R. I. Crawford, J. R. Miller, C. M. Ferreira, M. Nosrati, and M. Kashani-Sabet, 2002, Altered clinical course of malignant melanoma in HIV-positive patients: Arch Dermatol, v. 138, p. 765-70.

Rosenberg, S. A., M. T. Lotze, L. M. Muul, S. Leitman, A. E. Chang, S. E. Ettinghausen, Y. L. Matory, J. M. Skibber, E. Shiloni, and J. T. Vetto, 1985, Observations on the systemic administration of autologous lymphokine-activated killer cells and recombinant interleukin-2 to patients with metastatic cancer: N Engl J Med, v. 313, p. 1485-92.

Rosenberg, S. A., J. C. Yang, R. M. Sherry, U. S. Kammula, M. S. Hughes, G. Q. Phan, D. E. Citrin, N. P. Restifo, P. F. Robbins, J. R. Wunderlich, K. E. Morton, C. M. Laurencot, S. M. Steinberg, D. E. White, and M. E. Dudley, 2011, Durable complete responses in heavily pretreated patients with metastatic melanoma using T-cell transfer immunotherapy: Clin Cancer Res, v. 17, p. 4550-7.

Sasse, A. D., E. C. Sasse, L. G. Clark, L. Ulloa, and O. A. Clark, 2007, Chemoimmunotherapy versus chemotherapy for metastatic malignant melanoma: Cochrane Database Syst Rev, p. CD005413.

Satzger, I., A. Meier, F. Schenck, A. Kapp, A. Hauschild, and R. Gutzmer, 2007, Autoimmunity as a prognostic factor in melanoma patients treated with adjuvant low-dose interferon alpha: Int J Cancer, v. 121, p. 2562-6.

Schilling, B., A. Sucker, K. Griewank, F. Zhao, B. Weide, A. Görgens, B. Giebel, D. Schadendorf, and A. Paschen, 2013, Vemurafenib reverses immunosuppression by myeloid derived suppressor cells: Int J Cancer, v. 133, p. 1653-63.

Schreibelt, G., K. F. Bol, E. H. Aarntzen, W. R. Gerritsen, C. J. Punt, C. G. Figdor, and I. J. de Vries, 2013, Importance of helper T-cell activation in dendritic cell-based anticancer immunotherapy: Oncoimmunology, v. 2, p. e24440.

Semenza, G. L., 2003, Targeting HIF-1 for cancer therapy: Nat Rev Cancer, v. 3, p. 721-32.

Senzer, N. N., H. L. Kaufman, T. Amatruda, M. Nemunaitis, T. Reid, G. Daniels, R. Gonzalez, J. Glaspy, E. Whitman, K. Harrington, H. Goldsweig, T. Marshall, C. Love, R. Coffin, and J. J. Nemunaitis, 2009, Phase II clinical trial of a *granulocyte-macrophage colony-stimulating factor-encoding, second-generation oncolytic herpesvirus in patients with unresectable metastatic melanoma: J Clin Oncol, v. 27, p. 5763-71.*

Sevko, A., M. Sade-Feldman, J. Kanterman, T. Michels, C. S. Falk, L. Umansky, M. Ramacher, M. Kato, D. Schadendorf, M. Baniyash, and V. Umansky, 2013, Cyclophosphamide promotes chronic inflammation-dependent immunosuppression and prevents antitumor response in melanoma: J Invest Dermatol, v. 133, p. 1610-9.

Shang, B., Z. Cao, and Q. Zhou, 2012, Progress in tumor vascular normalization for anticancer therapy: challenges and perspectives: Front Med, v. 6, p. 67-78.

Silverberg, M. J., C. Chao, W. A. Leyden, L. Xu, M. A. Horberg, D. Klein, W. J. Towner, R. Dubrow, C. P. Quesenberry, R. S. Neugebauer, and D. I. Abrams, 2011, HIV infection, immunodeficiency, viral replication, and the risk of cancer: Cancer Epidemiol Biomarkers Prev, v. 20, p. 2551-9.

Sladden, M. J., C. Balch, D. A. Barzilai, D. Berg, A. Freiman, T. Handiside, S. Hollis, M. B. Lens, and J. F. Thompson, 2009, Surgical excision margins for primary cutaneous melanoma: Cochrane Database Syst Rev, p. CD004835.

Song, S., Y. Wang, J. Wang, W. Lian, S. Liu, Z. Zhang, F. Liu, and L. Wei, 2012, Tumour-derived IL-10 within tumour microenvironment represses the antitumour immunity of Socs1-silenced and sustained antigen expressing DCs: Eur J Cancer, v. 48, p. 2252-9.

Spano, J. P., D. Costagliola, C. Katlama, N. Mounier, E. Oksenhendler, and D. Khayat, 2008, AIDS-related malignancies: state of the art and therapeutic challenges: J Clin Oncol, v. 26, p. 4834-42.

Spanogle, J. P., C. A. Clarke, S. Aroner, and S. M. Swetter, 2010, Risk of second primary malignancies following cutaneous melanoma diagnosis: a population-based study: J Am Acad Dermatol, v. 62, p. 757-67.

Stein, C. A., S. Wu, A. M. Voskresenskiy, J. F. Zhou, J. Shin, P. Miller, N. Souleimanian, and L. Benimetskaya, 2009, G3139, an anti-Bcl-2 antisense oligomer that binds heparin-binding growth factors and collagen I, alters in vitro endothelial cell growth and tubular morphogenesis: Clin Cancer Res, v. 15, p. 2797-807.

Stockfleth, E., C. Ulrich, T. Meyer, and E. Christophers, 2002, Epithelial malignancies in organ transplant patients: clinical presentation and new methods of treatment: Recent Results Cancer Res, v. 160, p. 251-8.

Sully, K., O. Akinduro, M. P. Philpott, A. S. Naeem, C. A. Harwood, V. E. Reeve, R. F. O'Shaughnessy, and C. Byrne, 2013, The mTOR inhibitor rapamycin opposes carcinogenic changes to epidermal Akt1/PKBα isoform signaling: Oncogene, v. 32, p. 3254-62.

Tao, J., Y. Li, Y. Q. Liu, L. Li, J. Liu, X. Shen, G. X. Shen, and Y. T. Tu, 2008, Expression of transporters associated with antigen processing and human leucocyte antigen class I in malignant melanoma and its association with prognostic factors: Br J Dermatol, v. 158, p. 88-94.

Taube, J. M., R. A. Anders, G. D. Young, H. Xu, R. Sharma, T. L. McMiller, S. Chen, A. P. Klein, D. M. Pardoll, S. L. Topalian, and L. Chen, 2012, Colocalization of inflammatory response with B7-h1 expression in human melanocytic lesions supports an adaptive resistance mechanism of immune escape: Sci Transl Med, v. 4, p. 127ra37.

Thomadaki, H., and A. Scorilas, 2006, BCL2 family of apoptosis-related genes: functions and clinical implications in cancer: Crit Rev Clin Lab Sci, v. 43, p. 1-67.

Topalian, S. L., F. S. Hodi, J. R. Brahmer, S. N. Gettinger, D. C. Smith, D. F. McDermott, J. D. Powderly, R. D. Carvajal, J. A. Sosman, M. B. Atkins, P. D. Leming, D. R. Spigel, S. J. Antonia, L. Horn, C. G. Drake, D. M. Pardoll, L. Chen, W. H. Sharfman, R. A. Anders, J. M. Taube, T. L. McMiller, H. Xu, A. J. Korman, M. Jure-Kunkel, S. Agrawal, D. McDonald, G. D. Kollia, A. Gupta, J. M. Wigginton, and M. Sznol, 2012, Safety, activity, and immune correlates of anti-PD-1 antibody in cancer: N Engl J Med, v. 366, p. 2443-54.

Travis, L. B., R. E. Curtis, J. D. Boice, B. F. Hankey, and J. F. Fraumeni, 1991, Second cancers following non-Hodgkin's lymphoma: Cancer, v. 67, p. 2002-9.

Travis, L. B., R. E. Curtis, B. F. Hankey, and J. F. Fraumeni, 1992, Second cancers in patients with chronic lymphocytic leukemia: J Natl Cancer Inst, v. 84, p. 1422-7.

Tsimberidou, A. M., S. Wen, P. McLaughlin, S. O'Brien, W. G. Wierda, S. Lerner, S. Strom, E. J. Freireich, L. J. Medeiros, H. M. Kantarjian, and M. J. Keating, 2009, Other malignancies in chronic lymphocytic leukemia/small lymphocytic lymphoma: J Clin Oncol, v. 27, p. 904-10.

Turcotte, S., A. Gros, K. Hogan, E. Tran, C. S. Hinrichs, J. R. Wunderlich, M. E. Dudley, and S. A. Rosenberg, 2013, Phenotype and Function of T Cells Infiltrating Visceral Metastases from Gastrointestinal Cancers and Melanoma: Implications for Adoptive Cell Transfer Therapy: J Immunol.

Viguier, M., F. Lemaître, O. Verola, M. S. Cho, G. Gorochov, L. Dubertret, H. Bachelez, P. Kourilsky, and L. Ferradini, 2004, Foxp3 expressing CD4+CD25(high) regulatory T cells are overrepresented in human metastatic melanoma lymph nodes and inhibit the function of infiltrating T cells: J Immunol, v. 173, p. 1444-53.

Vucic, D., K. Deshayes, H. Ackerly, M. T. Pisabarro, S. Kadkhodayan, W. J. Fairbrother, and V. M. Dixit, 2002, SMAC negatively regulates the anti-apoptotic activity of melanoma inhibitor of apoptosis (ML-IAP): J Biol Chem, v. 277, p. 12275-9.

Wang, Z. E., S. L. Reiner, S. Zheng, D. K. Dalton, and R. M. Locksley, 1994, CD4+ effector cells default to the Th2 pathway in interferon gamma-deficient mice infected with Leishmania major: J Exp Med, v. 179, p. 1367-71.

Wasif, N., R. J. Gray, S. P. Bagaria, and B. A. Pockaj, 2013, Compliance with guidelines in the surgical management of cutaneous melanoma across the USA: Melanoma Res, v. 23, p. 276-82.

Wierda, W. G., M. J. Cantwell, S. J. Woods, L. Z. Rassenti, C. E. Prussak, and T. J. Kipps, 2000, CD40-ligand (CD154) gene therapy for chronic lymphocytic leukemia: Blood, v. 96, p. 2917-24.

Wilkins, K., R. Turner, J. C. Dolev, P. E. LeBoit, T. G. Berger, and T. A. Maurer, 2006, Cutaneous malignancy and human immunodeficiency virus disease: J Am Acad Dermatol, v. 54, p. 189-206; quiz 207-10.

Wisgerhof, H. C., J. R. Edelbroek, J. W. de Fijter, G. W. Haasnoot, F. H. Claas, R. Willemze, and J. N. Bavinck, 2010, Subsequent squamous- and basal-cell carcinomas in kidney-transplant recipients after the first skin cancer: cumulative incidence and risk factors: Transplantation, v. 89, p. 1231-8.

Wolchok, J. D., and Y. Saenger, 2008, The mechanism of anti-CTLA-4 activity and the negative regulation of T-cell activation: Oncologist, v. 13 Suppl 4, p. 2-9.

Wrzesinski, C., C. M. Paulos, A. Kaiser, P. Muranski, D. C. Palmer, L. Gattinoni, Z. Yu, S. A. Rosenberg, and N. P. Restifo, 2010, Increased intensity lymphodepletion enhances tumor treatment efficacy of adoptively transferred tumor-specific T cells: J Immunother, v. 33, p. 1-7.

Wu, R., M. A. Forget, J. Chacon, C. Bernatchez, C. Haymaker, J. Q. Chen, P. Hwu, and L. G. Radvanyi, 2012, Adoptive T-cell therapy using autologous tumor-infiltrating lymphocytes for metastatic melanoma: current status and future outlook: Cancer J, v. 18, p. 160-75.

Zavos, G., N. P. Karidis, G. Tsourouflis, J. Bokos, K. Diles, G. Sotirchos, E. Theodoropoulou, and A. Kostakis, 2011, Nonmelanoma skin cancer after renal transplantation: a single-center experience in 1736 transplantations: Int J Dermatol, v. 50, p. 1496-500.

Zhang, Q. J., R. P. Seipp, S. S. Chen, T. Z. Vitalis, X. L. Li, K. B. Choi, A. Jeffries, and W. A. Jefferies, 2007, TAP expression reduces IL-10 expressing tumor infiltrating lymphocytes and restores immunosurveillance against melanoma: Int J Cancer, v. 120, p. 1935-41.

Zheng, Y., M. T. Stephan, S. A. Gai, W. Abraham, A. Shearer, and D. J. Irvine, 2013, In vivo targeting of adoptively transferred T-cells with antibody- and cytokine-conjugated liposomes: J Control Release.

Zitelli, J. A., C. Brown, and B. H. Hanusa, 1997, Mohs micrographic surgery for the treatment of primary cutaneous melanoma: J Am Acad Dermatol, v. 37, p. 236-45.

Zwald, F. O., L. J. Christenson, E. M. Billingsley, N. C. Zeitouni, D. Ratner, J. Bordeaux, M. J. Patel, M. D. Brown, C. M. Proby, S. Euvrard, C. C. Otley, T. Stasko, and E. r. Melanoma Working Group of The International Transplant Skin Cancer Collaborative and Skin Care in Organ Transplant Patients, 2010, Melanoma in solid organ transplant recipients: Am J Transplant, v. 10, p. 1297-304.

A Local Comprehensive Evaluation of New Radiosurgery Technology:
An Analytical and Methodological Approach

Jeffrey Noah Greenspoon
Division of Radiation Oncology, Department of Oncology
McMaster University, Canada

1   Introduction

In Ontario radiation treatment delivery resources (megavoltage linear accelerators) are assigned to individual cancer centres based on population size and radiation treatment utilization, by Cancer Care Ontario (CCO). There are fourteen cancer centres in Ontario providing radiotherapy. Each cancer centre serves a different population and the capacity of each treatment centre ranges from two to seventeen linear accelerators. Each cancer centre has a relatively fixed number of linear accelerators and thus a fixed capacity to perform radiotherapy. In the year 2010 in Ontario the average number of radiation courses delivered by a megavoltage machine was 550 (Cancer Quality Council of Ontario) Radiation therapy wait times are also closely monitored by CCO. For non urgent cases it is expected that patients will begin radiotherapy within two weeks of the decision to proceed with treatment (Cancer Quality Council of Ontario). Due to the relatively fixed infrastructure capacity and the large capital investment that is required when allocating radiation oncology equipment local evaluation of substitutable technologies prior to technology adoption is typically not possible. Evaluation by CCO is typically done in retrospect to aid in future technology allocation decisions. To address the need to analytically evaluate substitutable technologies in Radiation Oncology we discuss a three part methodology that can function as a template for a health technology assessment of substitutable technology in Radiation Oncology. The first part of this evaluation of two radiotherapy technologies is a needs assessment to evaluate the local need for the new radiotherapy resource. If sufficient need is demonstrated to warrant the new technology then either a decision analytic model or a small prospective trial is performed to evaluate the variable costs of the new technology. There is no need to formally evaluate differences in fixed cost because these are known values e.g. purchase price, installation and setup. Finally a local cost-benefit analysis to evaluate the local societal benefit is performed using willingness-to-pay methodology. At the conclusion of this three part health technology assessment local decision makers will have enough information to make an explicit, community supported decision regarding new technology adoption when deciding between substitutable technologies. We will introduce this methodology and show its applicability using the example of dedicated robotic radiosurgery compared to standard flexible fixed gantry radiosurgery for the treatment of brain metastases.

2   Background-radiosurgery and Technology Evaluation

Radiosurgery is a rapidly emerging technology in Radiation Oncology in Ontario. It offers a non-invasive alternative to surgery in properly selected cases (Muacevic & Wowra 2008, Andrews *et al.*, 2004, Linskey *et al.*, 2010). Although the majority of patients treated with radiosurgery in Ontario are those with brain metastases from a primary tumour, the clinical indications for radiosurgery are expanding. Encouraging clinical trial results have been reported for the primary treatment of early stage lung cancer, prostate cancer, liver metastases, bone metastases and a number of benign tumours. (Roberge *et al.*, 2010). There are as well open clinical trials evaluating new indications for radiosurgery in Ontario. (Ryu, 2011, Lukka, 2011, Greenspoon, 2011). Although the treatment of brain metastases is with palliative intent, aggressive local management with radiosurgery has led to both improved survival and quality of life (Andrews *et al.*, 2004, Linskey ME *et al.*, 2010, Sperduto *et al.*, 2008). Although there are alternatives in the management of brain metastases (e.g. surgery, whole brain radiation therapy and supportive care) this evaluation focuses on providing a delivery method for radiosurgery once the decision between alternative treatments has been reached. (Roberge *et al.*, 2010, Sperduto *et al.*, 2008).

Radiosurgery can be delivered in two broad ways. Individual Cancer Centres can purchase equipment to modify a traditional linear accelerator to provide radiosurgery on a conventional machine. This flexible unit can then provide conventional radiotherapy when it is not performing radiosurgery (Boudreau *et al.*, 2009). Alternatively, a Cancer Centre can allocate a permanent part of its radiation treatment capacity to performing radiosurgery through the purchase of a new dedicated radiosurgery unit. Although this unit will be unable to perform conventional radiation treatments it has the ability to perform complex radiosurgery treatments (Boudreau *et al.*, 2009). A dedicated radiosurgery unit can likely provide radiosurgery in a shorter time than a flexible unit through streamlined treatment planning and machine quality assurance (Greenspoon, 2011, Boudreau *et al.*, 2009). We will highlight and discuss the advantages and limitations of this methodology by performing a pilot substitutable technology evaluation of a dedicated robotic radiosurgery unit compared to a standard fixed gantry radiosurgery unit for the treatment of brain metastases. Formal evaluation in a local environment would involve more depth in data collection and analysis.

3   An Analytical Methodology to Perform Technological Requirement Planning

3.1   Background

Using the framework for workforce planning by (Birch *et al.*) we can perform an explicit need based assessment for radiosurgery in Ontario. This method explicitly breaks down machine use into three interacting factors. The main strength of this methodology is the explicit evidence informed inputs that relate population size to technology need. The needs based approach to workforce planning can be described as follows:

$$N_t = (N/Q)_t \times (Q/H)_t \times (H/P)_t \times P_t$$

This equation relates current healthcare system need N_t to the size of the population P_t multiplied by three factors that relate population to need. H represents the level of health (or illness) in the population P_t. $(H/P)_t$ is an epidemiological term to describe the current average health status of individuals in the population. Explicitly defining an epidemiological term allows for needs adjustments due to a change in health status when planning between current populations. This term also allows for epidemiological changes when planning for the future population P_{t+1}. For example new surgical technique may significantly decrease local tumour recurrences and therefore decrease future illness (H_{t+1}). Thus despite a future population growth the average need per person of our future population would decrease $(H/P)_{t+1}$. Q_t represents the current quantity of health services delivered. $(Q/H)_t$ represents the quantity of service provided for a specific health state. This term allows for the explicit consideration of changes in the indications for care. For example, until recently patients with small lung tumours were not considered appropriate for radiosurgery. Recently, with the publication of clinical efficacy trials it is now known that selected patients with small lung tumours benefit from radiosurgery (Roberge *et al.*, 2010). Therefore, where ten years ago the planned amount of radiosurgery given for small lung tumour was $(Q/H)_{t-10} = 0$, there are now selected patients with small lung tumours where radiosurgery is the treatment of choice $(Q/H)_t > 0$. The third term in the equation relates to productivity of a treatment modality. For the purposes of this paper it is the inverse of the productivity of each radiosurgery method being examined $(N/Q)_t$. Thus as the productivity of a treatment modality increases the number of machines needed to fulfill the population need decreases assuming all other aspects of healthcare need are equal. Although there are currently no randomized comparisons of two radiosurgery techniques in the Ontario environment, subgroup analyses of a randomized trial has demonstrated equivalence in terms of efficacy (Andrews *et al.*, 2004) and there is an ongoing open randomized trial in Ontario (Greenspoon, 2011). This trial will compare the process of delivering radiosurgery for both a dedicated radiosurgery unit and a flexible unit. This will inform the community of the relative productivity of each unit which will enable more accurate needs assessments and future economic evaluations to be performed (Greenspoon, 2011).

3.2   An Application of the Analytical Approach to Radiosurgery Planning: Single Brain Metastases

Using the above method as a framework, we will explicitly describe each term in the above analytical model to describe the current need for radiosurgery for single brain metastases. We will also hypothesize how each term may change over the ten year life of capital radiotherapy technology in Ontario. The purpose of this example is to highlight the use of this methodology not to provide valid results.

The most straightforward term is P_t. The Ontario population in 2009 was approximately 13.0 million (Statistics Canada: 2009 Census). Using an estimated 1% population growth per year the Ontario population at the end of our ten year technology cycle would be 14.4 million.

The epidemiological term for need $(H/P)_t$ can be estimated using the current published literature. We do not believe that estimating the current need for radiosurgery based on use is appropriate. Current use may underestimate the current epidemiological need for two major reasons. First radiosurgery is a relatively new technology and some primary oncologists may not be aware of its indications. Second radiosurgical resources in Ontario are located exclusively in large urban cancer centres which may limit the access of some members of the population to this resource (Birch & Chambers, 1993). For these reasons we will rely on the published literature to assess the current epidemiological need.

Brain metastases are reported to occur in up to 50% of patients with the diagnosis of cancer (Pickren *et al.*, 1983, Posner & Chernik, 1978). Additionally, up to 40% of patients with brain metastasis will present with a single lesion (Posner & Chernik, 1978, Mheta *et al.*, 1997). It is estimated that there are approximately 60,000 new cancer cases per year in Ontario, resulting in up to 12,000 patients per year presenting with a single brain metastasis (Cancer Quality Council of Ontario). Approximately 50% of these patients will require an operative procedure for emergent symptom resolution or tissue diagnosis leaving 6,000 patients in Ontario every year for the elective management of a single brain metastasis from all primary tumour sites (CQCI, Mheta *et al.*, 1997, Caroli *et al.*, 2011). With the current size of the population of 13.0 million there are 6000 potential cases for radiosurgery for a single brain metastasis or 0.05% of the population. If one had access to high quality local data regarding the incidence of urgent and elective presentations of single brain metastases then one could substitute local data to calculate the above percentage.

This incidence of brain metastases is currently rising (Chang *et al.*, 2007). It has been hypothesized that a decrease in cancer specific mortality, improvements in systemic therapy and the relative protection of the brain from systemic therapy are responsible for the rising incidence of brain metastases (Linskey *et al.*, 2010, Roberge *et al.*, 2010, Chang *et al.*, 2007). We therefore hypothesize that the future epidemiological need for radiosurgery for single brain metastases will increase over time $((H/P)_{t+10} > (H/P)_t)$.

As described above approximately 6000 patients in Ontario are potentially eligible for radiosurgery for single brain metastases (potential $(Q/H)_t$). There are other treatments options available to patients with a single brain metastasis (neurosurgery, conventional radiation, supportive care). There are many patient and physician factors that are involved in treatment modality decisions. It is beyond the scope of this paper to estimate how this decision making may change over time. We will therefore not assume a change in patient and physician preference when estimating $(Q/H)_{t+10}$. Alternatively radiosurgery is a relatively new modality in Ontario. Within one year of the introduction of radiosurgery to the Juravinski Cancer Centre at McMaster University we have observed an increase in the referral rate for radiosurgery for a single brain metastasis (Schultz *et al.,* 2011). This is thought to be due to the education of community oncologists, the creation of multidisciplinary team care for metastatic disease and a population based focus on quality of life. Although there is likely a ceiling effect once most oncologists and patients are educated and informed of the treatment options, it seems reasonable to assume that the proportionate amount of radiosurgery performed for patients with a single brain metastasis will increase over the next ten years $((Q/H)_{t+10} > (Q/H)_t)$.

The final term to discuss is related to technical productivity. In radiosurgery the technical productivity $(Q/N)_t$ is measured as the number of courses of radiotherapy delivered per year. In Ontario CCO assumes a ten hour work day, five days a week. Technical productivity is a simple measure of a very complex process. Each patient requires immobilization device fitting, radiotherapy planning and quality assurance prior to beginning therapy. The average number of courses of radiotherapy delivered per unit yearly in Ontario is 550 $(Q/N)_t=550$ (Cancer Quality Council of Ontario). When planning for radiosurgical needs, as the technical productivity improves the number of physical units needed to deliver the necessary care decrease. Therefore, the term in the resource planning model is the inverse of the technical productivity $(N/Q)_t$. Although radiosurgery can be very time consuming and complex it is reasonable to assume that the technical productivity of radiosurgery will improve analogous to the technical productivity of all radiotherapy. In Ontario there has been a 9% improvement in technical productivity from 2008/2009 to 2009/2010 (Cancer Quality Council of Ontario). It seems unreasonable to plan for a continued 9% yearly productivity improvement. Decision makers would be in a better position to plan for future productivity; however for modeling purposed we will assume a 1% productivity improvement per year over the ten year life cycle of our radiosurgical equipment. This means that in ten years we could expect the average technical productivity to be 607 yearly courses/unit $(Q/N)_{t+10}$.

Decision makers should also use this methodology to perform sensitivity analyses by varying the values of each parameter in the model based on how they are predicted to change over time or where there is uncertainty in the result. Once this model has been completed using local data it will be clear if there is enough local need to justify the adoption of a dedicated radiosurgery unit. If there is not enough local demand for a dedicated radiosurgery unit then the evaluation can conclude that the adoption of (as per our example) a dedicated radiosurgery unit is not a responsible use of resources at the present time. Using the example of single brain metastases we have demonstrated that an explicit analytical model to estimate technology need is feasible to perform. The key strength of this methodology is the ability to explicitly define the model inputs. These variables can therefore be based on data from the local environment and meaningful multi-way or probabilistic sensitivity analyses can be performed (Birch *et al.,* 2007, Birch & Chambers, 1993, Buxton MJ *et al.,* 1997, Briggs AH 2000, Gafni A). If local need for a dedicated radiosurgery unit is demonstrated then either a local pragmatic comparison or a decision analytic model can be developed.

3.3   Application of the Analytical Model to Current Radiosurgical Requirement

Using the information above we are able to populate the analytical model introduced by (Birch *et al.*) to calculate the current radiosurgical need in Ontario for patients with a single brain metastasis. P_t = 13 million, $(H/P)_t$ = 0.05% = 0.0005, $(Q/H)_t$ = 50% (Range of Values Tested 25% – 75%) = 0.5(0.25 – 0.75), $(N/Q)_t$ = 1/550 (Range tested 1/400 – 1/650) = 0.0018 (0.0015 – 0.0025). Using the above values the number of full time radiosurgical units required in Ontario to meet the needs of patients with single brain metastases is N_t = 5.9. Performing an extreme value sensitivity analysis with the range of values above we see that the range of radiosurgical machine requirement for single brain metastases is from $N_{t(low)}$ = 2.5- $N_{t(high)}$ = 12.2. We have allowed one decimal point in our calculation of full time radiosurgery machine requirements because, as described above some linear accelerators have the flexibility to perform both conventional radiotherapy as well as radiosurgery. This large range is driven by the range of values tested for $(Q/H)_t$. To narrow this range one could seek local patient and physician preferences to accurately estimate the local $(Q/H)_t$. Using this model we can incorporate expected future changes to each term in the needs assessment to allow decision makers to plan for the future technology and human resource needs in radiosurgery in Ontario. For example if the population of patients with a single brain metastasis increases and radiosurgery machine productivity increases by a similar proportion there may not be a need to increase future radiosurgery capacity.

4   Evaluation of Variable Costs of Each Technology

Although the fixed cost is a large component of the cost per patient treated with radiosurgery, the variable cost is equally important when considering the total cost per patient treated to aid in resource allocation decisions (Cancer Quality Council of Ontario). Fixed costs will be assessed as part of the full economic evaluation introduced in section 3. In order to understand the differences in variable costs between two potential units two methods can be undertaken. An individual cancer centre that has access to both units can perform a pragmatic randomized trial (Greenspoon, 2011). This trial should be designed to evaluate the variable costs associated with performing radiosurgery on both units. Therefore the process of delivering radiosurgery on each unit should be explicitly outlined and time data should be gathered in as unbiased a way as possible given the limitations of not being able to blind either the patient or the treatment unit staff. At the Juravinski Cancer Centre we have developed a common process for radiosurgery planning and delivery designed to evaluate the variable costs associated with performing radiosurgery on both a flexible fixed gantry radiosurgery unit and a dedicated robotic radiosurgery unit. The process is broken down as follows: 1) Immobilization device fitting 2) CT simulation 3) Treatment planning 4) Treatment delivery. A small randomized trial designed to capture a meaningful difference in treatment planning/delivery time would provide the necessary data to model differences in the variable costs between both units. Breaking down the process into four component parts allows one to factor in differences in the expertise of the personnel required at each step in the process. For example, one could hypothesize that the total treatment process time of both units was identical but the treatment planning time was significantly longer using fixed gantry radiosurgery. With the breakdown of the total process into four component parts, this trial would capture a variable cost difference between the units because treatment planning involves the expertise of many professionals with relatively high salaries.

Many cancer centres in Canada will not have the capacity to compare two units because the community need will only require one unit. In these circumstances a decision analytic model can be developed with estimates for the time and resources required at each step in the radiosurgery treatment planning/delivery process (Buxton *et al.*, 1997). Multi-way sensitivity analyses should also be performed varying the time required at each step in the process within reasonable limits. Local data for many of the aspects of treatment planning and delivery will be available from analysis of current practice and can be used as a point estimate to populate the model. An individual cancer centre can further improve the validity of the model by seeking time and resource utilization data from other Canadian cancer centres with the new technology being evaluated to improve the validity of the results obtained. This modelling method provides more uncertainty in the estimate of variable cost than does a direct observation trial but may be the only method available to most Canadian Cancer Centres (Briggs, 2000).

The data gathered from either the trial or the model based comparison can be used to calculate the true incremental cost of a new substitutable Radiation Oncology technology e.g. dedicated robotic radiosurgery. The variable cost for both technologies is calculated from the trial or model can be combined with the known fixed cost. Using appropriate amortization rates and salary inflation one could then calculate the yearly incremental cost of providing the new technology in the local environment. If the process of delivering treatment is much more efficient with the newer expensive technology it is feasible that the incremental cost of the new technology could be $0 or even a cost savings. Using the incremental yearly cost calculated in this pragmatic comparison one can then proceed to perform a local economic evaluation.

5   Economic Evaluation: Cost-benefit Analysis using Willingness-to-pay

5.1   Background

A full economic evaluation of two technologies involves a comparison of both the cost and outcomes of two technologies (Gafni, 1996). A complete comparison of the cost and therefore the incremental cost is available from part 2) of the methodology described above. It is much more difficult to compare outcomes (both efficacy and quality of life) when evaluating two substitutable technologies in Radiation Oncology. Regarding clinical efficacy, current international protocols examining radiosurgery for brain metastases do not specify or suggest a specific method of delivery of radiosurgery (Brown *et al.*, 2008, Brown & Roberge, 2011). A large randomized trial and a matched pair analysis have shown no difference in clinical outcome for multiple methods of delivering radiosurgery for brain metastases (Andrews *et al.*, 2004, Wowra *et al.*, 2009). This equivalent efficacy is consistent with the physics and biology of radiosurgery. Radiosurgery delivers high dose, ablative radiotherapy with sub-millimetre accuracy. Any type of hardware that can deliver these high doses with precision will accomplish equivalent tumour ablation.

When comparing quality of life in an economic evaluation, utilities (preferences) are compared in a cost-utility analysis. However, the main difference between robotic and fixed gantry radiosurgery is patient comfort during a 1 – 2 hour procedure. It would be extremely difficult to capture differences in health utility scores that are typically averaged over a one year period (e.g. Quality Adjusted Life Years) (Rabin & Charro 2001). For that reason a cost-utility analysis would underestimate the quality of life benefit experienced with a two hour intervention. A cost comparison is able to evaluate differences in short term costs, long term costs and total budget impact, however, unlike cost-benefit and cost-effectiveness analyses it fails to consider patient or population preferences when selecting between available technologies (Gafni, 1996). When evaluating substitutable technologies in radiation oncology a cost-benefit analysis using decision boards and willingness to pay is an explicit method to help identify the societal benefit of a new technology and therefore the technology most suited to the local environment. Using this methodology incremental cost will be the difference in total cost (fixed+variable) between both technologies (Gafni, 1996). Benefit would be ascertained using local tax payer directed decision boards and willingness-to-pay methodology. Cost-benefit methodology provides a method to seek community involvement in directing decision makers when allocating resources between two substitutable technologies. By seeking tax-payer opinion different communities will have different thresholds to what is a cost-effective technology making this methodology transportable to any community. As an outline we will describe decision boards and the creation of a willingness-to-pay question as well as the strengths and weaknesses of this approach.

5.2   Cost

Both robotic radiosurgery and linear accelerator radiosurgery are physically interchangeable technologies. If a Cancer Centre elects to purchase a robotic linear accelerator to meet the need of the community they would not need to purchase a fixed gantry linear accelerator as well. The JCC at McMaster University is the third largest cancer centre in the province and it serves a region of 1.5 million residents (1.0 million tax payers) (Statistics Canada: 2009 Census). This large size has allowed the JCC to have the need to support both a robotic and fixed gantry radiosurgery linear accelerators. This allows us to have accurate local fixed and variable costs. Fixed costs consist of capital purchase, renovation, annual operations, immobilization device purchase and centre overhead. Variable costs include the human resource costs associated with immobilization device fitting, treatment planning, quality assurance, treatment delivery, nursing and physician costs. Direct cost data has been directly acquired from JCC purchase renovation and installation costs at the time of purchase of both units in 2009. Immobilization device unit costs were directly acquired from the JCC based on the centres current purchase and shipping price. The JCC employs an electronics and machinery department for annual operations and therefore does not purchase warranties from manufacturers. Variable costs were assumed to be the same for both robotic and fixed gantry radiosurgery. At the time of the publication of this report there was no data to suggest that the process of planning and delivering radiosurgery was different for each approach. The process of planning and delivering radiosurgery would influence the variable cost. There is an ongoing clinical trial based at the JCC evaluating the difference in process between robotic and fixed gantry radiosurgery to accurately estimate the variable cost associated with each approach for treating brain metastases. Preliminary data from this trial as well as expert opinion suggest that robotic radiosurgery can be delivered in a slightly shorter time that fixed gantry radiosurgery (Sperduto *et al.*, 2008).

     This evaluation is comparing robotic to fixed gantry radiosurgery, we are therefore interested in the incremental cost of providing robotic radiosurgery. Costs that are the same between both arms will cancel each other out when the incremental costs are calculated ($C_{robotic} - C_{fixed}$). As outlined above for this evaluation variable costs are assumed to be the same for both technologies. Among the fixed costs both centre overhead and annual operating costs were assumed to be equal for both technologies. Since these machines are substitutable for each other and they occupy the same physical space, centre overheads would be equal for both technologies. As well since the JCC has a dedicated robotics and machinery department, the annual operating cost would be the same for both units.

5.3   Utilization

A full time radiosurgery unit should treat 550 courses yearly as outlined by CCO. Using the CCO radiation utilization nomenclature each metastasis treated is one course of treatment, therefore when a patient has 1-3 brain metastases they may receive 1, 2 or 3 courses of radiotherapy (Cancer Quality Council of Ontario). Using JCC specific data since July 2010 among patients with 1 – 3 brain metastases treated, 45% had one lesion, 39% had two lesions, and 16% had three lesions (Schultz *et al.,* 2011). Using these numbers the average patient with 1 – 3 brain metastases received 1.7 courses of radiosurgery. Therefore, in order to deliver 550 courses of brain metastasis radiosurgery the JCC would need to treat 325 patients.

Fixed Cost Robotic Radiosurgery

Purchase Price = $4,300,000CAD

Renovation (JCC Specific) = $600,000CAD

TOTAL UPFRONT INVESTMENT = $4,900,000CAD

TOTAL YEARLY INVESTMENT (assuming 5% amortization and 10 year replacement) = $623,666CAD

Immobilization device unit cost = $35CAD

Yearly number of patients with 1 – 3 brain metastases treated on unit = 325

YEARLY IMMOBILIZATION COST = $11,375CAD = 325 × $35CAD

TOTAL YEARLY FIXED COST = $635,041CAD = $623,666CAD + $11,375CAD

Fixed Cost Fixed-Gantry Linear Accelerator

Purchase Price = $3,150,540CAD

Renovation Cost (JCC Specific) = $600,000CAD

TOTAL UPFRONT INVESTEMENT = $3,750,540CAD

TOTAL YEARLY INVESTMENT (assuming 5% amortization rate and 10 year replacement) = $477,364CAD

Immobilization device unit cost = $180CAD

Yearly number of patients with 1 – 3 brain metastases treated on unit = 325

YEARLY IMMOBILIZATION COST = $58,500CAD = 325 × $180CAD

TOTAL YEARLY FIXED COST = $535,864CAD = $477,364CAD + $58,500CAD

INCREMENTAL COST OF ROBOTIC COMPARED TO FIXED GANTRY RADIOSURGERY = $635,041CAD – $535,864CAD = $99,177CAD/year.

5.4   Tax-payer Directed Decision Board

Decision boards involve the creation of a decision aid to break down a complex decision into component parts. These aids have been shown to improve patient comprehension of complex decisions in oncology (Whelan *et al.,* 1999, Whelan *et al.,* 2004). Decision boards have been shown to improve patient under-standing and satisfaction with their decision in both complex radiotheraputic and chemotherapeutic deci-sions (Whelan *et al.,* 1999, Whelan *et al.,* 2004). By breaking down a complex decision, decision boards explicitly elicit patient preferences prior to making a decision (Whelan *et al.,* 1999). In the setting of sub-stitutable technologies in radiosurgery a decision board can be created that is presented to members of the local community to gain an understanding of the local societal preference. In the setting of substitutable technologies in Radiation Oncology decision board methodology can provide an unbiased representation of the local preference that can then be used to aid in the decision making process. We have outlined the layout for a decision board to be presented to lay members of society to ascertain preference for a substitutable radiosurgery technology to treat brain metastases.

A decision board can be created to summarize the clinical scenario of brain metastases to the general population. In the background section a brief description of cancer incidence and the lifetime risk of developing 1-3 brain metastases can be outlined. The next section of the decision board described the prognosis, treatment options and outcome when a patient is diagnosed with 1-3 brain metastases. A description of palliative nature of treatment, with a focus on quality-of-life as well as survival should then be outlined. Following this outline of brain metastases, the options regarding the radiosurgical treatment modality can be compared in a chart that compared the two treatment options in terms of immobilization device, patient comfort and treatment time. At the introduction of the two radiosurgery modalities both should be described as being equivalent in terms of efficacy (overall survival, local control) and toxicity (neurocognitive). At the conclusion of this section of the decision board participants should be informed that the cancer centre would be purchasing only one of these units with the intention of treating all eligible patients with brain metastases. This section should also describe radiotherapy units as having a ten year replacement and that each unit is critically appraised at the end of this period and at that time a replacement or different unit may be purchased. Participants should then be asked a closed end question as to which unit they preferred at their local cancer centre for the next ten years either 1) Robotic 2) Fixed-Gantry 3) either and were asked to circle one of the options.

5.5   Willingness-to-pay

Willingness to pay is a method to measure an individual's strength of preference (O'Brien *et al.*, 1998, Matthews *et al.*, 2002). The goal of a willingness-to-pay algorithm is to ascertain using a monetary question how much an individual prefers their stated option. If a representative sample of the population of interest is surveyed then the population preference and willingness-to-pay can be inferred from the sample (O'Brien *et al.*, 1998). Valid willingness-to-pay responses require the presentation of comprehensive alternatives and the implications of any financial commitment (opportunity cost) (Matthews *et al.*, 2002). Therefore using this Cost-benefit methodology the decision board must present the required information about the differences in the technology and the implications of directing extra funding to a new technology (Matthews *et al.*, 2002). In this example if participants preferred robotic radiosurgery they would enter a willingness-to-pay bidding algorithm. Participants who selected fixed-gantry or who had no preference did not continue to this section since they preferred the lower incremental cost option. The willingness-to-pay question was framed as a yearly tax that would be added to the municipal property tax bill of all local residents in the local cancer centre catchment area. This tax would finance the incremental cost of robotic radiosurgery compared to fixed gantry radiosurgery. Taxation based willingness-to-pay algorithms have been successfully used in the past to assess public willingness-to-pay for a healthcare intervention in a publically funded healthcare system (O'Brien *et al.*, 1998, Matthews *et al.*, 2002). Participants would be explicitly asked if they would support this local tax program. Participants who answered "yes" would be randomized to one of two potential bidding algorithms. One would have a low starting bid (e.g. $1) and the other had a high starting bid (e.g. $5).[Figure 1] The use of two starting points is a methodology that has been used in published literature to asses for starting point bias (O'Brien *et al.*, 1998 , Matthews *et al.*, 2002). Starting point bias implies that a participant's final willingness-to-pay for a new program is influenced by the starting bid and this hypothesis can be formally tested by having a random assignment of participants to two different starting bids. Participants would then be assigned a final willingness-to-pay based on their responses in the bidding game. Participants who selected "no" i.e. those who would not support a local tax program and those who preferred fixed-gantry or either option would be assigned a willingness-to-pay value of $0. Mean yearly willingness-to-pay was then calculated for all participants and a one sample t-test would be performed to evaluate the 95% confidence interval of this point estimate. To assess for starting point bias, mean willingness-to-pay would be individually calculated for participants randomized to both the low and high starting points. These mean values would then be compared using a two sample t-test. If the mean willingness for participants randomized to the high starting point was more than those randomized to the low starting point using a one sided $\alpha=0.05$ then one would conclude that there is a starting point bias (O'Brien et al., 1998; Matthews et al., 2002).

Net societal benefit would then calculated by subtracting mean yearly willingness to pay from the yearly incremental cost of robotic compared to fixed gantry radiosurgery. Using the upper and lower bound of our 95% confidence interval for mean willingness-to-pay one would then calculate a 95% confidence interval for net yearly societal benefit. If the point estimate of net societal benefit is positive and the 95% confidence interval does not encompass negative values then we will conclude that robotic radiosurgery is cost effective in the local environment. For example, after a comprehensive survey if a mean yearly willingness to pay was calculated as $2.30CAD with a 95% confidence interval of $0.23CAD-$4.38CAD then the population willingness to pay is $2,300,000CAD (1,000,000 tax payers x $2.30CAD) and a 95% confidence interval of ($230,000CAD-$4,300,000CAD). As described in the costing section the incremental cost of robotic radiosurgery is $99,177CAD. The mean net societal benefit of robotic radiosurgery would then be $2,300,000 CAD- $99,177CAD=$2,200,823CAD with a 95% confidence interval of $130,823CAD- $4,280,823CAD.

5.6   Limitations to Cost-benefit Analysis and Willingness-to-pay

There are two major limitations to cost-benefit analysis using willingness to pay methodology that are high lined in the above example. First, the description of a complex medical condition e.g. brain metastases is often difficult for the general public to understand (O'Brien & Gafni, 1996). Even if one can understand the clinical context it is even more difficult to empathize with patients that suffer from the condition if one does not have any experience with the condition. As a patient or health care provider in oncology one would develop an understanding of the complex condition of brain metastases both physically and psychosocially and therefore be able to empathize with patients with the condition. Unfortunately for a cost-benefit analysis to have validity in the population of interest one needs to survey the entire population not just patients and healthcare providers to ascertain societal willingness-to-pay (O'Brien et al., 1998, Matthews et al., 2002, O'Brien & Gafni, 1996). Second, when performing taxation based willingness-to-pay bidding algorithm seemingly small dollar amounts translate into large societal willingness-to-pay values. For example in the Hamilton-Burlington-Brant-Niagara Local Health Integration Network there are approximately 1,000,000 tax payers (Statistics Canada: 2009 Census). If the average willingness-to-pay is calculated at $1 the total taxpayer willingness-to-pay would be quite large i.e. $1,000,000 CAD. It may be difficult for the general public to fully understand the implications of opportunity cost and that the $1 willingness-to-pay for radiosurgery equates to $1 less spent on other social programs that are funded using municipal tax dollars. While the above limitations must be considered when using cost-benefit analysis and willingness-to-pay methodology the advantage of truly evaluating local societal strength of preference for a substitutable technology make it a very strong method to explicitly evaluate this type of technology in Radiation Oncology.

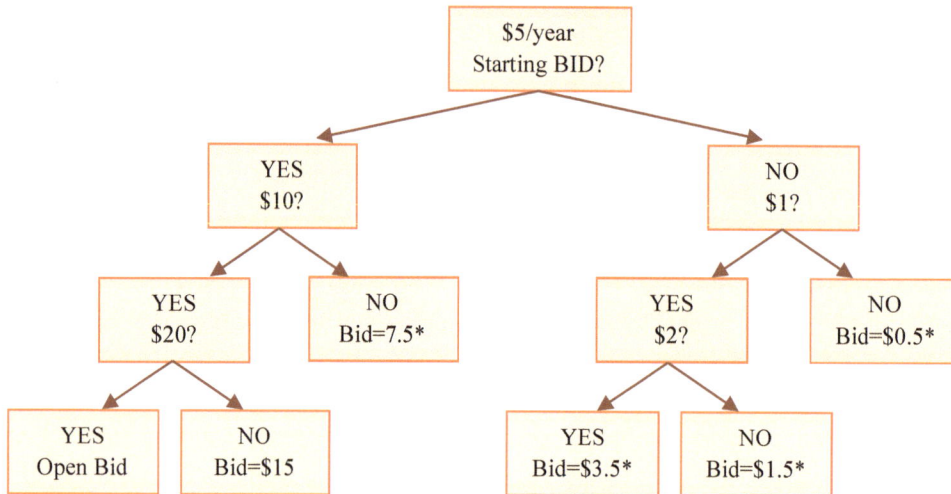

Figure 1: The bid algorithm for the $5/year (high) starting bid taxation based w willingness-to-pay. *represents calculated willingness-to-pay based on the mean of the willingness-to-pay interval.

Through the example of a dedicated as compared to a flexible radiosurgery unit we have described a method to perform a timely and pragmatic technology-assessment to evaluate substitutable technologies in Radiation Oncology. We have described the methodological and pragmatic limitations and strengths to two common methods to evaluate variable costs as well as cost-benefit and cost-utility analysis to perform an economic evaluation of the options. We have also explicitly described an explicit methodology to evaluate local need prior to the economic evaluation and how this methodology can be used to adjust for population, patient or provider trends over time.

6   Discussion

6.1   Planning for Radiosurgery (Technical Efficiency and Opportunity Cost)

There are fourteen cancer centres in Ontario providing radiotherapy. Each cancer centre serves a different population and the capacity of each treatment centre ranges from two to seventeen linear accelerators. Each cancer centre has a relatively fixed number of linear accelerators and thus a fixed capacity to perform radiotherapy. When a cancer centre replaces an existing flexible linear accelerator with a dedicated radiosurgery unit they are making a trade off. This trade off is known as the opportunity cost (Buxton *et al.*, 1997). The opportunity cost of increasing radiosurgery capacity is that the cancer centre will have a decreased capacity to provide conventional radiation over the next ten years. Each cancer centre could perform an explicit assessment of their current and future needs and examine different methods of meeting the radiosurgical needs of their community. For small catchment areas it may minimize the opportunity cost of providing radiosurgery by providing a limited flexible capacity for radiosurgery with one flexible linear accelerator and if the need for radiosurgery exceeds the local capacity patients could travel to centres with larger radiosurgery capacity.

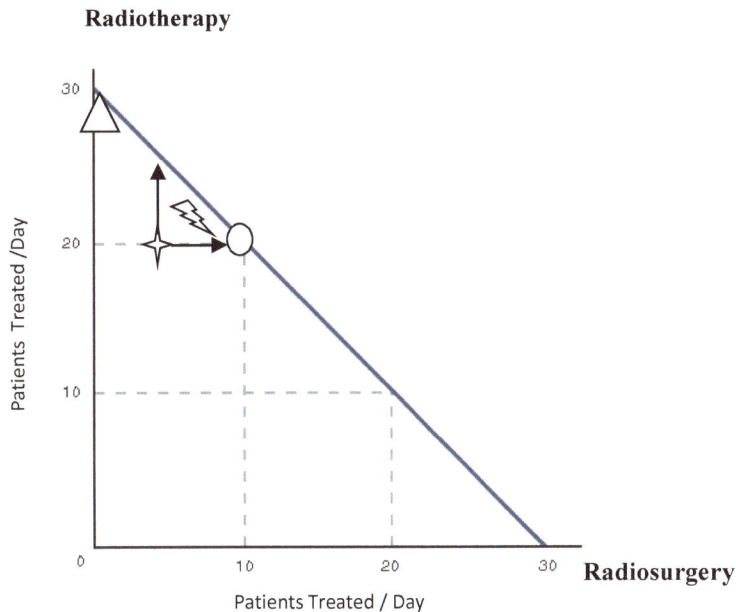

Figure 2: The Production Possibility Frontier for Radiotherapy and Radiosurgery. The circle represents the maximum production when one radiotherapy unit is substituted for a dedicated radiosurgery unit. The star represents a point of inefficient production. The area bounded by the two arrows (containing the lightning bolt) represents the area of improved efficiency over the star.

Figure 2 represents a production possibility frontier for a hypothetical cancer centre that has the capacity to treat one patient per hour per unit. A production possibility frontier represents the maximum number of cases treated daily using the available equipment (Morris *et al.*, 2007). The centre is equipped with three units and it is assumed that radiotherapy and radiosurgery are equally substitutable at all levels of production (hence the straight line negative slope for the production possibility frontier). Hypothetically, if this cancer centre replaces a conventional radiotherapy unit with a dedicated radiosurgery unit the maximum capacity for radiotherapy decreases from thirty patients daily to twenty patients daily and the maximum capacity for radiosurgery increases from zero patients daily to ten patients daily. This trade-off in case mix represents the opportunity cost of purchasing a dedicated radiosurgery unit. If this cancer centre had previously used its radiotherapy resources to their maximum capacity they would treat thirty patients daily (represented by the triangle on the production possibility frontier). If the cancer centre once it substitutes one conventional unit with a dedicated radiosurgery unit is able to treat twenty patients with conventional radiation daily and ten patients with radiosurgery daily this would represent a new point on the production possibilities frontier (circle). At this point the cancer centre has changed its production mix, however it continues to produce with maximum efficiency since both the triangle and circle are located on the frontier. If however the cancer centre replaces a conventional radiotherapy unit with a dedicated radiosurgery unit and is only treating five patients daily with radiosurgery the new point of production on the production possibilities frontier is represented by the star. At this point the cancer centre is producing less efficiently than either the triangle or the circle because the star is located within the frontier. The area bounded by the arrows and the frontier line (lightning bolt) represent points of improved efficiency over the star. The only point bounded by this area achievable with the dedicated radiosurgery machine is the circle. All other points (including those on the frontier) would only be achievable if the cancer centre had elected to purchase a flexible machine capable of producing both radiosurgery and conventional radiotherapy. This hypothetical example highlights the importance of performing a technology needs assessment prior to resource allocation decisions. A technology needs assessment has the ability to help minimize the opportunity cost of providing new treatment options in both publically funded and fee-based healthcare systems.

7   Conclusion

Oncology decision makers are increasingly being faced with difficult decisions regarding the adoption of new technology. Timely local needs assessments and economic evaluations would be valuable components of this decision making process (Greenspoon *et al.*, 2012). We have discussed a three part locally applicable evaluation of new technology in radiation oncology that combines 1) a local assessment of need 2) a local assessment of incremental cost and 3) a local assessment of tax-payer willingness-to-pay for a specific new technology. This methodology has the ability to provide a level of transparency and accountability when allocating limited Radiation Oncology capital healthcare resources.

Acknowledgement

This work has been partially funded through a grant from the Juravinski Cancer Centre Foundation.

References

Andrews DW et al 2004: Whole Brain Radiation Therapy With or Without Stereotactic Radiosurgery Boost for Patients with One to Three Brain Metastases: Phase III Results of the RTOG 9508 Randomized Trial. Lancet 363:1665-1672, 2004

Birch & Chambers 1993: To each according to their need: A community-based approach to allocating health care resources. Canadian Medical Association Journal 149:607-612, 1993

Birch S et al 2007: Human Resources Planning and the Production of Health: A Needs-Based Analytical Framework. Canadian Public Policy 33:S1-S16, 2007 (suppl)

Boudreau R et al. 2009: TomoTherapy, GammaKnife and CyberKnife Therapies for Patients with Tumours of the Lung, Central Nervous System, or Intra-abdomen: A Systematic Review of Clinical Effectiveness and Cost-Effectiveness. Ottawa: Canadian Agency for Drugs and Technologies in Health, 2009

Briggs AH 2000. Handling Uncertainty in Cost-Effectiveness Models. Pharmacoeconomics 17(5) 479-500, 2000

Brown P et al 2008: Phase III Randomized Trial of the Role of Whole Brain Radiation Therapy in Addition to Radiosurgery in Patients with One to Three Cerebral Metastases. August 2008. Available at http://ncctg.mayo.edu/

Brown P & Roberge D 2011: A Phase III Trial of Post-Surgical Stereotactic Radiosurgery (SRS) Compared with Whole Brain Radiotherapy (WBRT) for Resected Metastatic Brain Disease. July 2011. Available at http://ncctg.mayo.edu/

Buxton MJ et al 1997: *Modeling in Economic Evaluation: An Unavoidable Fact of Life. Health Economics 6:217-227, 1997*

Cancer Quality Council of Ontario: *Radiation Machine Efficiency. www.csqi.on.ca*

Caroli M et al 2011: *Surgical Brain Metastases: Management and Outcome Related to Prognostic Indexes: A Critical Review of a Ten-Year Series. ISRN Surg 2011: 207103, 2011*

Chang JE et al 2007: *Therapeutic advances in the treatment of brain metastases. Clin Adv Hematol Oncol 5(1):54-64, 2007*

Gafni A. 1996 *Economic Evaluation of Health Care Interventions: An Economist's Perspective. ACP Journal Club 124:A12-A14, 1996*

Greenspoon et al 2012: *Technology Resource Planning in Radiation Oncology: An Application of a Needs Based Analytical Framework to Radiosurgery Planning in Ontario. Journal of Oncology Practice; e-pub July 24, 2012*

Greenspoon JN 2011: *Robotic Compared to Fixed Gantry Radiosurgery for Brain Metastases (TRICK). Clinical Trials Registry 2011. NCT01353573. www.clinicaltrials.gov*

Linskey ME et al 2010: *The Role of Stereotactic Radiosurgery in the Management of Patients with Newly Diagnosed Brain Metastases: A Systematic Review and Evidence-Based Clinical Practice Guideline. J Neurooncol 96:45-68, 2010*

Lukka H 2011: *A Randomized Phase II Trial of Hypofractionated Radiotherapy for Favourable Risk Prostate Cancer. Clinical Trials Registry 2011. NCT01434290. www.clinicaltrials.gov*

Matthews et al 2002: *Putting your money where your mouth is: Willingness-to-pay for dental gel. Pharmacoeconomics 2002; 20:245-255*

Mheta M et al 1997: *A Cost-Effectiveness and Cost-Utility Analysis of Radiosurgery VS. Resection for Single-Brain Metastases. Int J Radiation Oncology Biol Phys 39:445-454, 1997*

Morris et al. 2007: *Economic Analysis in Health Care (ed 2). West Sussex, England, Wiley, 2007*

Muacevic & Wowra 2008: *Microsurgery Plus Whole Brain Irradiation Versus Gamma Knife Surgery Alone for Treatment of Single Metastases to the Brain: A Randomized Controlled Multicentre Phase III Trial. J Neurooncol 87:299-307, 2008*

O'Brien & Gafni 1996: *When Do the "Dollars" Make Sense? Toward a Conceptual Framework for Contingent Valuation Studies in Health Care. Med Decis Making 1996;16:288-299.*

O'Brien et al 1998: *Assessing the value of a new pharmaceutical: a feasibility study of contingent valuation in managed care. Medical Care 1998;36:370-384*

Pickren et al 1983: *Brain Metastases: An autopsy study. Cancer Treat Symp 2:295-313, 1983*

Posner & Chernik 1978: *Intracranial metastases from systemic cancer. Adv Neurol 19:579-592, 1978*

Rabin & Charro 2001: *EQ-5D: A Measure of Health Status from the EuroQol Group. Ann Med. 2001; 33:337-343*

Roberge D et al 2010: *Radiosurgery Scope of Practice in Canada: a report of the Canadian association of radiation oncology (CARO) radiosurgery advisory committee. Radiother Oncol 95(1): 122-128, 2010*

Ryu S 2011: *Image-Guided Radiosurgery or Stereotactic Body Radiation Therapy in Treating Patients With Localized Spine Metastases. Clinical Trials Registry 2011. NCT00922974. www.clinicaltrials.gov*

Schultz C et al 2011: *Stereotactic Radiosurgery and Radiation Therapy Experience at the Juravinski Cancer Centre. Presented at the Canadian Radiation Oncology Annual Scientific Meeting, Winnipeg, MB, September 14-17, 2011*

Sperduto PW et al 2008: *A New Prognostic Index and Comparison to Three Other Indices for Patients With Brain Metastases: An Analysis of 1,960 Patients in the RTOG Database. Int J Radiation Oncology Biol Phys 70:510-514, 2008*

Statistics Canada: *2009 Census. www.statcan.gc.ca*

Whelan et al 1999. Mastectomy or Lumpectomy? Helping Women Make Informed Choices. J Clin Oncol 1999; 17(6):1727-1735

Whelan et al 2004: Effect of a Decision Aid on Knowledge and Treatment Decision Making for Breast Cancer Surgery: A Randomized Trial. JAMA 2004;292:435-441

Whelan, et al 2003: Helping Patients Make Informed Choices: A Randomized Trial of a Decision Aid for Adjuvant Chemotherapy in Lymph Node-Negative Breast Cancer. J Natl Cancer Inst 2003;95:581-587

Wowra B et al.2009 Quality of radiosurgery for single brain metastases with respect to treatment technology: a matched-pair analysis. J Neurooncol 2009; 94:69-77

Carbon Monoxide and the Brain

Vicki L. Mahan
Department of Pediatric Cardiothoracic Surgery
St. Christopher's Hospital for Children
Drexel University College of Medicine, United States

Leo E. Otterbein
Department of Surgery
Beth Israel Deaconess Medical Center
Harvard Medical School, United States

1   Introduction

As a neurotransmitter, endogenous carbon monoxide (CO) is critical for normal brain function and neuroprotection and, thus, agents affecting the synthesis, transactions, and disposition of the gas have clinical relevance. Production originates from oxidative degradation of iron protoporphyrin IX (from senescing red blood cells and ineffective erythropoiesis, myoglobin, catalase, peroxidases, and cytochromes) and heme-independent sources including auto- and enzymatic oxidation of phenols, photo-oxidation of organic compounds, iron-ascorbate-catalyzed lipid peroxidation of microsomal lipids and phospholipids, and reduction of cytochrome b_5 (Wu & Wang, 2005; Kajimura *et al.*, 2010; Kirkby & Adin, 2006; Ryter & Choi, 2013; Rodgers *et al.*, 1994). Heme oxygenase isozymes catalyze the metabolism of heme, the primary source of CO, to iron, biliverdin, and CO. Cytoprotective effects have been attributed to the production of CO and bilirubin (Ryter *et al.*, 2004; Ryter & Otterbein, 2004; Ryter *et al.*, 2002; Kim *et al.*, 2006; Chung *et al.*, 2008; Soares *et al.*, 2002). The majority of CO formed is taken up in the cytosol before being released and combined with hemoglobin and, thus, correlation of carboxyhemoglobin (COHb) levels with biological changes induced by CO and remnant effects of CO after COHb elimination is poor. Quantifying tissue CO levels using measurements of expired CO has been used as a marker of inducible HO-1 activity, but is also imprecise. A new method for measuring the rate of endogenous CO production in humans described by Coburn and colleagues allows calculation of the rate of heme catabolism with a precision of ± 2 µmol/h and is applicable as a diagnostic and therapeutic tool in neurophysiology, neurometabolism, and neurologic pathologies (Coburn, 1973; Coburn, 2012).

2   Heme Oxygenase Systems

In 1894, Gréhant found that normal dog blood contained a small amount of combustible gas and assumed that it was CO (Gréhant, 1894). Saint-Martin and Nicloux later suggested endogenous production of CO and Sjöstrand and colleagues, in the 1950's, provided experimental evidence for the existence of CO in the human body (decomposition of hemoglobin in vivo produced endogenous CO) and that its production could be regulated (Sjöstrand, 1950; Sjöstrand, 1952). Further studies by Coburn *et al.* determined that at least part of the endogenous production of CO is from hemoglobin catabolism and that an increase in heme metabolism results in increased CO production (Coburn *et al.*, 1963). In 1968, Tenhunen and colleagues concluded that an enzyme system in microsomes that required molecular oxygen and NADPH and that was inhibited by carbon monoxide (microsomal heme oxygenase) was important in heme turnover in rats (Tenhunen, 1968; Tenhunen, 1969). The inducible form heme-oxygenase 1 (HO-1) was identified in 1974 (Maines & Kappas, 1974; Yoshida *et al.*, 1974), the constitutive heme-oxygenase 2 (HO-2) in 1986 (Maines *et al.*, 1986), and the constitutive heme-oxygenase 3 (HO-3) in 1997 (McCoubrey *et al*, 1997). A fourth heme-oxygenase, heme-oxygenase 4 (HO-4), has been identified in plants (Emborg *et al.*, 2006).

HO-1 is primarily localized in endoplasmic reticulum, but has been isolated in cytoplasm, nuclear matrix, mitochondria, and peroxisomes (Kim *et al.*, 2011; Gottlieb *et al.*, 2012; Kim *et al.*, 2004). Under basal conditions, tissues not involved in red blood cell or hemoglobin metabolism have low to undetectable levels, but the enzyme is ubiquitously induced (Schipper *et al.*, 2009; Barbagallo *et al.*, 2013; Sass *et al.*, 2012; Deshane *et al.*, 2005; Cheng *et al.*, 2013). HO-2 proteins are primarily anchored to the endoplasmic reticulum. Testes and brain have the highest expression of HO-2, but the protein is also present in abundant amounts in other systemic tissues (Ewing & Maines, 1997; Xia *et al.*, 2002; Andres & Luszczki, 2004, Baum *et al.*, 2000). Hayashi and colleagues studied the structure of the third isoform (heme oxygenase-3) in the rat with genomic PRC and found two HO-3-related genes (HO-3a and HO-3b). The authors suggest that HO-3 is nonfunctional and that the HO-3a and HO-3b genes are processed pseudogenes derived from HO-2 transcripts (Hayashi *et al.*, 2004). Although HO-3 is not catalytically active, it is thought to work in oxygen sensing. Its' subcellular localization is unclear (Maines, 1997; Maines, 1992).

HO-1 and HO-2 represent the products of distinct genes (ho-1, ho-2, also specified as hmox1, hmox2) and are principally responsible for the catalysis of heme into bilirubin. Both catalyze three successive monooxygenation steps to convert heme to CO, Fe^{2+} and biliverdin in the presence of reducing equivalents. Biliverdin is rapidly converted to bilirubin by biliverdin reductase while the iron is sequestered into ferritin. Historically, the CO generated was considered a waste product with no physiologic function that was exhaled through the lung, scavenged in cytoplasm, or oxidized. Recent efforts have identified this gasotransmitter as a biologically active molecule that modulates a number of signaling pathways and is the primary mechanism by which HO-1 and HO-2 impart cytoprotective effects in animals.

Several authors have shown endogenous CO has the ability to regulate the inflammatory response and act as a regulatory molecule in a number of pathophysiological responses (El-Sayed *et al.*, 2012; Nako *et al.*, 2006; Ozaki *et al.*, 2012; Rivier, 1998; Schallner *et al.*, 2012; Nuhn *et al.*, 2013; Naito *et al.*, 2012; Parfenova *et al.*, 2006; Chang *et al.*, 2003; Vukomanovic *et al.*, 2011; Namiranian *et al.*, 2005; Wang *et al.*, 2006; Wang & Doré, 2008). In mammals, CO has a high affinity for binding to hemoglobin, myoglobin, and neuroglobin. The latter is neuroprotective against hypoxic-ischemic injury. The gas reversibly binds to molecular targets, almost exclusively to transition metals (iron, manganese, vanadium, cobalt, tungsten, copper, nickel, and molybdenum) present in structural and functional proteins (Boczkowski *et al.*, 2006; Desmard *et al.*, 2007; Watts *et al.*, 2012). By binding to a heme prosthetic group, CO regulates components of cell signaling that include BK(Ca) channels, guanylyl cyclase, NADPH oxidase and the mitochondrial respiratory cycles. Binding of CO to heme proteins generally inhibits their function with the exception of soluble guanylate cyclase (sGC) which is activated and responsible for CO-induced activation of neurotransmission and vasodilation (Gullotta *et al.*, 2012; Zhong *et al.*, 2011; Dennery, 2013; Schallner *et al.*, 2013). CO activates the nitric oxide synthases (NOS2/NOS3). Activation of nNOS, which has not been tested, might therefore be responsible for mediating glutamate action at metabotropic receptors directly or via a cGMP-dependent pathway (Bilban *et al.*, 2008; Morse *et al.*, 2002; Dulak & Józkowicz, 2003; Piantadosi, 2008; Choi *et al.*, 2012; Wilkinson & Kemp, 2011; Maines, 1980).

3 Production and Neuroprotective Effects of Endogenous Carbon Monoxide

Endogenous formation of neuronal CO is dependent on the expression of brain heme oxygenases. HO-1 and HO-2 have been extensively investigated in animal models (Schallner *et al.*, 2013; Laitinen & Juvonen, 1995; Sutherland *et al.*, 2009; Colombrita *et al.*, 2003; Calabrese *et al.*, 2002). Isoforms in the rat brain assessed by real-time quantitative RT-PCR are greatest for HO-2 seen throughout the brain at much higher levels than HO-1 and HO-3. Whether this same pattern of expression occurs in humans has not been tested. The highest levels of expression are in the cerebellum and the hippocampus. HO-1 and HO-2 are detectable in both cortical neurons and type I astrocytes (Scapagnini *et al.*, 2002). The isoform HO-1 is highly expressed in select neurons in the hilus of the dentate gyrus, hypothalamus, cerebellum, and brainstem whereas HO-2 is more widely expressed in mitral cells in the olfactory bulb, pyramidal cells in the cortex and hippocampus, granule cells in the dentate gyrus, and many neurons in the thalamus, hypothalamus, cerebellum and caudal brainstem (Vincent *et al.*, 1994). Under normal conditions, the HO-2 constitutive isoform accounts for nearly all of brain heme oxygenase activity and therefore CO production. Physiologic functions in the brain attributed to endogenous CO include regulation of the hypothalamic-pituitary-adrenal axis, memory processes, carotid body chemoreception, control of respiration, circadian rhythm control, odor response adaptation, nociception and chemoreception regulation, hearing, learning, long-term potentiation, synaptic plasticity, neuroendocrine regulation, behavior modification, memory, and vision (hanafy *et al.*, 2013; Boehning & Snyder, 2002; Prabhakar *et al.*, 1995; Brann *et al.*, 1997; Mancuso *et al.*, 1999; Ingi & Ronnett, 1995; Prabhakar, 1998).

The functions of HO-2 in the central nervous system have been defined using HO-2 gene deletion and pharmacological inhibitors/activators of the enzyme in animal models and cultured cells of neurons, astrocytes, and cerebral vascular endothelial cells (Parfenova *et al.*, 2006; Chang *et al.*, 2003; Vukomanovic *et al.*, 2011; Wang *et al.*, 2006; Wang & Doré, 2008; Vukomanovic *et al.*, 2010; Basuroy *et al.*, 2011; Yoneyama-Sarnecky *et al.*, 2010; Fan *et al.*, 2008). Activation results in an increase in CO. As a gasotransmitter, CO cannot be stored in synaptic vesicles so that it must be formed on demand. CO preferentially targets heme-containing proteins and has been shown to activate and inhibit enzyme activity (Piantadosi, 2002; Fukoto *et al.*, 2012; Deng *et al.*, 2014). Studies by Doré and colleagues showed that HO-2 deletion with resultant reduction in CO results in increased neurotoxicity in cultured brain cells and increased damage following transient cerebral ischemia in mice (Doré *et al.*, 2000). Several authors have shown that pharmacologic inhibition or gene deletion of brain HO-2 exacerbates oxidative stress induced by seizures, glutamate, and inflammatory cytokines, and causes cerebral vascular injury (Basuroy *et al.*, 2011; Parfenova & Leffler, 2008). Exposure of cortical neurons to glutamate increases HO-2 activity and CO production by calcium-calmodulin in a calcium-dependent manner, a process that occurs in milliseconds (Boehning *et al.*, 2004). Heme oxygenase-2 is also activated during neuronal stimulation by phosphorylation by CK2 and may be more long-term (Boehning *et al.*, 2003). Stimulation of metabotropic and ionotropic glutamate receptors lead to increased CO production as well (Glaum *et al.*, 1993; Parfenova *et al.*, 2012; Gomperts *et al.*, 2000; Nathanson *et al.*, 1995; Lin *et al.*, 2004). Brain homeostasis and neuronal survival during seizures, hypoxia and hypotension correspond to upregulation of HO-2 expression with CO production and resulting neuroprotection while absence of HO-2 is cytoprotective (Parfenova & Leffler, 2008; Kim & Doré, 2005).

The inducible isoform HO-1 has been targeted for neuroprotection and neuroinflammation in several neurodegenerative diseases (Schipper *et al.*, 2009; Jazwa & Cuadrado, 2010; Cuadrado & Royo, 2008; Bastianetto & Quirion, 2010; Chien *et al.*, 2011; Colin-González *et al.*, 2013; Innamorato *et al.*, 2009; Innamorato *et al.*, 2009). Evidence suggests that the pathogenesis of Parkinson's disease, Alzheimer's disease, Friedreich's ataxia, multiple sclerosis, amyotrophic lateral sclerosis, and Huntington's disease may be due to formation of reactive oxygen species and/or reactive nitrogen species with mitochondrial dysfunction (Hegde *et al.*, 2011; Sabens Liedhegner *et al.*, 2012; Koppula *et al.*, 2012; Hegde *et al.*, 2012; Fujita *et al.*, 2012). Lack of HO-1 activity and formation of CO would enhance susceptibility to oxidative injury (Calabrese *et al.*, 2010; Calabrese *et al.*, 2005; Calabrese *et al.*, 2006; Noda *et al.*, 2011).

4   Exogenous Carbon Monoxide as a Neuroprotector

Neuroprotection using exogenous CO as inhaled carbon monoxide (CO) or injectable carbon monoxide releasing molecules (CORM) is a novel and underexplored strategy. Well known as a toxin at high doses, exogenous CO also has critical physiologic and cytoprotective properties at low concentrations and has known anti-apoptotic, anti-inflammatory, antiproliferative, and metabolic properties (Ryter & Choi, 2007; Wen et al., 2012; Moody & Calvert, 2011; Takagi et al., 2011; Tsui et al., 2007; Hoetzel et al., 2008; Scott et al., 2009; Bechman et al., 2009; Takagi et al., 2010; Hoetzel et al., 2007; Zhou et al., 2010; Goebel et al., 2011). What is sorely lacking are critical dosing regimens to optimize the benefit and limit the exposure times to achieve the minimal effective dose. Studies by Vieira and colleagues showed that the preconditioning of murine primary cerebellar granule cells with exogenous CO prevented neuronal apoptosis induced by excitotoxicity and oxidative stress (Vieira et al., 2008). Zeynalov and colleagues evaluated the role of inhaled CO following 90-minutes of transient focal brain ischemia in a mouse model. Inhalation of 125 parts per million (ppm) or 250 ppm CO begun immediately at the onset of reperfusion resulted in reduction of hemispheric infarct volume, improved neurological deficit scores, and limited brain edema. Inhalation of 250 ppm CO begun 1 to 3 hours after ischemia resulted in reduction of infarct volume and improved neurological deficit scores (Zeynalov & Doré, 2009). Wang et al exposed male wild-type and Nrf2-knockout mice to 250 ppm CO or control air for 18 hours immediately after permanent middle cerebral artery occlusion. Nrf2 is the principle transcription factor responsible for regulating HO-1 expression. CO neuroprotection was completely abolished in Nrf2-knockout mice suggesting that the beneficial effect of inhaled CO is at least partially be mediated through the Nrf2 pathway and therefore likely HO-1 (Wang et al., 2011). Inhaled CO is being primarily delivered via a mask, sealed mask, or ventilator for 1 to 2 hour intervals depending on the study protocol. Critical here is the regulation of the delivered dose which if by mask is completely dependent on the respiratory rate and volume of each breath. Delivery through the ventilator obviates the need to monitor the breathing patterns and will provide a more stable carboxyhemoglobin level. The delivery as a gas is problematic since it relies on patient compliance and proper control of volume and gas concentrations and monitoring. Motterlini and others circumvented this by inventing molecules that release CO. CO releasing molecules (CORMs) have proven to be very effective modalities by which to deliver CO into the body. Orally bioavailable CO will make the inhaled gas mode of administration obsolete as the control of dosing will be much more precise. Pretreatment with the CORM ALF186 in a rat model of ischemia-reperfusion injury of retinal ganglion cells abrogated injury via the soluble guanylate cyclase-cGMP pathway (Schallner et al., 2013). In a rat model of hemorrhagic stroke, Yabluchanskiy et al showed that pretreatment with CORM-5 minutes before injury significantly decreased the injury, treatment 3 hours after brain damage exacerbated the injury, and treatment 3 days after injury resulted in partial protection suggesting that the timing of CORM-3 administration is critical (Yabluchanskiy et al., 2012). In our recent report we found that piglets preconditioned with inhaled CO had less apoptosis in the neocortex/striatum and hippocampus after cardiopulmonary bypass (CPB) and deep hypothermic circulatory arrest (DHCA). Moreover animals treated with CO demonstrated a change in metabolic substrate utilization that correlated with neuroprotection (Mahan et al., 2012).

5   Exogenous Carbon Monoxide may Change Neurometabolism that Results in Neuroprotection

The neuroenergetics of the brain is dependent on complex metabolic interactions between cell types and energy requirements are high (Aubert & Costalat, 2005; Pelleri & Magistretti, 2004; Attwell & Gibb, 2005; Pellerin et al., 2007; Bélanger et al., 2011; Harris et al., 2012; MacAskill et al., 2010; Jolivet et al., 2009). Neurons account for most of the energy consumption during brain activation. About 85% of glucose consumed during brain activation is initiated by aerobic glycolysis in astrocytes triggered by the demand for glycolytically derived energy for Na^+-dependent accumulation of transmitter glutamate and its amidation to glutamine. Suggested mechanisms regulating the distribution of energy metabolism among the different cell types include the canonical sodium conductance mechanism (Hodgkin & Huxley, 1952; Laughlin et al., 1998), the glutamate-lactate exchange mechanism (Sibson et al., 1998; Magistretti et al., 1999), and the diffusion-limited delivery of oxygen to brain tissue (Buxton & Frank, 1997). Neurons possess highly oxidative metabolism and are susceptible to ischemia whereas astrocytes depend more on glycolysis and metabolism associated with synthesis of intermediates. Distribution of energy substrates from the systemic circulation into neurons is principally determined by astrocytes and the dependence of cerebral function on blood glucose as a fuel does not exclude lactate or other substrates as an energy source. Lactate is used as a metabolic substrate by the brain, but the blood-brain transport of lactate is limited. At physiologically occurring lactate concentrations, lactate uptake is at most 25% of the rate of glucose oxidation. In the unstimulated adult brain, glucose is the primary energy source under basal conditions due to high concentrations in plasma and the ability of glucose transporters to carry glucose across the blood-brain barrier. With increasing stimulation, oxidative metabolism declines, oxygen-to-glucose index (OGI) decreases and brain lactate increases. Sibson and colleagues suggest that lactate generated by glycolysis in astrocytes undergoes oxidation in neurons which is dictated by the functional activity (Sibson et al., 1998).

Modulation of neurometabolic pathways by exogenous CO with resultant neuroprotection is likely dependent on the dose and timing of administration, either pre, peri, and/or post stressor. The challenge is to effect safe and effective CO concentrations in neural tissues without producing deleterious effects and to define the neural cellular targets and metabolic pathways. Recently, Queiroga and colleagues concluded that CO controls mitochondrial functioning, oxidative metabolism, and substrate utilization (Queiroga et al., 2012). Exogenous CO may result in a change in metabolic substrate in the brain and may define the role of exogenous CO in neurometabolism and, subsequent, neuroprotection. This will be dependent as well on the availability of specific metabolic substrates.

Several studies show that lactate may be the preferred energy substrate of activated neurons and is neuroprotective (Rasmussen et al., 2011; Ivanov et al., 2011; Schurr et al., 1999; Schurr & Gozal, 2011; Won et al., 2012; Neves et al., 2012; Herzog et al., 2013) and lactate may be a major substrate for the mitochondrial tricarboxylic acid cycle (Dienel & Hertz, 2001; Dienel, 2012). Lactate preserves neuronal function in experimental models of excitotoxicity, posthypoxic recovery, cerebral ischemia, and energy deprivation and can sustain neuronal integrity as an alternative energy substrate. In newborn piglets with intrauterine growth restriction (IUGR), Moxon-Lester et al showed that during hypoxia brain lactate in some IUGR piglets were higher than in other IUGR piglets and normal weight piglets and that apoptosis in the frontal cortex and thalamus of IUGR piglets with high brain lactate were lower than IUGR piglets with low brain lactate. The authors concluded that increased brain lactate during hypoxia may be neuroprotective in IUGR piglets (Moxon-Lester et al., 2007). In a rat model of acute/severe hypoglycemia,

Won and colleagues concluded that supplementation of glucose with lactate reduced neuronal death in the hippocampus and hypothesized that increasing brain lactate in this model offsets the decrease in NAD^+ due to overactivation of PARP-1 by acting as an alternative energy substrate that can effectively bypass glycolysis and be fed directly to the citric acid cycle to maintain cellular ATP levels (Won *et al.*, 2012). Our results in newborn piglets preconditioned with inhaled CO before CPB/DHCA are also consistent with a change to lactate as the metabolic substrate and resulting neuroprotection (Mahan *et al.*, 2012).

CO is able to regulate several classes of ion channels (Boycott *et al.*, 2013; Riddle & Walker, 2012; Decaluwé *et al.*, 2012; Pouokam *et al.*, 2011; Dallas *et al.*, 2011; Hou *et al.*, 2009) including calcium activated K(+), voltage-activaged K(+) and Ca(2+) channel families, ligand-gated P2X receptors, tandem P domain K(+) and channels and epithelial Na(+) channel (Figure 1).

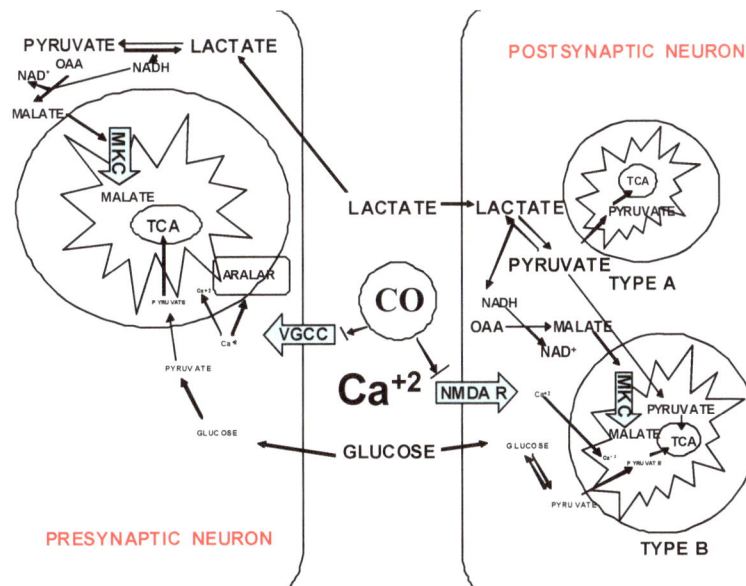

Figure 1: Proposed mechanisms of effect of CO on presynaptic neurons and postsynaptic-neurons on change to lactate as metabolic substrate. Ca^{2+} signaling has been proposed as the primary determiner of change from glucose to lactate metabolism in the brain. CO could block both NMDA R and VGCC allowing less Ca^{2+} to reach the cytoplasm. This would decrease the amount of glucose available for the mitochondrial TCA cycle in both the presynaptic and postsynaptic neurons. Physiologic cystosol Ca^{2+} also binds to aralar which allows an increase in malate transfer into the mitochondria and a change to the CiMASH pathway.

Ca^{2+} signaling might therefore control the switch between glucose and lactate utilization during synaptic activity. Intermittent rises in intracellular Ca^{2+} during synaptic activation causes influx of Ca^{2+} into the mitochondria resulting in activation of the tricarboxylic acid cyle dehydrogenases. This leads to a lower activity of the malate-aspartate shuttle and results in lactate production. Bak and colleagues showed that glucose utilizations is positively correlated with intracellular Ca^{2+} whereas lactate utilization is not (Bak *et al.*, 2012).

The calcium-activated potassium channels (BK(Ca)) are distributed in both excitable and non-excitable cells and are involved in action potential repolarization, neuronal excitability, neurotransmitter release, hormone section, tuning of cochlear hair cells, innate immunity, and modulation of smooth muscle tone. These channels are highly sensitive to intracellular calcium concentrations and voltage. The mechanisms by which CO regulates the calcium channels are unclear, remain controversial, and requires further study. However, Telezhkin and colleagues found that cystein residue 91 in the C-terminal tail of human BK(Ca)α subunit is important for activation by CO (Telezhkin *et al.*, 2011). In cultured mouse glutamatergic neurons, Bak *et al* evaluated the effect of an ionomycin-induced increase in intracellular Ca^{2+} on glucose and lactate metabolism and concluded that glucose utilization is positively correlated with intracellular Ca^{2+} but that lactate utilization is not. The authors proposed a compartmentalized Ci-MASH (Ca^{2+}-induced limitation of the malate-aspartate shuttle) that defines pre- and post-synaptic compartments metabolizing glucose and glucose plus lactate in whitch the latter displays a positive correlation between oxidative metabolism of glucose and Ca^{2+} signaling (Bak *et al.*, 2012).

Almeida and colleagues studied the effects of CO exposure on primary cultures of astrocytes and showed that CO prevented apoptosis, increased ATP, improved oxidative metabolism, decreased lactate production, reduced glucose use, increased cytochrome c oxidase enzymatic specific activity, stimulated mitochondrial biogenesis and enhanced Bcl-2 expression (Almeida *et al.*, 2012). Pretreatment with CO protected neurons from glutamate-induced apoptosis. The authors propose that exogenous CO induces intracellular ROS generation which activates NOS (increased NO production) that in turn activates sGC leading to increased levels of cGMP and the opening of ATP-dependent mitoK$_{ATP}$ (important for neuronal cell protection) (Vieira *et al.*, 2012).

6   Clinical Application of Inhaled Carbon Monoxide for Neuroprotection

Inhaled CO is an important therapeutic option and has entered clinical trials (www.clinicaltrials.gov). These include "Carbon Monoxide Therapy for Severe Pulmonary Arterial Hypertension," "The Safety and Adverse Reaction Study of Neonatal to Carbon Monoxide," "Safety Study of Inhaled Carbon Monoxide in Healthy Volunteers," "Study of Inhaling Carbon Monoxide to Treat Patients with Intestinal Paralysis After Colon Surgery," "Carbon Monoxide to Prevent Lung Inflammation," "Modification of Chronic Inflammation by Inhaled Carbon Monoxide in Patients with Stable Chronic Obstructive Pulmonary Disease (COPD)," "Study of Inhaled Carbon Monoxide to Treat Idiopathic Pulmonary Fibrosis," and "CO Mitochondrial Biogenesis," "Studies in humans performed by INO Therapeutics LLC evaluated the safety and tolerability of inhaled single doses of carbon monoxide when administered as an inhaled gas for approximately 1 hour to healthy males (randomized, single blind, placebo controlled in parallel groups). Doses of 0.2, 0.75, 2.0, and 2.3 mg/kg/hr resulted in mean total maximum COHb levels of 2.0%, 3.4%, 7.7%, and 8.8%, respectively. All doses were well tolerated. Analyses of neurocognitive test data could not detect evidence of any acute or delayed differences in response between exposure to any of the carbon monoxide doses. The second study in humans performed by INO Therapeutics LLC was a randomized, single-blind study conducted in four panels of subjects. A total number of 12 healthy male volunteers received carbon monoxide or placebo by inhalation (ten subjects receiving CO and 2 subjects receiving placebo). In Panel 1, 12 subjects were given repeated doses of 2.3 mg CO/kg or placebo during 1 hour for 10 consecutive days. Panel 2 included 12 subjects receiving a single dose of 3.0 mg CO/kg or placebo. Panel 3 included 12 subjects given repeated doses of 3.0 mg CO/kg or placebo during 1 hour for

10 consecutive days. Panel 4 was a crossover study that included 12 subjects receiving a 3.0 mg CO/kg single dose sourced from a 5.97 mg/L drug product and a 3.0 mg CO/kg single dose sourced from a 12 mg/L drug product. The highest level of COHb measured was 13.9% in the 3.0 mg/kg/hour dose. These studies indicate that inhaled CO is safe and tolerable in humans. Clinical application in neurological disorders remains unexplored however anecdotal data suggest that smokers have a very low incidence of Alzheimers disease (Chang *et al.*, 2012).

Preclinical studies of protective conditioning, a powerful laboratory strategy used to evaluate metabolic pathways and cell death, using many different stimuli show less pathology in models of epilepsy, stroke, hypoxia-ischemia, traumatic brain injury, and craniocerebral tumor resection (Mergenthaler & Dirnagl, 2011; Koch *et al.*, 2012; Severino *et al.*, 2011; Sanders *et al.*, 2010; Lim & Hausenloy, 2012; Zhao *et al.*, 2012; Rybnikova *et al.*, 2012; Segal *et al.*, 2012; Hahn *et al.*, 2011; Gao *et al.*, 2012; Zeng *et al.*, 2012). Clinical application of inhaled CO as a neuroprotective agent (the agent does not have to be the same as the potentially lethal insult) could be as a preconditioning agent, postconditioning agent, periconditioning agent, or agent used intraoperatively and may benefit patients undergoing cardiopulmonary bypass for heart surgery, extracorporeal membrane oxygenation, resection of brain tumors/abscesses or vascular malformations, deep hypothermic circulatory arrest, radiation or chemotherapy for brain tumors, traumatic brain injury, hypoxic injury of the newborn, stroke, epilepsy, and neurodegenerative diseases. Timing and dosing for maximum effect and safety needs to be evaluated in clinical trials for these indications.

The role of CO in the brain and central nervous system (CNS) has historically been negative, however recent data as presented in this chapter suggest that this dogma needs to be reevaluated. Endogenous CO is critical for normal brain function. Clearly CO is produced in the brain as a neurotransmitter and regulates memory and circadian rhythms. Therefore how can it also be so potently toxic? The answer is, of course, the dose and duration of exposure. The reports of the beneficial effects of CO in the brain and CNS continue to emerge and serve as a call for this simple gas to be reevaluated. Indeed, CO is currently being tested in clinical trials after passing rigorous safety testing. CO, like NO before it, may prove to be a therapeutic option and a new and novel approach to various neuropathologies. Clearly the time has come to reassess this simple gas as one cannot ignore the remarkable data that continues to be reported. The role for CO as a neurotherapeutic based on compelling animal data necessitates further testing in humans.

References

Almeida, A. S, Queiroga, C. S. F., Sousa, M. F. Q., Alves, P. M., & Vieira, H. L. A. (2012). Carbon monoxide modulates apoptosis by reinforcing oxidative metabolism in astrocytes: Role of Bcl-2. *Journal of Biological Chemistry, 287(14),* 10761-10770.

Andres, M. M. & Luszczki, J. J. (2004). Modified western blot technique in fast detection of heme oxygenase (HO-1/HO-2) in various tissues and organs of experimental animals. *Annales Universitatis Mariae Curie-Sklodowska. Section D: Medecina, 59(2),* 298-302.

Attwell, D. & Gibb, A. (2005). Neuroenergetics and the kinetic design of excitatory synapses. *Nature Reviews. Neuroscience, 6(11),* 841-849.

Aubert, A. & Costalat, R. (2005). Interaction between astrocytes and neurons studied using a mathematical model of compartmentalized energy metabolism. *Journal of Cerebral Blood Flow & Metabolism, 25(11),* 1476-1490.

Bak, L. K., Obel, L. F., Walls, A. B., Schousboe, A., Faek, S. A. A., Jajo, F. S., & Waagepetersen HS. (2012). Novel model of neuronal bioenergetics: Postsynaptic utilization of glucose but not lactate correlates positively with Ca^{2+} signalling in cultured mouse glutamatergic neurons. ASN Neuro, 4(3), e00083.

Barbagallo, I., Galvano, F., Frigiola, A., Cappello, F., Riccioni, G., Murabito, P., D'Orazio, N., Torella, M., Gazzolo, D., & Li Volti, G. (2013). Potential therapeutic effects of natural heme oxygenase-1 inducers in cardiovascular diseases. Antioxidants and Redox Signaling, 18(5), 507-521.

Bastianetto, S. & Quirion, R. (2010). Heme oxygenase 1: Another possible target to explain the neuroprotective action of resveratrol, a multifaceted nutrient-based molecule. Experimental Neurology, 225(2). 237-239.

Basuroy, S., Tcheranova, D., Bhattacharya, S., Leffler, C. W., & Parfenova, H. (2011). Nox4 NADPH oxidase-derived reactive oxygen ppecies, via endogenous carbon monoxide, promote survival of brain endothelial cells during TNF-α-induced apoptosis. American Journal of Physioogy. Cell Physiology, 300(2), C256-265.

Baum, O., Feussner, M., Richter, H., &Gossrau, R. (2000). Heme oxygenase-2 is present in the sarcolemma region of skeletal muscle fibers and is non-continuously co-localized with nitric oxide synthase-1. Acta Histochemica, 102(3):281-298.

Beckman, J. D., Belcher, J. D., Vineyard, J. V., Chen, C., Nguyen, J., Nwaneri, M. O., O'Sullivan, M. G., Gulbahce, E., Hebbel, R. P., & Vercellotti, G. M. (2009). Inhaled carbon monoxide reduces leukocytosis in a murine model of sickle cell disease. American Journal of Physiology. Heart and Circulatory Physiology, 297(4), H1243-H1253.

Bélanger, M., Allaman, I., & Magistretti, P. J. (2011). Brain energy metabolism: Focus on astrocyte-neuron metabolic cooperation. Cell Metabolism, 14(6), 724-738.

Bilban, M., Haschemi, A., Wegiel, B., Chin, B. Y., Wagner, O., & Otterbein, L. E. (2008). Heme oxygenase and carbon monoxide initiate homeostatic signaling. Journal of Molecular Medicine, 86, 267-279.

Boczkowski, J., Poderoso, J. J., & Motterlini, R. (2006). CO-metal interaction: Vital signaling from a lethal gas. Trends in Biochemical Sciences, (11), 614-621.

Boehning, D. & Snyder, S. H. (2002). Circadian rhythms. Carbon monoxide and clocks. Science, 298(5602), 2339-2340.

Boehning, D., Moon, C., Sharma, S., Hurt, K. J., Hester, L. D., Ronnett, G. V., Shugar, D., & Snyder, S. H. (2003). Carbon monoxide neurotransmission activated by CK2 phosphorylation of heme oxygenase-2. Neuron, 40(1), 129-137.

Boehning, D., Sedaghat, L., Sedlak, T. W., & Snyder, S. H. (2004). Heme oxygenase-2 is activated by calcium-calmodulin. Journal of Biological Chemistry, 279(30), 30927-30930.

Boycott, H. E., Dallas, M. L., Elies, J., Pettinger, L., Boyle, J. P., Scragg, J. L., Gamper, N., & Peers, C. (2013). Carbon monoxide inhibition of Cav3.2 T-type Ca2+ channels reveals tonic modulation by tioredoxin. FASEB Journal, 27(8), 3395-3407.

Brann, D. W., Bhat, G. K., Lamar, C. A., & Mahesh, V. B. (1997). Gaseous transmitters and neuroendocrine regulation. Neuroendocrinology, 65(6), 385-395.

Buxton, R. B. & Frank, L. R. (1997). A model for the coupling between cerebral blood flow and oxygen metabolism during neural stimulation. Journal of Cerebral Blood Flow & Metabolism, 17, 64-72.

Calabrese, V., Scapagnini, G., Ravagna, A., Fariello, R. G., Giuffrida Stella, A. M., & Abraham, N. G. (2002). Regional distribution of heme oxygenase, HSP70, and glutathione in brain: Relevance for endogenous oxidant/antioxidant balance and stress tolerance. Journal of Neuroscience Research, 68(1), 65-75.

Calabrese, V., Lodi, R., Tonon, C., D'Agata, V., Sapienza, M., Scapagnin, G., Mangiameli, A., Pennisi, G., Stella, A. M., & Butterfield, D. A. (2005). Oxidative stress, mitochondrial dysfunction and cellular stress response in Friedreich's Ataxia. Journal of the Neurological Sciences, 233(1-2), 145-162.

Calabrese, V., Butterfield, D. A., Scapagnini, G., Stella, A. M., & Maines, M. D. (2006). Redox regulation of heat shock protein expression by signaling involving nitric oxide and carbon monoxide: Relevance to brain aging, neurodegenerative disorders, and longevity." Antioxidants & Redox Signaling, 8(3-4), 444-477.

Calabrese, V., Cornelius, C., Dinkova-Kostova, A. T., Calabrese, E. J., & Mattson, M. P. (2010). Cellular stress responses, the hormesis paradigm, and vitagenes: Novel targets for therapeutic intervention in neurodegenerative disorders. Antioxidants & Redox Signaling, 13(11), 1763-1811.

Chang, C. H., Zhao, Y., Lee, C., & Ganguli, M. (2012). Smoking, death, and alzheimer disease: A case of competing risks. Alzheimer Disease and Associated Disorders, 26, 300-306.

Chang, E. F., Wong, R. F., Vreman, H. J., Igarashi, T., Galo, E., Sharp, F. R., Stevenson, D. K., & Noble-Haeusslein, L. J. (2003). Heme oxygenase-2 protects against lipid peroxidation-mediated cell loss and impaired motor recovery after traumatic brain injury. Journal of Neuroscence, 23(9), 3689-3696.

Chaverri, J., Barrera-Oviedo, D., & Maldonado, P. D. (2013). Heme oxygenase-1 (HO-1) upregulation delays morphological and oxidative damage induced in an excitotoxic/pro-oxidant model in the rat striatum. Neuroscience, 231, 91-101.

Cheng, X., Ku, C. H., & Siow, R. C. (2013). Regulation of the Nrf2 antioxidant pathway by microRNAs: New players in micromanaging redox homeostasis. Free Radical Biology and Medicine, 64, 4-11.

Chien, W. L., Lee, T. R., Hung, S. Y., Kang, K. H., Lee, M. J., & Fu, W. M. (2011). Impairment of oxidative stress-induced heme oxygenase-1 expression by the defect of parkinson-related gene of PINK1. Journal of Neurochemistry, 117(4), 643-653.

Choi, Y. K., Por, E. D., Kwon, Y. G., & Kim, Y. M. (2012). Regulation of ROS production and vascular function by carbon monoxide. Oxidative Medicine and Cellular Longevity, 2012, 794237.

Chung, H. T., Choi, B. M., Kwon, Y. G., & Kim, Y. M. (2008). Interactive relations between nitric oxide (NO) and carbon monoxide (CO): Heme oxygenase-1/CO pathway is a key modulator in NO-mediated antiapoptosis and anti-inflammation. Methods in Enzymology, 441, 329-338.

Coburn, R. F., Blakemore, W. S., & Forster, R. E. (1963). Endogenous carbon monoxide production in man. Journal of Clinical Investigation, 42(7), 1172-1178.

Coburn, R. F. (1973). Endogenous carbon monoxide metabolism. Annual Review of Medicine, 24, 241-250.

Coburn, R. F. (2012) The measurement of endogenous carbon monoxide production. Journal of Applied Physiology, 112(11), 1949-1955.

Colin-González, A. L., Orozco-Ibarra, M., Chánez-Cárdenas, M. E., Rangel-López, E., Santamaria, A., Pedraza-Innamorato, N. G., Lastres-Becker, I., & Cuadrado, A. (2009). Role of microglial redox balance in modulation of neuroinflammation. Current Opinion in Neuroogy, 22(3):308-314.

Colombrita, C., Calabrese, V., Stella, A. M., Mattei, F., Alkon, D. L., & Scapagnini, G. (2003). Regional rat brain distribution of heme oxygenase-1 and manganese superoxide dismutase mRNA: Relevance of redox homeostasis in the aging process. Experimental Biology and Medicine (Maywood), 228(5), 517-524.

Cuadrado, A. & Rojo, A. I. (2008). Heme oxygenase-1 as a therpeutic target in neurodegenerative diseases and brain infections. Curr ent Pharmaceutical Design, 14(5), 429-442.

Dallas, M. L., Boyle, J. P., Milligan, C. J., Sayer, R., Kerrigan, T. L., McKinstry, C., Lu, P., Mankouri, J., Harris, M., Scragg, J. L., Pearson, H. A., & Peers, C. (2011). Carbon monoxide protects against oxidant-induced apoptosis via inhibition of Kv2.1. FASEB Journal, 25(5), 1519-1530.

Decaluwé, K., Pauweis, B., Verpoest, S., & Van de Voorde, J. (2012). Divergent mechanisms involved in CO and CORM-2 induced vasorelaxation. European Journal of Pharmacology, 674(2-3), 370-377.

Deng, J., Lei, C., Chen, Y., Fang, Z., Yang, Q., Zhang, H., Cai, M., Shi, L., Dong, H., & Xiong, L. (2014). Neuroprotective gases – fantasy or reality for clinical use. Progress in Neurobiology, pii, S0301-0082(14)00011-2. doi: 10.1016/j.penurobiol.2014.01.001. [Epub ahead of print].

Dennery, P. A. (2013). Signaling function of heme oxygenase proteins. Antioxidants & Redox Signaling, [Epub ahead of print].

Deshane, J., Wright, M., & Agarwal, A. (2005). Heme oxygenase-1 expression in disease states. Acta Biochimica Polonica, 52(2), 273-284.

Desmard, M, Boczkowski, J., Poderoso, J., & Motterlini, R. (2007). Mitochondrial and cellular heme-dependent proteins as targets for the bioactive function of the heme oxygenase/carbon monoxide system. Antioxidants & Redox Signaling, 9(12), 2139-2155.

Dienel, G. A. & Hertz, L. (2001). Glucose and lactate metabolism during brain activation. Journal of Neuroscience Research, 66(5), 824-838.

Dienel, G. A. (2012). Fueling and imaging brain activation. ASN Neuro, 4(5), e00093.

Doré, S., Goto, S., Sampei, K., Blackshaw, S., Hester, L. D., Ingi, T., Sawa, A., Traystman, R. J., Koehle, R.C., & Snyder, S. H. (2000). Heme oxygenase-2 acts to prevent neuronal death in brain cultures and following transient cerebral ischemia. Neuroscience, 99(4), 587-592.

Dulak, J. & Józkowicz, A. (2003). Carbon monoxide – a "new" gaseous modulator of gene expression. Acta Biochimica Polonica, 50(1), 31-47.

Emborg, T. J., Walker, J. M., Noh, B., & Vierstra, R. D. (2006). Multiple heme oxygenasefFamily members contribute to the biosynthesis of the phytochrome chromophore in Arabidopsis. Plant Physiology, 140, 856-868.

El-Sayed, S., Hassan, M., Ibrahim, M., Elbassuoni, E., & Aziz, N. (2012). Modified endogenous carbon monoxide production through modulation of heme oxygenase activity alters some aspects of the cold restraint stress response in male albino rats. Endocrine Regulations, 46(4), 205-215.

Ewing, J. F. & Maines, M. D. (1997). Histochemical localization of heme oxygenase-2 protein and mRNA expression in rat brain. Brain Research. Brain Research Protocols, 1(2), 165-174.

Fan, W., Dong, W., Leng, S., Li, D., Cheng, S., Li, C., Qu, H., & He, H. (2008). Expression and colocalization of NADPH-diaphorase and heme oxygenase-2 in trigeminal ganglion and mesencephalic trigeminal nucleus of the rat. Journal of Molecular Histology, 39(4), 427-433.

Fujita, K., Yamafuji, M., Nakabeppu, Y., & Noda, M. (2012). Therapeutic approach to neurodegenerative diseases by medical gases: Focusing on redox signaling and related antioxidant enzymes. Oxidative Medicine and Cellular Longevity, Article ID 324256.

Fukoto, J. M., Carrington, S. J., Tantillo, D. J., Harrison, J. G., Ignarro, L. J., Freeman, B. A., Chen, A., & Wink, D. A. (2012). Small molecule signaling agents: The integrated chemistry and biochemistry of nitrogen oxides, oxides of carbon, dioxygen, hydrogen sulfide, and their derived species. Chemical Research in Toxicology, 25(4), 769-793.

Gao, C. J., Niu, L., Ren, P. C., Wang, W., Zhu, C., Li, Y. Q., Chai, W., & Sun, X. D. (2012). Hypoxic preconditioning attenuates global cerebral ischemic injury following asphyxial cardiac arrest through regulation of delta opioid receptor system. Neuroscience, 202, 352-362.

Glaum, S. R. & Miller, R. J. (1993). Zinc protoporhyrin-IX blocks the effects of metabotropic glutamate receptor activation in the rat nucleus tractus solitarii. Molecular Pharmacology, 43(6), 965-969.

Goebel, U., Siepe, M., Schwer, C. I., Schibilsky, D., Brehm, K., Priebe, H. J., Schlensak, C., & Loop, T. (2011). Postconditioning of the lungs with inhaled carbon monoxide after cardiopulmonary bypass in pigs. Anesthesia and Analgesia. 112(2), 282-291.

Gomperts, S. N., Carroll, R., Malenka, R. C., & Nicoli, R. A. (2000). Distinct roles for ionotropic and metabotropic glutamate receptors in the maturation of excitatory synapses. Journal of Neuroscience, 20(6), 2229-2237.

Gottlieb, Y, Truman, M., Cohen, L. A., Leichtmann-Bardoogo, Y., & Meyron-Holz, E. G. (2012). Endoplasmic reticulum anchored heme-oxygenase 1 faces the cytosol. Haematologicam 97(10), 1489-1493.

Gréhant, N. (1894) Les Gaz du Sang. Paris, G. Masson.

Gullotta, F., di Masi, A., Coletta, M., & Ascenzi, P. (2012). CO metabolism, sensing, and signaling. BioFactors (Oxford, England), 38(1), 1-13.

Hahn, C. D., Manlhiot, C., Schmidt, M. R., Nielsen, T. T., & Redington, A. N. (2011). Remote ischemic per-conditioning: A novel therapy for acute stroke? Stroke, 42(10), 2960-2962.

Hanafy, K. A., Oh, J., & Otterbein, L. E. (2013). Carbon monoxide and the brain: Time to rethink the dogma. Curr ent Pharmaceutical Dessign, 19(15), 2771-2775.

Harris, J, J,, Jolivet, R., & Attwell, D. (2012). Synaptic energy use and supply. Neuron, 75(5), 762-777.

Hayashi, S., Omata, Y., Sakamoto, H., Higashimoto, Y., Hara, T., Sagara, Y., & Noguchi, M. (2004). Characterization of rat heme oxygenase-3 gene. Implication of processed pseudogenes derived from heme oxygenase-2 gene. Gene, 336(2), 241-250.

Hegde, M. L., Hegde, P. M., Rao, K. S. J., & Mitra, S. (2011). Oxidative genome damage and its repair in neurodegenerative diseases: Function of transition metals as a double-edged sword. Journal of Alzheimer's Disease, 240(Suppl 2), 183-198.

Hegde, M. L., Mantha, A. K., Hazra, T. K., Bhakat, K. K., Mitra, S., & Szczesny, B. (2012). Oxidative genome damage and its repair: Implications in aging and neurodegenerative disease. Mechanisms of Ageing and Development, 133(4), 157-168.

Herzog, R. I., Jiang, L., Herman, P., Zhao, C., Sanganahalli, B. G., Mason, G. F., Hyder, F., Rothman, D. L., Sherwin, R.S., & Behar, K. L. (2013). Lactate preserves neuronal metabolism and function following antecedent recurrent hypoglycemia. Journal of Clinical Investigation, 123(5), 1988-1998.

Hodgkin, A. L. & Huxley, A. F. (1952). A quantitative description of membrane current and its application to conduction and excitation in nerve. Journal of Physiology, 117, 500-544.

Hoetzel, A., Dolinay, T., Schmidt, R., Choi, A. M., & Ryter, S. W. (2007). Carbon monoxide in sepsis. Antioxidants and Redox Signaling, 9(11), 2013-2026.

Hoetzel, A., Dolinay, T., Vallbracht, S., Zhang, Y., Kim, H. P., Ifedigbo, E., Alber, S., Kaynar, A. M., Schmidt, R., Ryter, S. W., & Choi, A. M. (2008). Carbon monoxide protects against ventilator-induced lung injury via PPAR-gamma and inhibition of Egr-1. American Journal of Respiratory and Critical Care Medicine, 177(11), 1223-1232.

Hou, S., Heinemann, S. H., & Hoshi, T. (2009). Modulation of BK_{Ca} channel gating by endogenous signaling molecules. Physiology, 24, 26-35.

Ingi, T. & Ronnett, G. V. (1995). Direct demonstration of a physiological role for carbon monoxide in olfactory receptor neurons. Journal of Neuroscience, 15(12), 8214-8222.

Innamorato, N. G., Rojo, A. I., Garcia-Yagüe, A. J., Yamamoto, M., de Ceballos, M. L., & Cuadrado, A. (2008). The transcription factor Nrf2 is a therapeutic target against brain inflammation. Journal of Immunology, 181(1), 680-689.

Ivanov, A., Mukhtarov, M., Bregestovski, P., & Zilberter, Y. (2011). Lactate effectively covers energy demands during neuronal network activity in neonatal hippocampal slices. Frontiers in Neuroenergetics, 3, 2.

Jazwa, A. & Cuadrado, A. (2010). Targeting heme oxygenase-1 for neuroprotection and neuroinflammation in neurodegenerative diseases. Current Drug Targets, 11(12), 1517-1531.

Jolivet, R., Magistretti, P. J., & Weber, B. (2009). Deciphering neuron-glia compartmentalization in cortical energy metabolism. Frontiers in Neuroenergetics, 1, 1-10.

Kajimura, M., Fukuda, R., Bateman, R. M., Yamamoto, T., & Suematsu M. (2010). Interactions of multiple gas-transducing systems: Hallmarks and uncertainties of CO, NO, and H_2S gas biology. Antioxidants & Redox Signaling, 13, 157-192.

Kim, H. P., Want, X., Galbiati, F., Ryter, S. W., & Choi, A. M. K. (2004). Caveolae compartmentalization of heme oxygenase-1 in endothelial cells. FASEB Journal, 28, 1080-1089.

Kim, H. P., Ryter, S. W., & Choi,A. M. K. (2006). CO as a cellular signaling molecule. Annual Review of Pharmacology and Toxicology, 46, 411-449.

Kim, H. P., Pae, H., Back, S. H., Chung, S. W., Woo, J. M., Son, Y., & Chung, H. (2011). Heme oxygenase-1 comes back to endoplasmic reticulum. Biochemical and Biophysical Research Communication. 2011;404:1-5.

Kim, Y. S. & Doré, S. (2005). Catalytically inactive heme oxygenase-2 mutant is cytoprotective. Free Radical Biology & Medicine, 39(4), 558-564.

Kirkby, K. A. & Adin, C. A. (2006). Products of heme oxygenase and their potential therapeutic applications. American Journal of Physiology – Renal Physiology, 290(3), F563-F571.

Koch, S., Sacco, R. L., & Perez-Pinzon, M. A. (2012). Preconditioning the brain: Moving on to the next frontier of neuro-therapeutics. Stroke, 43(6), 1455-1457.

Koppula, S., Kumar, H., Kim, I. S., & Choi, D. (2012). Reactive oxygen species and inhibitors of inflammatory enzymes, NADPH oxidase, and iNOS in experimental models of parkinson's disease. Mediators of Inflammation, 2012, 823902.

Laitinen, J. T. & Juvonen, R. O. (1995). A sensitive microassay reveals marked regional differences in the capacity of rat brain to generate carbon monoxide. Brain Research, 694(1-2), 246-252.

Laughlin, S. B., de Ruyter van Steveninck, R. R., & Anderson, J. C. (1998). The metabolic cost of neural information. Nat Neurosci, 1, 36-41.

Lim, S. Y. & Hausenloy, D. J. (2012). Remote ischemic conditioning: From bench to bedside. Frontiers in Physiology, 3, 27.

Lin, C. H., Lo, W. C., Hsiao, M., Tung, C. S., & Tseng, C. J. (2004). Interactions of carbon monoxide and metabotropic glutamate receptor groups in the nucleus tractus solitarii of rats. Journal of Pharmacology and Experimental Therapeutics, 308(3), 1213-1218.

MacAskill, A. F., Atkin, T. A., & Kittler, J. T. (2010). Mitochondrial trafficking and the provision of energy and calcium buffering at excitatory synapses. European Journal of Neuroscience, 32(2), 231-240.

Magistretti, P. J., Pellerin, L., Rothman, D. L., & Shulman, R. G. (1999). "Energy on Demand." Science, 283, 496-497.

Mahan, V. L., Zurakowski, D., Otterbein, L. E., & Pigula, F. A. (2012). Inhaled carbon monoxide provides cerebral cyto-protection in pigs. PLoS One, 7(8), e41982.

Maines, M. D. & Kappa, A. (1974). Cobalt induction of hepatic heme oxygenase: With evidence that Cyt P450 is not essential for this enzyme activity. Proceedings of the National Academy of Sciences of the United States of America, 71, 4293-4297.

Maines, M. D. (1980). Regional distribution of the enzymes of haem biosynthesis and the inhibition of 5-aminolaevulinate synthase by manganese in the rat brain. Biochemical Journal, 190(2), 315-321.

Maines, M. D., Trakshel, G. M., & Kutty, R. K. (1986). Characterization of two constitutive forms of rat liver microsomal heme oxygenase: Only one molecular species of the enzyme is inducible. Journal of Biological Chemistry, 261, 411-419.

Maines, M. D. (1992). Heme oxygenase: In Clinical Applications and Functions. Boca Rotan, FL: CRC Press.

Maines, M. D. (1997). The heme oxygenase system: A regulator of second messenger gases. Annual Review of Pharmacology and Toxicology, 37, 517-554.

Mancuso, C., Perluigi, M., Cini, C., De Marco, C., Giuffrida Stella, A. M., & Calabrese, V. (2006). Heme oxygenase and cyclooxygenase in the central nervous system: A functional interplay. Journal of Neuroscience Research, 84(7), 1385-1391.

McCoubrey, W. K. Jr, Huang, T. J., & Maines, M. D. (1997). Isolation and characterization of a cDNA from the rat brain that encodes hemoprotein heme oxygenase-3. European Journal of Biochemistry, 247(2), 725-732.

Mergenthaler, P. & Dirnagl, U. (2011). Protective conditioning of the brain: Expressway or roadblock? Journal of Physiology, 589(Pt 17), 4147-4155.

Moody, B. F. & Calvert, J. W. (2011). Emergent role of gasotransmitters in ischemia-reperfusion injury. Medical Gas Research, 1, 3.

Morse, D., Sethi, J., & Choi, A. M. K. (2002). Carbon monoxide-dependent signaling. Critical Care Medicine, 30(1), S12-S17.

Moxon-Lester, L., Sinclair, K., Burke, C., Cowin, G. J., Rose, S. E., & Colditz, P. (2007). Increased cerebral lactate during hypoxia may be neuroprotective in newborn piglets with intrauterine growth restriction. Brain Research, 1179, 79-88.

Naito, Y., Uchiyama, K., Takagi, T., & Youshikawa, T. (2012). Therapeutic potential of carbon monoxide (CO) for intestinal inflammation. Current Medicinal Chemistry, 19(1), 70-76.

Nako, A., Choi, A. M., & Murase, N. (2006). Protective effect of carbon monoxide in transplantation. Journal of Cellular and Molecular. Medicine, 10(3), 650-671.

Namiranian, K., Koehler, R. C., Sapirstein, A., & Doré, S. (2005). Stroke outcomes in mice lacking the genes for neuronal heme oxygenase-2 and nitric oxide synthase. Current Neurovascular Research, 2(1), 23-27.

Nathanson, J. A., Scavone, C., Scanlon, C., & McKee, M. (1995). The cellular Na^+ pump as a site of action for carbon monoxide and glutamate: A mechanism for long-term modulation of cellular activity. Neuron, 14(4), 781-794.

Neves, A., Costalat, R., & Pellerin, L. (2012). Determinants of brain cell metabolic phenotypes and energy substrate utilization unraveled with a modeling approach. PLoS Computational Biology, 8(9), e1002686.

Noda, M., Fujita, K., Lee, C. H., & Yoshioka, T. (2011). The principle and the potential approach to ROS-dependent cytotoxicity by non-pharmaceutical therapies: Optimal use of medical gases with antioxidant properties. Current Pharmaceutical Design, 17(22), 2253-2263.

Nuhn, P., Mitkus, T., Ceyhan, G. O., Künzli, B. M., Bergmann, F., Fischer, L., Giese, N., Friess, H., & Berberat, P. O. Heme oxygenase 1-generated carbon monoxide and biliverdin attenuate the course of experimental necrotizing pancreatitis. Pancreas, 42(2), 265-271.

Ozaki, K. S., Kimura, S., & Murase, N. (2012). Use of carbon monoxide in minimizing ischemia/reperfusion injury in transplantation. Transplantation Reviews (Orlando), 26(2), 125-139.

Parfenova, H., Basuroy, S., Bhattacharya, S., Tcheranova, D., Qu, Y., Regan, R. F., & Leffler, C. W. (2006). Glutamate induces oxidative stress and apoptosis in cerebral vascular endothelial cells: Contributions of HO-1 and HO-2 to cytoprotection. American Journal of Physiology. Cell Physiology, 290(5), C1399-1410.

Parfenova, H. & Leffler, C. W. (2008). Cerebroprotective functions of HO-2. Current Pharmaceutical Design, 14(5), 443-453.

Parfenova, H., Tcheranova, D., Basuroy, S., Fedinec, A. L., Liu, J., & Leffler, C. W. (2012). Functional role of astrocyte glutamate receptors and carbon monoxide in cerebral vasodilation response to glutamate. American Journal of Physiology. Heart and Circulatory Physiology, 302(1), H2257-H2266.

Pellerin, L. & Magistretti, P. J. (2004). Neuroenergetics: Calling upon astrocytes to satisfy hungry neurons. Neuroscientist, 10(1), 53-62.

Pellerin, L., Bouzier-Sore, A. K., Aubert, A., Serres, S., Merle, M., Costalat, R., & Magistretti, P. J. (2007). Activity-dependent regulation of energy metabolism by astrocytes: An update. Glia, 55(12), 1251-1262.

Piantadosi, C. A. (2002). Biological chemistry of carbon monoxide. Antioxidants & Redox Signaling, 4(2),259-270.

Piantadosi, C. A. (2008). Carbon monoxide, reactive oxygen signaling, and oxidative stress. Free Radical Biology and Medicine, 45(5), 562-569.

Pouokam, E., Steidle, J., & Diener, M. (2011). Regulation of colonic ion transport by gasotransmitters. Biological & Pharmaceutical Bulletin, 34(6), 789-793.

Prabhakar, N. R., Dinerman, J. L., Agani, F. H., & Snyder, S. H. (1995). Carbon monoxide: A role in carotid body chemoreception. Proceedings of the National Academy of Sciences of the United States of America, 92, 1994-1997.

Prabhakar, N. R. (1998). *Endogenous carbon monoxide in control of respiration. Respiration Physiology, 114(1), 57-64.*

Prabhakar, N. R. (1999). *NO and CO as second messengers in oxygen sensing in the carotid body. Respiration Physiology, 115(2), 161-168.*

Queiroga, C. S., Almeida, A. S., & Vieira, H. L. (2012). *Carbon monoxide targeting mitochondria. Biochem Res Int, 2012, 749845.*

Rasmussen, P., Wyss, M. T., & Lundby, C. (2011). *Cerebral glucose and lactate consumption during cerebral activation by physical activity in humans. FASEB Journal, 25(9), 2865-2873.*

Riddle, M. A. & Walker, B. R. (2012). *Regulation of endothelial BK channels by heme oxygenase-derived carbon monoxide and caveolin-1. American Journal of Physiology. Cell Physiology, 303(1), C92-C101.*

Rivier, C. (1998). *Role of nitric oxide and carbon monoxide in modulating the ACTH response to immune and nonimmune signals. Neuroimmunomodulation, 5(3-4), 203-213.*

Rodgers, P. A., Vreman, H. J., Dennery, P. A., & Stevenson, D. K. (1994). *Sources of carbon monoxide (CO) in biological systems and applications of CO detection technologies. Seminars of Perinatology, 18(1), 2-10.*

Rybnikova, E., Vorobyev, M., Pivina, S., & Samoilov, M. (2012). *Postconditioning by mild hypoxic exposures reduces rat brain injury caused by severe hypoxia. Neuroscience Letters, 513(1), 100-105.*

Ryter, S. W., Otterbein, L. E., Morse, D., & Choi, A. M. (2002). *Heme oxygenase/carbon monoxide signaling pathways: Regulation and functional significance. Molecular and Cellular Biochemistry, 234-235(1-2), 249-263.*

Ryter, S. W., Morse, D., & Choi, A. M. K. (2004). *Carbon monoxide: To boldly go where NO has gone before. Science Siganaling The Signal Transduction Knowledge Environment, 230, re6.*

Ryter, S. W. & Otterbein, L. E. (2004). *Carbon monoxide in biology and medicine. BioEssays, 26(3), 270-280.*

Ryter, S. W. & Choi, A. M. (2007). *Cytoprotective and anti-inflammatory actions of carbon monoxide in organ injury and sepsis models. Novartis Foundation Symposium, 280, 165-175.*

Ryter, S. W. & Choi, A. M. K. (2013). *Carbon monoxide: Present and future indications for a medical gas. Korean Journal of Internal Medicine, 28, 123-140.*

Sabens Liedhegner, E. A., Gao, X., & Mieyal, J. J. (2012). *Mechanisms of altered redox regulation in neurodegenerative diseases – focus on s-glutathionylation. Antioxidants & Redox Signaling, 16(6), 543-566.*

Sanders, R. D, Manning, H. J., Robertson, N. J., Ma, D., Edwards, A. D., Hagberg, H., & Maze, M. (2010). *Preconditioning and postinsult therapies for perinatal hypoxic-ischemic injury at term. Anesthesiology, 113(1), 233-249.*

Sass, G., Barikbin, R., & Tiegs, G. (2012). *The multiple functions of heme oxygenase-1 in the liver. Zeitschrift für Gastroenterologie, 50(1), 34-40.*

Scapagnini, G., D'Agata, V., Calabrese, V., Pascale, A., Colombrita, C., Alkon, D., & Cavallaro, S. (2002). *Gene expression profiles of heme oxygenase isoforms in the rat brain. Brain Research, 954, 51-59.*

Schallner, N., Fuchs, M., Schwer, C. I., Loop, T., Buerkle, H., Lagrèze, W. A., van Oterendorp, C., Biermann, J., & Goebel, U. (2012). *Postconditioning with inhaled carbon monoxide counteracts apoptosis and neuroinflammation in the ischemic rat retina. PLoS One, 7(9), e46479.*

Schallner, N., Romão, C. C, Biermann, J., Lagrèze, W. A., Otterbein, L. E., Buerkle, H., Loop, T., & Goebel, U. (2013). *Carbon monoxide abrogates ischemic insult to neuronal cells via the soluble guanylate cyclase-cGMP pathway. PloS One, 8(4), e60672.*

Schipper, H. M., Song, W., Zukor, H., Hascalovic, J. R., & Zeligman, D. (2009). *Heme oxygenase-1 and neurodegeneration: Expanding frontiers of engagement. Journal of Neurochemistry, 110, 469-485.*

Schurr, A., Miller, J. J., Payne, R. S., & Rigor, B. M. (1999). *An increase in lactate output by brain tissue serves to meet the energy needs of glutamate-activated neurons. Journal of Neuroscience, 19(1), 34-39.*

Schurr, A. & Gozal, E. (2011). Aerobic production and ttilization of lactate satisfy increased energy demands upon neuronal activation in hippocampal slices and provide neuroprotection against oxidative stress. Frontiers in Pharmacology, 2, 96.

Scott, J. R., Cukiernik, M. A., Ott, M. C., Bihari, A., Badhwar, A., Gray, D. K., Harris, K. A., Parry, N. G., & Potter, R. F. (2009). Low-dose inhaled carbon monoxide attenuates the remote intestinal inflammatory response elicited by hindlimb ischemia-reperfusion. American Journal of Physiology. Gastrointestinal and Liver Physiology, 296(1), G9-G14.

Segal, N., Matsuura, T., Caldwell, E., Sarraf, M., McKnite, S., Zviman, M., Aufderheide, T. P., Halperin, H. R., Lurie, K. G., & Yannopoulos, D. (2012). Ischemic postconditioning at the initiation of cardiopulmonary resuscitation facilitates functional cardiac and cerebral recovery after prolonged untreated ventricular fibrillation. Resuscitation, 83(11), 1397-1403.

Severino, P. C., Muller Gdo, A., Vandresen-Filho, S., & Tasca, C. I. (2011). Cell signaling in NMDA preconditioning and neuroprotection in convulsions induced by quinolinic acid. Life Sciences, 89(15-16), 570-576.

Sibson, N. R., Dhankhar, A., Mason, G. F., Rothman, D. L., Behar, K. L., & Shulman, R. G. (1998). Stoichiometric coupling of brain glucose metabolism and glutamatergic neuronal activity. Proceedings of the National Academy of Sciences in the United States of America, 95, 316-321.

Sjöstrand, T. (1950). Endogenous formation of carbon monoxide. Acta Physiologica Scandinavica, 22, 137-141.

Sjöstrand, T. (1952). The formation of carbon monoxide by the decomposition of haemoglobin in vivo. Acta Physiologica Scandinavica, 26(4), 338-344.

Soares, M. P., Usheva, A., Brouard, S., Berberat, P. O., Gunter, L., Tobiasch, E., & Bach, F. H. (2002). Modulation of endothelial cell apoptosis by heme xygenase-1-derived carbon monoxide. Antioxidants and Redox Signaling, 4(2), 321-329.

Sutherland, B. A., Rahman, R. M., Clarkson, A. N., Shaw, O. M., Nair, S. M., & Appleton, I. (2009). Cerebral heme oxygenase 1 and 2 spatial distributiuon is modulated following injury from hypoxia-ischemia and middle cerebral artery occlusion in rats. Neuroscience Research, 65(4), 326-334.

Takagi, T., Naito, Y., Mizushima, K., Akagiri, S., Suzuki, T., Hirata, I., Omatsu, T., Handa, O., Kokura, S., Ichikawa, H., & Yoshikawa, T. (2010). Inhalation of carbon monoxide ameliorates TNBS-induced colitis in mice through the inhibition of TNF-α expression. Digestive Diseases and Sciences, 55(10), 2797-2804.

Takagi, T., Naito, Y., Uchiyama, K., Suzuki, T., Hirata, I., Mizushima, K., Tsuboi, H., Hayashi, N., Handa, O., Ishikawa, T., Yagi, N., Kokura, S., Ichikawa, H., & Yoshikawa, T. (2011). Carbon monoxide liberated from carbon monoxide-releasing molecule exerts an anti-inflammatory effect on dextran sulfate sodium-induced colitis in mice. Digestive Diseases and Sciences, 56(6), 1663-1671.

Telezhkin, V., Brazier, S. P., Mears, R., Müller, C. T., Riccardi, D., & Kemp, P. J. (2011). Cysteine residue 911 in c-terminal tail of human BK(Ca)α channel subunit is crucial for its activation by carbon monoxide. Pflugers Archiv-European Journal of Physiology, 461(6), 665-675.

Tenhunen, R., Marver ,H. S., & Schmid, R. (1968). The enzymatic conversion of heme to bilirubin by microsomal heme oxygenase. Proceedings of the National Academy of Sciences of the United States of America, 61, 748-755.

Tenhunen, R., Marver, H. S., & Schmid, R. (1969). Microsomal heme oxygenase: Characterization of the enzyme. Journal of Biological Chemistry, 244, 6388-6394.

Tsui, T. Y., Obed, A., Siu, Y. T., Yet, S. F., Prantl, L. Schiltt, H. J., & Fan, S. T. (2007). Carbon monoxide inhalation rescues mice from fulminant hepatitis through improving hepatic energy metabolism. Shock, 27(2), 165-171.

Vieira, H. L., Queiroga, C. S., & Alves, P. M. (2008). Pre-conditioning induced by carbon monoxide provides neuronal protection against apoptosis. Journal of Neurochemistry, 107(2), 375-384.

Vincent, S. R., Das, S., & Maines, M. D. (1994). Brain heme oxygenase isoenzymes and nitric oxide synthase are co-localized in select neurons. Neuroscience, 63(1), 223-231.

Vukomanovic, D., McLaughlin, B., Rahman, M. N., Vlahakis, J. Z., Roman, G., Dercho, R. A., Kinobe, R. T., Hum, M., Brien, J. F., Jia, Z., Szarek, W. A., & Nakatsu, K. (2010). Recombinant truncated and microsoma heme oxygenase-1 and -2: Differential sensitivity to inhibitors. Canadian Journal of Physiology and Pharmacology, 88(4), 480-486.

Vukomanovic, D., McLaughlin, B. E., Rahman, M. N., Szarek, W. A., Brien, J. F., Jia, Z., & Nakatsu, K. (2011). Selective activation of heme oxygenase-2 by menadione. Canadian Journal of Physioogy and Pharmacology, 89, 861-864.

Wang, B., Cao, W., Biswal, S., & Doré, S. (2011). Carbon monoxide – activated Nrf2 pathway leads to protection against permanent focal cerebral ischemia. Stroke, 42, 2605-2610.

Wang, J., Zhuang, H., & Doré S. (2006). Heme oxygenase 2 is neuroprotective against intracerebral hemorrhage. Neurobiology of Disease, 22(3), 473-476.

Wang J and Doré, S. (2008). Heme oxygenase 2 deficiency increases brain swelling and inflammation after intracerebral hemorrhage. Neuroscience, 155(4), 1133-1141.

Watts, R. N., Ponka, P., & Richardson, D. R. (2003). Effects of nitrogen monoxide and carbon monoxide on molecular and cellular iron metabolism: Mirror-image effector molecules that target iron. Biochemical Journal, 369(Pt 3), 429-440.

Wen, Z., Liu, Y., Li, F., & Wen, T. (2012). Low dose of carbon monoxide intraperitonealiInjection provides potent protection against GalN/LPS-induced acute liver injury in mice. Journal of Applied Toxicology, (33(12), 1424-1432.

Wilkinson, W. J. & Kemp, P. J. (2011). Carbon monoxide: An emerging regulator of ion channels. Journal of Physiology, 589(13), 3055-3062.

Won, S. J., Jang, B. G., Yoo, B. H., Sohn, M., Lee, M. W., Choi, B. Y., Kim, J. H., Song, H. K., & Suh S. W. (2012). Prevention of acute/severe hypoglycemia-induced neuron death by lactate administration. Journal of Cerebral Blood Flow & Metabolism, 32(6), 1086-1096.

Wu, L. & Wang, R. (2005). Carbon monoxide: Endogenous production, physiological functions, and pharmacological applications. Pharmacological Reviews, 57(4), 585-630.

Xia, Z. W., Cui, W. J., Zhang, X. H., Shen, Q. X., Want, J., Li, Y. Z., Chen, S. N., & Yu, S.C. (2002). Analysis of heme oxygenase isomers in rat. World Journal of Gastroenterology, 8(6), 1123-1128.

Yabluchanskiy, A., Sawle, P., Homer-Vanniasinkam, S., Green, C. J., Foresti, R., & Motterlini, R. (2012). CORM-3, a carbon monoxide-releasing molecule, alters the inflammatory response and reduces brain damage in a rat model of hemorrhagic stroke. Critical Care Medicine, 40(2), 544-552.

Yoneyama-Sarnecky, T., Olivas, A. D., Azari, S., Ferriero, D. M., Manvelyan, H. M., & Noble-Haeusslein, L. J. (2010). Heme oxygenase-2 modulates early pathogenesis after traumatic injury to the immature brain. Developmental Neuroscience, 32(1), 81-90.

Yoshida, T., Takahashi, S., & Kikuchi, G. (1974). Partial purification and reconstruction of the heme oxygenase system from pig spleen microsomes. Journal of Biochemistry (Tokyo), 75. 1187-1191.

Zeng, Y., Xie, K., Dong, H., Zhang, H., Wang, F., Li, Y., & Xiong L. (2012). Hyperbaric oxygen preconditioning protects cortical neurons against oxygen-glucose deprivation injury: Role of peroxisome proliferator-activated receptor-gamma. Brain Research, 1452, 140-150.

Zeynalov, E. & Doré, S. (2009). Low oses of carbon monoxide protect against experimental focal brain ischemia. Neurotoxicity Research, 15(2), 133-137.

Zhao, H., Ren, C., Chen, X., & Shen J. (2012). From rapid to delayed and remote postconditioning: The evolving concept of ischemic postconditioning in brain ischemia. Current Drug Targets, 13(2), 173-187.

Zhong, F., Pan, J., Liu, X., Wang, H., Ying, T., Su, J., Huang, Z. X., & Tan, X. (2011). A novel insight into the heme and NO/CO binding mechanism of the alpha subunit of human soluble guanylate cyclase. Journal of Biological Inorganic Chemistry, 16(8), 1227-1239.

Zhou, H., Liu, J., Pan, P., Jin, D., Ding, W., & Li, W. (2010). Carbon monoxide inhalation decreased lung injury via anti-inflammatory and anti-apoptotic effects in brain death rats. *Experimental Biology and Medicine (Maywood)*, *235(10)*, 1236-1243.

Miliary Brain Metastases

Bora Gürer

Department of Neurosurgery
Diskapi Yildirim Beyazit Education and Research Hospital, Turkey

Ramazan Kahveci

Department of Neurosurgery
Kirikkale Yuksek Ihtisas Hospital, Turkey

1   Introduction

Postmortem examinations (Ogawa *et al.*, 2007) showed that the brain metastasis covers approximately 12-25% of the cancer patients. Metastasis is being the most common brain tumor; where up to 40% of all the brain neoplasms are developed from metastatic origin (Nemzek *et al.*, 1993). About 65-86% of all metastatic brain tumors are multiple, but almost always their number is less than five (Weisberg, 1979).

Most brain metastases are macroscopic parenchymal mass lesions with surrounding edema, and occur at the gray-white matter junction (Weisberg, 1979). Leptomeningeal carcinomatosis resulting from diffuse infiltration in the subarachnoid space also occurs in about 3% of the patients with lung, breast or gastric carcinomas (Ogawa *et al.*, 2007). On the other hand, there is an extremely rare form of brain metastases which are characterized by the presence of tumoral spreading into the perivascular Virchow-Robin spaces, parenchyma, and as well as meninges. Several terms were proposed to describe this rare form of the brain metastasis, such as "miliary carcinoma", miliary brain metastases", "metastatic meningoencephalic carcinomatosis without tunefaction". In 1951, Madow and Alpers, proposed the expression "carcinomatosis encephalitis" as the most adequate term. We, the authors of this chapter preferred to use the term "miliary brain metastases" because this term referred in the most recent publication and accepted by us as it defines the condition with clear terminology.

Miliary brain metastases are extremely rare conditions with poor prognosis. To our knowledge, in the English literature, there had been only 25 cases reported till today (Ara Callizo *et al.*, 1989; Bhushan, 1997; Bugalho *et al.*, 2005; Falk *et al.*, 2012; Floeter *et al.*, 1987; Fukuda *et al.*, 1988; Iguchi *et al.*, 2007; Inomata *et al.*, 2012; Kahveci *et al.*, 2012; Madow and Alpers, 1951; Mochizuki *et al.*, 2012; Nakamura *et al.*, 2001; Nemzek *et al.*, 1993; Ogawa *et al.*, 2007; Olsen *et al.*, 1987; Ribeiro *et al.*, 2007; Rivas *et al.*, 2005; Ruppert *et al.*, 2010; Shirai *et al.*, 1997; Wong *et al.*, 2007; Yamazaki *et al.*, 1993). The aim of this chapter is to provide detailed information on this condition and review the recent literature.

2   Clinical Manifestations

Clinical manifestations of the miliary brain metastases vary widely. Clinically, miliary brain metastases are usually silent and the symptoms differ from patient to patient. Despite this silent clinical presentation some may present with various signs and symptoms of the central nervous system at the onset. The patients who were suffering from miliary brain metastases frequently demonstrate an organic mental syndrome, dementia in a subacute fashion, hemiparesis and convulsions (Ogawa *et al.*, 2007; Rivas *et al.*, 2005; Shirai *et al.*, 1997). Early onset, rapidly progressing dementia is always prominent in the clinical course at an early point and may be a warning sign of this pathology.

However, neurological findings can strongly be minimal in majority of patients with miliary brain metastases. This indistinct clinical course may be due to weak edematous effect of the masses (Bhushan, 1997). Also speech abnormalities, gait disturbance can be the initial symptoms of miliary brain metastases. On the other hand, some patients do not have any neurological symptoms and were incidentally diagnosed during routine follow-up radiologic studies (Kahveci *et al.*, 2012).

3   Radiological Diagnosis

Plain skull x-rays and brain computed tomography (CT) have very limited diagnostic value in miliary brain metastases. In some calcified lesions, CT can easily detect multiple calcified lesions in the central nervous system (Ara Callizo *et al.*, 1989; Fukuda *et al.*, 1988; Yamazaki *et al.*, 1993). Furthermore, brain CT scan with contrast enhancement may demonstrate numerous tiny lesions (Floeter *et al.*, 1987; Olsen *et al.*, 1987). Also, the brain edema caused by multiple metastatic lesions can be evident in CT (Figure 1). Hydrocephalus that may result from meningeal and periventricular damage alters cerebrospinal fluid circulation can easily be detected by non-contrast CT.

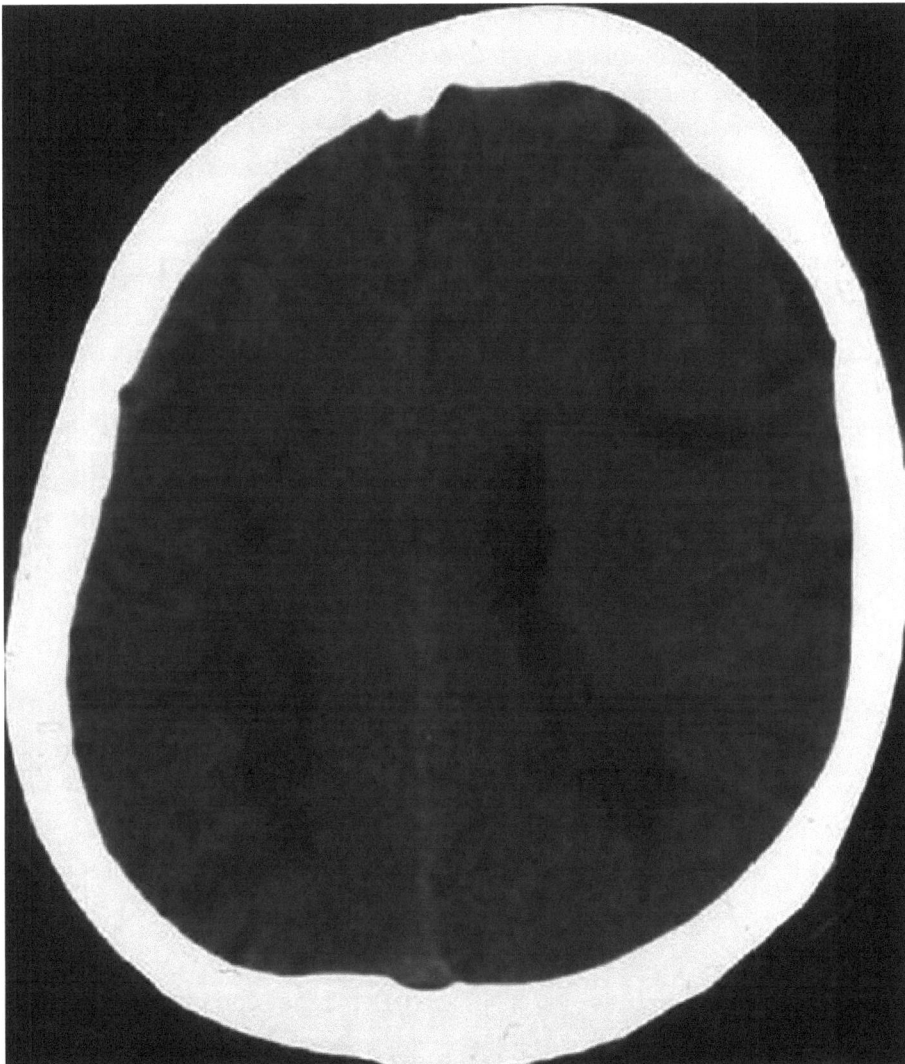

Figure 1: Brain CT of a patient with miliary brain metastases revealing the edematous regions

Prior to magnetic resonance imaging (MRI), delayed double-dose contrast enhanced CT scans were consulted to be the optimal method to evaluate metastatic disease of the central nervous system (Shalen *et al.*, 1981). Nowadays, MRI has proven to be more sensitive than CT in detection of any central nervous system pathology, and contrast enhanced MRI is the test of choice to evaluate metastatic disease of the brain and spinal cord (Brant-Zawadzki *et al.*, 1984). Magnetic resonance imaging with gadolinium enhancement was further improved lesion detection especially for metastatic disease (Hesselink and Press, 1988; Sze *et al.*, 1990).

Miliary metastasis are seen as nodular, tiny, multiple lesions with perivascular spreading; showing iso-to low intensity on T1 and high intensity signals on T2-weighted sequences of MRI and may present a nodular or peripheral (ring-like) contrast enhancement following gadolinium injection (Iguchi *et al.*, 2007) (Figure 2). In some cases in which brain MRI were performed did not show any abnormalities (McGuigan *et al.*, 2005; Nakamura *et al.*, 2001; Ogawa *et al.*, 2007; Rivas *et al.*, 2005). Furthermore some miliary brain metastases did not enhance with contrast media (McGuigan *et al.*, 2005; Nakamura *et al.*, 2001; Nemzek *et al.*, 1993; Yamazaki *et al.*, 1993). It is speculated that the contrast-enhanced MRI could fail to delineate the metastatic lesions because the blood-brain barrier remains intact at the early stages of the clinical course (Inomata *et al.*, 2012; Nemzek *et al.*, 1993; Ogawa *et al.*, 2007).

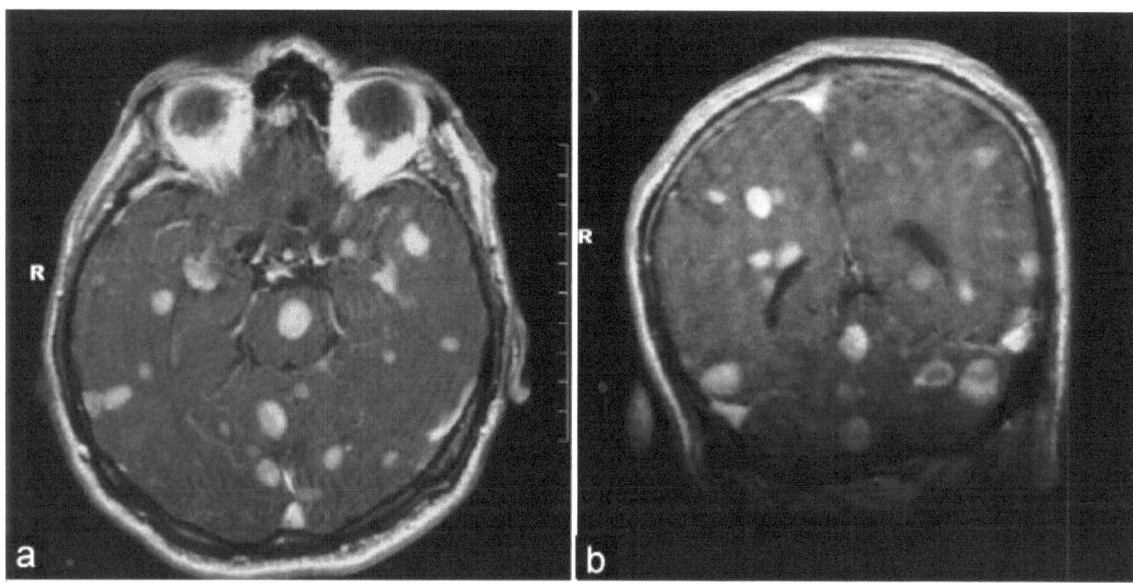

Figure 2: Gadolinium-enhanced axial, and coronal T1-weighted MRI section revealed multiple millimetric nodular lesions with homogenous enhancement in both cerebral hemispheres and the brainstem

On the other hand, a large number of infectious and non-infectious diseases such as miliary tuberculosis, neurocysticercosis or toxoplasmosis, can cause multiple enhancing lesions in the brain, and mimic miliary brain metastases (Garg and Sinha, 2010). So, differential diagnosis with proper imaging techniques is mandatory.

Proton magnetic resonance spectroscopy (MRS) is a potent instrument to analyze tissue metabolism noninvasively. It reflects alterations of the intracellular metabolite concentrations such as choline (Cho), creatine (Cr), N-acetylaspartate (NAA), lipids and lactate on pathological tissues (Hollingworth *et al.*, 2006). This technique may help to distinguish pathological tissue from normal brain tissue in means of differences of the intracellular metabolites (Hollingworth *et al.*, 2006). On proton MRS imaging, non-neoplastic lesions such as cerebral infractions and brain abscess have noticeable decreases in Cho, Cr and NAA levels. While tumors have generally elevated Cho and decreased levels of Cr and NAA, it had been shown that intracranial metastatic lesions showed strong elevations in levels of lipids. This elevation of the levels of lipids in metastatic tumors was significantly higher than any brain lesion except tuberculosis, abscess and toxoplasmosis (Möller-Hartmann *et al.*, 2002). On the other hand Cho, Cr and NAA levels were shown to decrease in tuberculosis, abscess and toxoplasmosis may help to distinguish infectious pathologies from miliary brain metastases (Kahveci *et al.*, 2012) (Figure 3). Kahveci *et al.* (2012) reported that Cho levels were increased with elevated Cho/NAA and decreased NAA/Cr ratios on proton MRS in a patient with miliary brain metastases. Proton MRS may contribute to make differential diagnosis of the miliary enhanced lesions of the central nervous system.

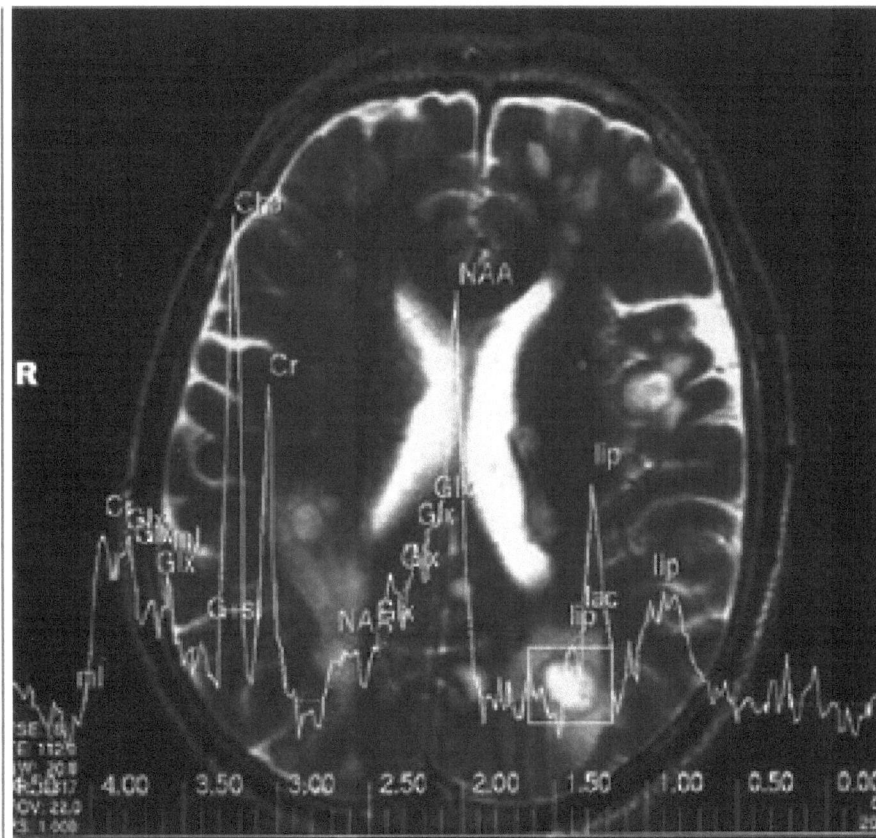

Figure 3: Proton MRS showed an increase in choline peak

4   Pathological Features

Parenchymal cerebral metastases are usually characterized by nodules or single masses in white and gray matter junction, as a result of hematogenic dissemination. It is estimated that up to 30% of patients with solid cancer have cerebral metastasis at the time of death (Ribeiro *et al.*, 2007). Miliary metastatic pattern describes the occurrence of several disseminated nodules in the brain parenchyma. It is quite uncommon and invades the perivascular Virchow-Robin spaces, parenchyma and meninges (Ribeiro *et al.*, 2007).

Since the clinical features are frequently non-specific and radiological studies often fail to make a correct diagnosis, neuropathological examination is essential to establish the diagnosis. In histopathologically proved cases, the most common site of metastasis to the brain in miliary brain metastases was the lung and the most common pathology was adenocarcinoma (Table 1). Although in macroscopic examination the gross evidence of tumor involvement is usually minimal. Light microscopic examination generally reveals outnumbered foci of metastases with a perivascular distribution (Figure 4).

The metastatic cascade, whereby cancer cells escape from the primary tumor site, invade surrounding tissue, intravasate into the bloodstream or lymphatics, and arrest, extravasate, survive and proliferate within a secondary site is an inherently inefficient process. Certain tumor types demonstrate an organ-specific pattern of spread (Talmadge and Fidler, 2010). Once metastatic cancer cells enter the brain circulation, they might arrest in sites of slow flow within the capillary bed at vascular branch points. The arrested cancer cells encounter brain vascular endothelial cells, which seems to promote metastatic tumor cell growth and invasion (Kienast *et al.*, 2010)

Kienast *et al.* (2010) used multiphoton laser scanning microscopy and a mouse cranial window model to follow in real time brain metastasis formation from both lung cancer and melanoma cell lines. After extravasation, there was a persistent correlation between tumor cells with micro-vessels, and either vessel co-option (with melanoma) or angiogenesis (with lung carcinoma). Previous studies showed a similar association between metastasizing tumor cells and blood vessels.

Recently, the importance of cellular adhesion molecules, which attach carcinoma cells to vascular endothelium, has been identified in metastatic processes. Ogawa *et al.* (2007), reported that in a miliary brain metastases case adhesion molecules were expressed abnormally and caused to trap carcinoma cells in the vessels. It has been hypothesized that perivascular pial sheath (adventitia) plays an important role for the development of the miliary brain metastases.

5   Differential Diagnosis

In the differential diagnosis of the miliary brain metastases, the diagnosis of paraneoplastic encephalopathy, vascular dementia, infectious encephalitis, and adverse effects of chemotherapy must be considered. The main MRI differential diagnosis is meningitis by Criptococcus sp because of the distribution pattern of the lesions in the perivascular spaces of Virchow-Robin in the diencephalon, centrum semiovale, leptomeninges, and the presence of hydrocephalus. But cerebrospinal fluid analysis of the miliary brain metastases patients is generally non-specific (Ribeiro *et al.*, 2007).

A variety of infective and non-infective etiologies can produce multiple ring-like enhancing lesions of the brain. It is a diagnostic challenge to make a correct diagnosis in such situations (el-Sonbaty *et al.*, 1995; Garg *et al.*, 2000; 2008; Oncul *et al.*, 2005; Tosomeen *et al.*, 1998). Also it is observed that infectious pathology is the most common etiology in patients with multiple ring enhancing lesions of the brain (Garg *et al.*, 2008). Of these infectious etiologies, tuberculosis and neurocysticecosis are the most common infections. Furthermore, metastatic etiology is the commonest of the non-infectious etiology (el-Sonbaty *et al.*, 1995; Garg *et al.*, 2000; 2008; Oncul *et al.*, 2005; Tosomeen *et al.*, 1998).

Author, Year	Age, Sex	Primary Site	Histology	Symptoms	Imaging of Diagnosis	Diagnosed by	Survival
Madow & Alpers, 1951	55, M	Lung	Adenocarcinoma	Psychiatric symptoms, Hemiparesis, Aphasia, Cerebellar signs, Convulsion	None	Autopsy	24m (?)
	48, M	Not identified	Adenocarcinoma	Psychiatric symptoms, Convulsion	None	Autopsy	1m (?)
	47, M	Lung	Adenocarcinoma	Psychiatric symptoms, Hemiparesis, Convulsion	None	Autopsy	15m
	31, F	Lung	Adenocarcinoma	Psychiatric symptoms, Convulsion, Headache	None	Autopsy	18m
Olsen et al., 1987	60, F	Unknown	Papillary adenocarcinoma	Unconsciousness	Contrast CT, Non-contrast MRI	Biopsy	Not reported
Floeter et al., 1987	60, F	Unknown	Papillary adenocarcinoma	Unconsciousness	Contrast CT, Contrast MRI	Biopsy	2m
Fukuda et al., 1988	60, F	Lung	Adenocarcinoma	Speech disturbance, Hemiparesis, Mild dementia	Non-contrast CT	Clinically	9m
Ara Callizo et al., 1989	61, M	Pancreas	Acinar cell carcinoma	Confusion, Hemiparesis	Non-contrast CT	Autopsy	7d
Nemzek et al., 1993	59, F	Lung	Small cell carcinoma	Lethargy, Slow speech, Convulsion	Non-contrast MRI	Autopsy	2m
Yamazaki et al., 1993	58, M	Lung	Adenocarcinoma	Dementia	Non-contrast CT	Biopsy	8m
Bhushan, 1997	69, M	Unknown	Undifferentiated adenocarcinoma	Dizziness, Gait disturbance	Contrast MRI	Biopsy	4m
Shirai et al., 1997	68, M	Heterotopic salivary	Adenocarcinoma	Stupor, Headache, Hemiparesis, Convulsion	Contrast MRI	Autopsy	7m

	Age, Sex	Primary site	Histology	Symptoms	Imaging	Diagnosis	Survival
Nakamura et al., 2001	44, M	Lung	Adenocarcinoma	Stupor; Psychiatric symptoms	Contrast MRI	Autopsy	2m
Rivas et al., 2005	79, F	Unknown	Papillary adenocarcinoma	Dementia; Visual hallucinations; Extrapyramidal signs	Normal radiology	Autopsy	6m
Bugalho et al., 2005	77, M	Stomach	Small cell gastric carcinoma	Cognitive deterioration; Gait disturbance; Urinary incontinence	Contrast MRI	Biopsy	4m
Ogawa et al., 2007	82, F	Lung	Papillary adenocarcinoma	Dementia; Mutism	Normal radiology	Autopsy	5m
Iguchi et al., 2007	66, M	Lung	Papillary adenocarcinoma	Hemiparesis; Dysathria	Contrast MRI	Autopsy	11m
Ribeiro et al., 2007	76, F	Lung	Adenocarcinoma	Confusion; Somnolence; Headache; Diplopia	Contrast MRI	Autopsy	14d
Wong et al., 2007	39, F	Lung	Small cell carcinoma	Confusion; Headache	Contrast MRI		Not available
Ruppert et al., 2010	55, M	Lung	Adenocarcinoma	Gait disturbance; Cerebellar signs	Non-contrast MRI	Autopsy	6 weeks
Falk et al., 2012	37, F	Lung	Adenocarcinoma	No symptoms	Contrast MRI	Radiologic	4m
Inomata et al., 2012	68, F	Lung	Adenocarcinoma	Headache; Nausea; Gait disturbance	Contrast MRI	Autopsy	3m
Mochizuki et al., 2012	37, F	Lung	Adenocarcinoma	Confusion; Dementia	Contrast MRI	Clinically	20m
	64, F	Lung	Adenocarcinoma	No symptoms	Contrast MRI	Clinically	18m
Kahveci et al., 2012	52, M	Lung	Adenocarcinoma	Seizure; Unconsciousness	Contrast MRI; Proton MR-spectroscopy	Biopsy	1m

Table: Presented cases of miliary metastases in the English literature.

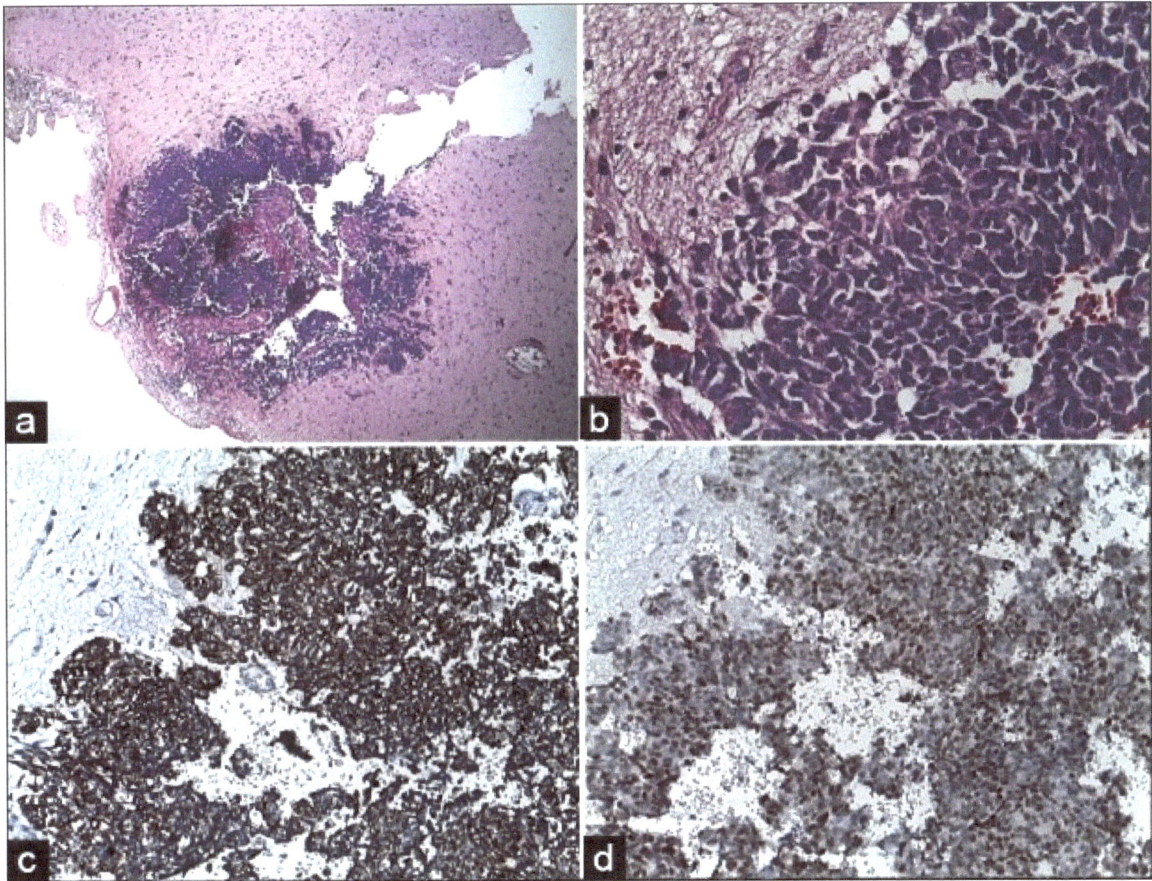

Figure 4: Pathologic specimen of cerebral biopsy of a patient with miliary brain metastases originating from lung adenocarcinoma. Microscopic examination with H and E staining revealed infiltrating glial tissue by neoplastic cells (original magnification ×4) (a), Microscopic examination with H and E staining revealed solid nests of atypical cells having pleomorphic nuclei and eosinophilic cytoplasm (original magnification ×40) (b), Immunohistochemical examination of tissue sections showed neoplastic cells cytoplasms staining positively for cytokeratin 7, and nuclear TTF-1 expression of neoplastic cells (c, d)

In HIV-infected patients, infections like toxoplasmosis, cryptococcosis, progressive multifocal leukoencephalopaty and certain neoplastic disease must be considered in the differential diagnosis (Porter and Sande, 1992; Thurnher *et al.*, 2001). Even so, no possible cause can be determined of an approximately 40% of patients with multiple ring enhancing brain lesions (Garg *et al.*, 2008).

As the most common presenting symptom of the miliary brain metastases is progressive dementia, a precise diagnosis is mandatory for clinical assessment and treatment. Dementia with Lewy bodies, Crutzfeldt-Jakop disease or Alzheimer Disease must be considered in differential diagnosis of miliary brain metastases.

6   Treatment

Prognosis of miliary brain metastases is poor without a significant effect attributed to chemotherapy or radiotherapy. When the paucity of the cases is considered, it is natural that there is not a standard treatment regimen for miliary brain metastases.

Whole brain radiation at 300 cGy per fraction X 10 fractions is the standard treatment for patients with brain metastases, particularly for those patients with poor performance status.

Gefitinib, a small molecule tyrosine kinase inhibitor of epidermal growth factor receptor (EGFR), has significant antitumor activity in advanced non-small-cell lung carcinoma. Gefitinib achieves dramatic radiologic and clinical regression in 10% of patients with non-small-cell lung carcinoma (Kris *et al.*, 2003). Partial response with gefitinib is associated with sensitivity mutation of EGFR. Epidermal growth factor receptor tyrosine kinase inhibitor treatment may be thought to be having some beneficial effects in treating miliary brain metastases (Wong *et al.*, 2007). The authors think that combination of whole brain radiation and gefitinib may be the only treatment of miliary brain metastases to our recent knowledge.

7   Outcome

Miliary brain metastasis is a seldom reported condition. To the best of our knowledge only 25 cases had been reported in English literature until mid-2013s (Ara Callizo *et al.*, 1989; Bhushan, 1997; Bugalho *et al.*, 2005; Falk *et al.*, 2012; Floeter *et al.*, 1987; Fukuda *et al.*, 1988; Iguchi *et al.*, 2007; Inomata *et al.*, 2012; Kahveci *et al.*, 2012; Madow and Alpers, 1951; Mochizuki *et al.*, 2012; Nakamura *et al.*, 2001; Nemzek *et al.*, 1993; Ogawa *et al.*, 2007; Olsen *et al.*, 1987; Ribeiro *et al.*, 2007; Rivas *et al.*, 2005; Ruppert *et al.*, 2010; Shirai *et al.*, 1997; Wong *et al.*, 2007; Yamazaki *et al.*, 1993) (Table). Prognosis of this uncommon condition is poor. The overall survival was reported to be as high as 24 months and as low as 14 days from the initial diagnosis. All reported cases of the miliary brain metastases were summarized in the Table.

8   Conclusion

Miliary brain metastases are somehow uncommon pattern of cerebral neoplastic metastasis which are difficult to diagnose the condition. This poor-prognosed disease must be considered in the differential diagnosis of progressive dementia and multiple enhancing lesions of the central nervous system.

References

Ara Callizo, J.R., Gimenez-Mas, J.A., Martin, J., & Lacasa, J. (1989). Calcified brain metastases from acinar-cell carcinoma of pancreas. Neuroradiology, 31(2), 200.

Bhushan, C. (1997). "Miliary" metastatic tumors in the brain. Case report. J Neurosurg, 86(3), 564-566.

Brant-Zawadzki, M., Badami, J.P., Mills, C.M., Norman, D., & Newton, T.H. (1984). Primary intracranial tumor imaging: a comparison of magnetic resonance and CT. Radiology, 150(2), 435-440.

Bugalho, P., Chorão, M., & Fontoura, P. (2005). Miliary brain metastases from primary gastric small cell carcinoma: illustrating the seed and soil hypothesis. J Neurooncol, 73(1), 53-56.

el-Sonbaty, M.R., Abdul-Ghaffar, N.U., & Marafy, A.A. (1995). Multiple intracranial tuberculomas mimicking brain metastases. Tuber Lung Dis, 76(3), 271-272.

Falk, A.T., Poudenx, M., Otto, J., Ghalloussi, H., & Barrière, J. (2012). Adenocarcinoma of the lung with miliary brain and pulmonary metastases with echinoderm microtubule-associated protein like 4-anaplastic lymphoma kinase translocation treated with crizotinib: a case report. Lung Cancer, 78(3), 282-284.

Floeter, M.K., So, Y.T., Ross, D.A., & Greenberg, D. (1987). Miliary metastasis to the brain: clinical and radiologic features. Neurology, 37(11), 1817-1818.

Fukuda, Y., Homma, T., Kohga, H., Uki, J., & Shisa, H. (1988). A lung cancer case with numerous calcified metastatic nodules of the brain. Neuroradiology, 30(3), 265-268.

Garg, R.K., Desai, P., Kar, M., & Kar, A.M. (2008). Multiple ring enhancing brain lesions on computed tomography: an Indian perspective. J Neurol Sci, 266(1-2), 92-96.

Garg, R.K., Kar, A.M., & Kumar, T. (2000). Neurocysticercosis like presentation in a case of CNS tuberculosis. Neurol India, 48(3), 260-262.

Garg, R.K., & Sinha, M.K. (2010). Multiple ring-enhancing lesions of the brain. J Postgrad Med, 56(4), 307-316

Hesselink, J.R., & Press, G.A. (1988). MR contrast enhancement of intracranial lesions with Gd-DTPA. Radiol Clin North Am, 26(4), 873-887.

Hollingworth, W., Medina, L.S., Lenkinski, R.E., Shibata, D.K., Bernal, B., Zurakowski, D., Comstock, B., & Jarvik, J.G. (2006). A systematic literature review of magnetic resonance spectroscopy for the characterization of brain tumors. AJNR Am J Neuroradiol, 27(7), 1404-1411.

Iguchi, Y., Mano, K., Goto, Y., Nakano, T., Nomura, F., Shimokata, T., Iwamizu-Watanabe, S., & Hashizume, Y. (2007). Miliary brain metastases from adenocarcinoma of the lung: MR imaging findings with clinical and post-mortem histopathologic correlation. Neuroradiology, 49(1), 35-39.

Inomata, M., Hayashi, R., Kambara, K., Okazawa, S., Imanishi, S., Ichikawa, T., Suzuki, K., Yamada, T., Miwa, T., Kashii, T., Matsui, S., Tobe, K., & Sasahara, M. (2012). Miliary brain metastasis presenting with calcification in a patient with lung cancer: a case report. J Med Case Rep, 6(1), 279.

Kahveci, R., Gürer, B., Kaygusuz, G., & Sekerci, Z. (2012). Miliary brain metastases from occult lung adenocarcinoma: Radiologic and histopathologic confirmation. J Neurosci Rural Pract, 3(3), 386-389.

Kienast, Y., von Baumgarten, L., Fuhrmann, M., Klinkert, W.E., Goldbrunner, R., Herms, J., & Winkler, F. (2010). Real-time imaging reveals the single steps of brain metastasis formation. Nat Med, 16(1), 116-122.

Kris, M.G., Natale, R.B., Herbst, R.S., Lynch, T.J. Jr., Prager, D., Belani, C.P., Schiller, J.H., Kelly, K., Spiridonidis, H., Sandler, A., Albain, K.S., Cella, D., Wolf, M.K., Averbuch, S.D., Ochs, J.J., & Kay, A.C. (2003). Efficacy of gefitinib, an inhibitor of the epidermal growth factor receptor tyrosine kinase, in symptomatic patients with non-small cell lung cancer: a randomized trial. JAMA, 290(16), 2149-2158.

Madow, L., & Alpers, B.J. (1951). Encephalitic form of metastatic carcinoma. AMA Arch Neurol Psychiatry, 65(2), 161-173.

McGuigan, C., Bigham, S., Johnston, D., & Hart, P.E. (2005). Encephalopathy in a patient with previous malignancy but normal brain imaging. Neurology, 65(1), 165.

Mochizuki, S., Nishimura, N., Inoue, A., Murakami, K., Nukiwa, T., & Chohnabayashi, N. (2012). Miliary brain metastases in 2 cases with advanced non-small cell lung cancer harboring EGFR mutation during gefitinib treatment. Respir Investig, 50(3), 117-121.

Möller-Hartmann, W., Herminghaus, S., Krings, T., Marquardt, G., Lanfermann, H., Pilatus, U., & Zanella, F.E. (2002). Clinical application of proton magnetic resonance spectroscopy in the diagnosis of intracranial mass lesions. Neuroradiology, 44(5), 371-381.

Nakamura, H., Toyama, M., Uezu, K., Nakamoto, A., Toda, T., & Saito, A. (2001). *Diagnostic dilemmas in oncology: case 1. Lung cancer with miliary brain metastases undetected by imaging studies. J Clin Oncol, 19(23), 4340-4341.*

Nemzek, W., Poirier, V., Salamat, M.S., & Yu, T. (1993). *Carcinomatous encephalitis (miliary metastases): lack of contrast enhancement. AJNR Am J Neuroradiol, 14(3), 540-542.*

Ogawa, M., Kurahashi, K., Ebina, A., Kaimori, M., & Wakabayashi, K. (2007). *Miliary brain metastasis presenting with dementia: progression pattern of cancer metastases in the cerebral cortex. Neuropathology, 27(4), 390-395.*

Olsen, W.L., Winkler, M.L., & Ross, D.A. (1987). *Carcinomatous encephalitis: CT and MR findings. AJNR Am J Neuroradiol, 8(3), 553-554.*

Oncul, O., Baylan, O., Mutlu, H., Cavuslu, S., & Doganci, L. (2005). *Tuberculous meningitis with multiple intracranial tuberculomas mimicking neurocysticercosis clinical and radiological findings. Jpn J Infect Dis, 58(6), 387-389.*

Porter, S.B., & Sande, M.A. (1992). *Toxoplasmosis of the central nervous system in the acquired immunodeficiency syndrome. N Engl J Med, 327(23), 1643-1648.*

Ribeiro, H.B., Paiva, T.F. Jr., Mamprin, G.P., Gorzoni, M.L., Rocha, A.J., & Lancellotti, C.L. (2007). *Carcinomatous encephalitis as clinical presentation of occult lung adenocarcinoma: case report. Arq Neuropsiquiatr, 65(3B), 841-844.*

Rivas, E., Sanchez-Herrero, J., Alonso, M., Alvarez, M.J., Teijeira, S., Ballestín, C., Tardio, A., & Navarro, C. (2005). *Miliary brain metastases presenting as rapidly progressive dementia. Neuropathology, 25(2), 153-158.*

Ruppert, A.M., Stankoff, B., Lavolé, A., Gounant, V., Milleron, B., & Seilhean, D. (2010). *Miliary brain metastases in lung cancer. J Clin Oncol, 28(34), e714-716.*

Shalen, P.R., Hayman, L.A., Wallace, S., & Handel, S.F. (1981). *Protocol for delayed contrast enhancement in computed tomography of cerebral neoplasia. Radiology, 139(2), 397-402.*

Shirai, H., Imai, S., Kajihara, Y., Tamada, T., Gyoten, M., Kamei, T., Hata, T., & Shirabe, T. (1997). *MRI in carcinomatous encephalitis. Neuroradiology, 39(6), 437-440.*

Sze, G., Milano, E., Johnson, C., & Heier, L. (1990). *Detection of brain metastases: comparison of contrast-enhanced MR with unenhanced MR and enhanced CT. AJNR Am J Neuroradiol, 11(4), 785-791.*

Talmadge, J.E., & Fidler, I.J., (2010). *AACR centennial series: the biology of cancer metastasis: historical perspective. Cancer Res, 70, 5649-5669.*

Thurnher, M.M., Rieger, A., Kleibl-Popov, C., Settinek, U., Henk, C., Haberler, C., & Schindler, E. (2001). *Primary central nervous system lymphoma in AIDS: a wider spectrum of CT and MRI findings. Neuroradiology, 43(1), 29-35.*

Tosomeen, A.H., Berbari, E.F., Levy, N.T., McClure, R.F., Krecke, K.N., & Osmon, D.R. (1998). *Instructive case report. A 26-year-old Indian woman with seizures and multiple intracranial mass lesions. J Med Liban, 46(6), 349-352.*

Weisberg, L.A. (1979). *Computerized tomography in intracranial metastases. Arch Neurol, 36(10), 630-634.*

Wong, E.T., Wu, J.K., & Mahadevan, A. (2007). *Gefitinib and high-dose fractionated radiotherapy for carcinomatous encephalitis from non-small cell lung carcinoma. Biologics, 1(3), 321-324.*

Yamazaki, T., Harigaya, Y., Noguchi, O., Okamoto, K., & Hirai, S. (1993). *Calcified miliary brain metastases with mitochondrial inclusion bodies. J Neurol Neurosurg Psychiatry, 56(1), 110-111.*

The Role of Computational Epidemiology and Risk Analysis in the Fight against HIV/AIDS

Berhanu Tameru, David Nganwa, Asseged B. Dibaba, Vinaida Robnett,
Center for Computational Epidemiology, Bioinformatics and Risk Analysis (CCEBRA)
College of Veterinary Medicine, Nursing and Allied Health (CVMNAH)
Tuskegee University, Tuskegee, Alabama, USA

Gemechu B. Gerbi
Epidemiology and Surveillance Branch, Division of Viral Hepatitis, NCHHSTP
Centers for Disease Control and Prevention, Atlanta, Georgia, USA

Tsegaye Habtemariam
Center for Computational Epidemiology, Bioinformatics and Risk Analysis (CCEBRA)
College of Veterinary Medicine, Nursing and Allied Health (CVMNAH)
Tuskegee University, Tuskegee, Alabama, USA

1   Introduction

The devastating effects of the HIV/AIDS pandemic are compounded by its complex patterns of transmission and spread. The rate of its transmission and the demographic spread of the disease both in time and space are influenced not only by direct factors such as age, gender, marital status, number of sexual partners, sexual preferences, frequency of extramarital liaisons, etc., but indirectly by factors such as psychosocial, socioeconomic, HIV/AIDS risky behaviors and ultimately by the complex interactions and interplay between all these factors. It is these aforementioned interactions and their evolution over time that provides a major difficulty in trying to predict the spread and social impact of the disease (Tameru *et al.*, 2012; Gerbi *et al.*, 2012; Diaz *et al.*, 1994). Teasing out these various factors using the epidemiologic problem oriented approach methodology will greatly facilitate in developing knowledge bases that are an integral part in incorporating these factors in the different models developed.

In general a model can be considered as a pattern, plan, representation (especially in miniature), or description designed to show the main object or workings of an object, system, or concept. In Scientific modeling, modeling is considered as being the process of generating abstract, conceptual, graphical and or mathematical models which are implemented in computer models to study the behavior of a complex system by computer simulations. Science offers a growing collection of methods, techniques and theories about all kinds of specialized scientific modeling. Modeling is an essential and inseparable part of all scientific activity, and many scientific disciplines have their own ideas about specific types of modeling. Several researchers have developed computational tools and mathematical approaches to study the effects of various mitigation methods on HIV/AIDS at different population levels, in vivo or in vitro, macro to micro levels, just to name a few (Ho *et al.*, 1995; Perlson & Nelson, 1999; Habtemariam *et al.*, 2001; Tam *et al.*, 2008; Tameru *et al.*, 2012). The approaches range from compartmental models represented by sets of differential equations (Anderson & May, 1992; Rvachev & Longini, 1985; Sattenspiel & Simon, 1988); to highly complex individual-based models which represent daily activities and interconnections of individuals via transmission networks (Eubank *et al.*, 2004). Compartmental models can be easily solved, but they cannot model adaptive behaviors of individuals and complex interactions of different groups of populations during disease outbreaks. While individual-based models like Agent Based Modeling can capture the spread of diseases with high-fidelity, modeling large populations often requires utilization of supercomputers and makes it impractical for quick what-if analyses of interventions or treatments under varying different conditions.

This volume which is an update review chapter provides a synthesis of our collective knowledge regarding the application of computational epidemiologic modeling and risk analysis in addressing HIV/AIDS pandemic in both macro and micro settings undergirded by sound epidemiology. Numerous case examples with different approaches for modeling the AIDS pandemic and the HIV pathogenesis in HIV infected individuals are given. The role and importance of computational epidemiologic modeling are discussed. A new avenue of research, involving the application of risk assessment in solving public health problems in general and its suitability in modeling HIV/AIDS dynamics in particular is explored.

1.1   Computational Epidemiologic Models

The use of computational epidemiologic models, undergirded by sound epidemiologic and mathematical principles, has brought a substantial progress in the understanding of HIV and CD4 cell dynamics. In its early stages, the applications of these models were based on relatively simple mathematical templates that considered the body as a one compartment system. In spite of being very attractive, from the experimental and/or mathematical standpoint of view, the underlying simplification means that a lot of factors that significantly affect the population dynamics both at macro (human) and micro (cellular) population levels are effectively avoided. This simplification also affects the kinetics linked to the infection, immunology, and chemotherapy dynamics throughout the host. As epidemiologic research involves a complex set of host, environment and agent factors as they interact to impact health in any given population (whether biotic or abiotic), generating large datasets which require the use of more advanced computational methods is a necessity. Computational epidemiologic methods are useful for studying such large and complex models (Habtemariam *et al.* 2001; Wai-Yuan & Hulin, 2008; Tameru *et al.*, 2012). Another dimension of the challenges faced by the public health decision makers is epitomized by the emerging/re-emerging diseases, as they have to face and deal with a lot of uncertainty at the early stages of new disease outbreaks.

1.2   Risk Analysis

Epidemiologic problem-solving and decision-making often proceeds in the face of uncertainties and limited information. Emerging diseases are one such challenging problem to public health decision makers since they encounter a lot of uncertainty even at the early stages of disease outbreaks. Risk analysis is a process for decision making under uncertainty that consists of three fundamental tasks: risk management, risk assessment, and risk communication. Risk analysis can be considered as the process of examining the whole of a risk holistically by assessing the risk and its related relevant uncertainties for the purpose of its efficacious management, facilitated by effective communication skills about the risk. It is a systematic way of gathering, recording, and evaluating information that can lead to recommendations for a decision or action in response to an identified hazard or opportunity for gain. Risk analysis is not a science rather science based; it is not certain (usually expressed in probability distributions & confidence intervals), it is not a solution (from all possible options, the best one is picked under the pertinent available information at that point in time); and it is not static (needs to be updated whenever new information is available). In the context of public health, Quantitative Risk Assessment is the process that quantifies the likelihood of the introduction of infection, it's establishment, or spread of a pathogen or disease in a given susceptible population. Standard epidemiological procedures are utilized to systematically evaluate health risks from the combined effects of multiple factors that lead to the identified hazard scenarios for each step in the process; mathematical and computing methods are utilized to assess the magnitude of the risk and mitigations effect. The ultimate goal is to support and facilitate public health officials in making informed decisions based on organized science based analyses.

1.3   The Epidemiologic Framework to Risk Analysis

Definitions of epidemiology and risk analysis as pertains to this book chapter are that: Epidemiology is defined as the study of the dynamics of health/ill health processes in a given population. It is often directed at problem solving and decision or policy making at the population level. On the other hand, risk analysis is defined as the practice of decision making based on scientific evidence (Risk Newsletter, 2000). Like epidemiology, risk analysis is often focused on population-based studies although both methodologies can be applied to any population such as cellular, molecular, genomes and others. This is because in epidemiology, the population under study can be groups of animals (*e.g.,* herd health), humans (*e.g.,* public health), plants (phytoepidemiology), cellular and molecular populations (molecular epidemiology), or populations of genes (genetic epidemiology). Epidemiology is a discipline that can be applied to the study of population dynamics from the molecular (microepidemiology) to higher levels (macroepidemiology) of population dynamics. This breadth of epidemiology provides risk analysis with the framework for its application in a vast array of population-based studies from genomics and biotechnology to even global health/international trade. The link between epidemiology and risk analysis is rational and intuitive. The two areas complement and supplement each other. In epidemiology, the basis for reasoning and explanation, the opportunity for dealing with choices, risks or benefits especially in the face of uncertainties, and the need to analyze and manage imperfect data are common occurrences. The same applies to risk analysis. The dilemma is that the paucity, incompleteness and uncertainty of available data further complicate quantitative models. Yet, epidemiologic problem solving and decision-making as well as risk analysis often must proceed in the face of uncertainties and limited knowledge. A risk assessment is never complete nor is it static. As more knowledge and information is gained over time, a risk analysis particularly the risk assessment component can be revised and updated as appropriate. To handle the types of challenges described above, computer modeling (Risk Analysis and Epidemiologic Modelling) provides a powerful alternative tool to traditional empirical (field or laboratory based) studies. Computational epidemiology provides a mechanism for approximating biological interactions, via bio-mathematical expressions that can be tested using computer models as the experimental medium. This new approach is the realm of computational science (Pool, 1992). Computational science integrates the two traditional areas of empirical and theoretical sciences. It also builds upon and extends the methods and tools available to research by exploiting computational resources. Computational epidemiology and risk analysis now provide alternative avenues where systems, which may be complex, too large, and not feasible because the information is scanty and uncertain; or the cost is too prohibitive, can be approximated and simulated realistically.

2   History of Computational Epidemiology and Risk Analysis Models

Computational epidemiologic models and simulations are emerging as vital research tools in epidemiology, biology, and various other fields in advancing the bench (wet) lab and public health policy research agenda. Scientists are recognizing the huge potential of these tools in solving some of today's biggest health problems. Computational epidemiology is a multidisciplinary field utilizing techniques from computer science, mathematics, geographic information sciences and public health to develop tools and models to aid epidemiologists and other scientists in their studies of the temporal-spatial spread of diseases. Research in computational epidemiology is now considered to be an exponentially expanding arena of scientific exploration. In particular the HIV/AIDS pandemic, where more than 25 million people have so far died from the disease since 1981, making it amongst the most serious threats to global health that we face today. Epidemic models of infectious diseases date back to Daniel Bernoulli's mathematical analysis of smallpox in 1760 and have been developed extensively since the early 1900s. Mathematical epidemiologic modeling, with the help of computational tools, has provided new insights on such important issues as drug resistance, rate of spread of infections, epidemic trends, and effects of interventions such as treatment and vaccination.

The term computational epidemiology was first coined by Professor Tsegaye Habtemariam (a founding member of the Center for Computational Epidemiology, Bioinformatics and Risk Analysis (CCEBRA) at Tuskegee University)) (Habtemariam *et al.*, 1988) to better understand the complex biomedical systems in diseases like the HIV/AIDS pandemic. Computational epidemiology enables infectious and non-infectious diseases and risk agents of plants, animals and humans to be examined and investigated without jeopardizing lives or creating hazards. This relatively young strand of computational science is being used to understand a range of problems from soybean and wheat rust to HIV/AIDS, swine influenza, foot and mouth disease, rift valley fever and bioterrorism to name a few. In light of this, computational epidemiology has the potential to influence global issues that both directly and indirectly affect human, animal, plant health and the environment, representing a milestone in modern science (Tameru *et al.*, 2012). The CCEBRA is a unique facility that has been involved since the early 1980s in groundbreaking work in this niche of science, that of Computational Science. Epidemiologic research involves the study of a complex set of host, environment and causative agent factors, with the most advanced of these efforts focusing on micro (cellular/molecular) and macro (host) population levels.

Computational epidemiologic models of HIV/AIDS provide important insights in population dynamics through studies at the molecular and cellular levels as well as at the human population level (Ho *et al.*, 1995; Habtemariam *et al.*, 2001; and Tameru *et al.*, 2008). As of today, wet lab science has not yet achieved a level of success to produce a viable vaccine or effective medication for preventing or treating HIV/AIDS. The alternative research approach of computational modeling (the so called the third dimension of science), has also been a priority for researchers in other disciplines.

While risk analysis especially the risk assessment component has existed in various forms for many years, the process used by US Environmental Protection Agency (EPA) and others was formalized in the pivotal 1983 National Research Council (NRC) report known as the "Red Book" (National Research Council, 1983). The Red Book codified the well-known four steps of risk assessment (hazard identification, exposure assessment, dose-response assessment, and risk characterization) and it emphasized the necessity of a conceptual distinction between risk assessment, risk management and risk communication. Over the intervening quarter-century, risk assessment has evolved substantially, driven in part by additional NRC reports, EPA, World Trade Organization, and other agency guidelines, and publications in the peer-reviewed literature. There are two major types of risk assessments namely Qualitative Risk Assessments and Quantitative Risk Assessments (Probabilistic Risk Assessment (PRA)). The PRA is used to estimate risk by computing probability distributions to determine what can go wrong, how likely is it to happen, and what are its consequences. Health (human, animal and plant) PRA provides insights into how the risk propagates from the source to the end point (Scenario tree); how likely is each scenario to happen; what will be the consequence (*e.g.*, the number of people potentially infected or killed); the efficacies and weaknesses of different mitigations to reduce the risk and associated consequences. However, there is a need in expanding the use of PRA in human health as most of the human health risk assessments are of environmental and food safety in nature.

3 The Steps Utilized in Developing Computational Epidemiologic Models

Systems dynamic modelling (SDM), a tool widely used in epidemiological and mathematical modelling, allows researchers and scientists to study and develop a holistic way to assess not only the behavior of the system, but the relationships and interactions between different entities within the system so that scientists can predict what will happen if these systems behaviors persist over time into the future.

Systems dynamic modelling is a concept based on systems thinking whereby dynamic interactions between the elements of the system is considered in order to study the behavior of the system as a whole. This methodology, introduced in the mid-1950s by Forrester and first described at length in his book "Industrial Dynamics) (Forester, 1961) with some additional principles presented in his later works (Forrester, 1985), involves development of causal diagrams and computer simulation models that are unique to each problem setting. A central principle of SDM is that the complex behaviors of organizational and social systems are the result of ongoing accumulations of people, material or financial assets, information, or even biological or psychological states. Both balancing and reinforcing feedback mechanisms and the concepts of accumulation and feedback have been discussed in various forms for centuries. However, SDM uniquely enables the practical application of these concepts in the form of computerized models so that alternative policies and scenarios can be tested in a systematic way that answers the questions of "what if" and "why".

The systems analysis approach to model development consists of seven major steps which are all interlinked and we will follow these seven steps in sequence to illustrate how to develop computational epidemiologic (risk assessment) models.

- Step 1: Develop the Epidemiologic Problem Oriented Approach (EPOA) methodology, (to collect, synthesize and organize the epidemiologic data).

- Step 2: Create a conceptual systems model diagram based on the EPOA. This involves defining the subsystems in the model and conceptualizing their relationships and interactions with each other (see Figure 2).

- Step 3: (i) Dynamic model development - the systems dynamics and the underlying structure for the mathematical formulations will be described by means of differential (difference) and partial differential equations (ii) risk assessment model development: (a) identifying the hazard (*i.e.,* HIV/AIDS); (b) developing a scenario tree which outlines a series of mitigations and all the failures which could occur, culminating in the occurrence of the identified hazard; (c) gathering and documenting the evidence.

- Step 4: Develop a Mathematical Model

- Step 5: Develop a Computer Simulation Model (A simulation model)

- Step 6: Test, Validate, Perform Sensitivity Analysis, and update the model (update the knowledge base). Compare the models' response/behavior/performance to reality, other models, or published works

- Step 7: Implement the Model.

As an example a systems dynamics model for HIV/AIDS identifies links between the sub-systems, state variables, rate variables, parameters and constants in a system. The developed models can be used to provide important insights in population dynamics at the macro (human) population level and at the micro (cellular) population level and helps in giving insight for alternative HIV/AIDS control and prevention strategies.

3.1   Knowledge Base: The Epidemiologic Problem Oriented Approach (EPOA) Methodology

In the epidemiologic modeling of HIV/AIDS and other diseases, the Epidemiologic Problem Oriented Approach (EPOA) methodology facilitates the development of systematic and structured knowledge bases, which are crucial for development of computational epidemiologic models (Nganwa *et al.*, 2010). A detailed analytic understanding of the epidemiology of a population under study and a decomposition of all relevant determinants of health and disease provides the essential framework for the development of computational epidemiologic and risk assessment models and enables the laying out of the comprehensive and fundamental structures for the models. The method of decomposition of any epidemiologic or risk assessment task relies heavily on EPOA. As in any problem solving and decision making exercise, the EPOA essentially consists of a problem identification/definition/characterization component, followed by a problem management/solution/mitigation component. We use the classical epidemiologic triad (epidemiologic triplet) consisting of host, agent and environment interactions, and examination of agent transmission pathways and spread of disease both in time and space as the first key step to computational epidemiology or risk assessment (problem identification triad). Rational intervention strategies (mitigations) that minimize the risk of transmission and introduction of a disease or pest are then integrated into such an epidemiologic framework. The second set of triad, composed of prevention/control, treatment or therapeutics to eliminate a risk agent and health maintenance/promotion is the decision making step (problem/management /solution/mitigation triad).

The two triads are interlinked by diagnostic linkage procedures used in identifying and characterizing the risk agent when possible. The individual pillars of each triad are interlinked and intertwined. Each pillar of the triads is decomposed into its respective variables and parameters.

The first triad the Problem Identification/Characterization Triad: The agent pillar; identifies the agent and its characteristics like infective dose and route(s) of infection, survival under different conditions, pathogenicity, life cycle, transmission pathways etc. The host pillar; identifies and characterizes the characteristics of all possible hosts whether they are definitive, intermediate, reservoir or paratenic. Host characteristics are identified in detail including intrinsic and extrinsic factors. The environment pillar; characterizes the physical (abiotic), biological (biotic) and socio-economic environments for both the host and agent and how they interplay. Psychosocial factors and determinants are considered. In the second triad Problem Management/Solution/Mitigation Triad: The therapeutics/treatment pillar; considers if the disease is treatable curatively, palliatively or for secondary problems. Options, ease of availability and accessibility to treatment are taken into consideration; Prevention/control pillar; considers if prevention is primary, secondary or tertiary; and the Health Maintenance/Health Promotion pillar; considers in general the health maintenance of the population mainly after a disease or condition has already occurred and is geared towards lowering the prevalence and incidence rates to their lowest level coupled with prevention, control strategies and eventual eradication of the disease being the ultimate goal.

Although the generic term risk analysis is composed of: a) risk assessment, b) risk management, and, c) risk communication, our emphasis in this chapter is on risk assessment. These components viewed through the EPOA methodology are part of the classical problem solving steps of: a) problem identification and characterization (risk assessment), and, b) problem management (risk management and risk communication). It is noteworthy to emphasize that both risk management and risk communication rely on sound risk assessments, which may be qualitative or quantitative in nature.

Risk mitigation in this chapter is broadly defined to include all activities and resources required to: a) prevent introduction of risk agents, b) eliminate the risk agent if possible, and/or c) manage the risk event by taking steps to minimize or reduce the risk of spread once introduced into a disease free population (for macro on population level modeling) or susceptible individual (for micro modeling). We contend that effective approaches to risk management rely upon: a) sound science-based risk assessment which in turn depends on a detailed understanding and decomposition of the epidemiologic factors and the transmission pathways for the risk agent under study, and, b) education and information sharing (nationally and internationally).

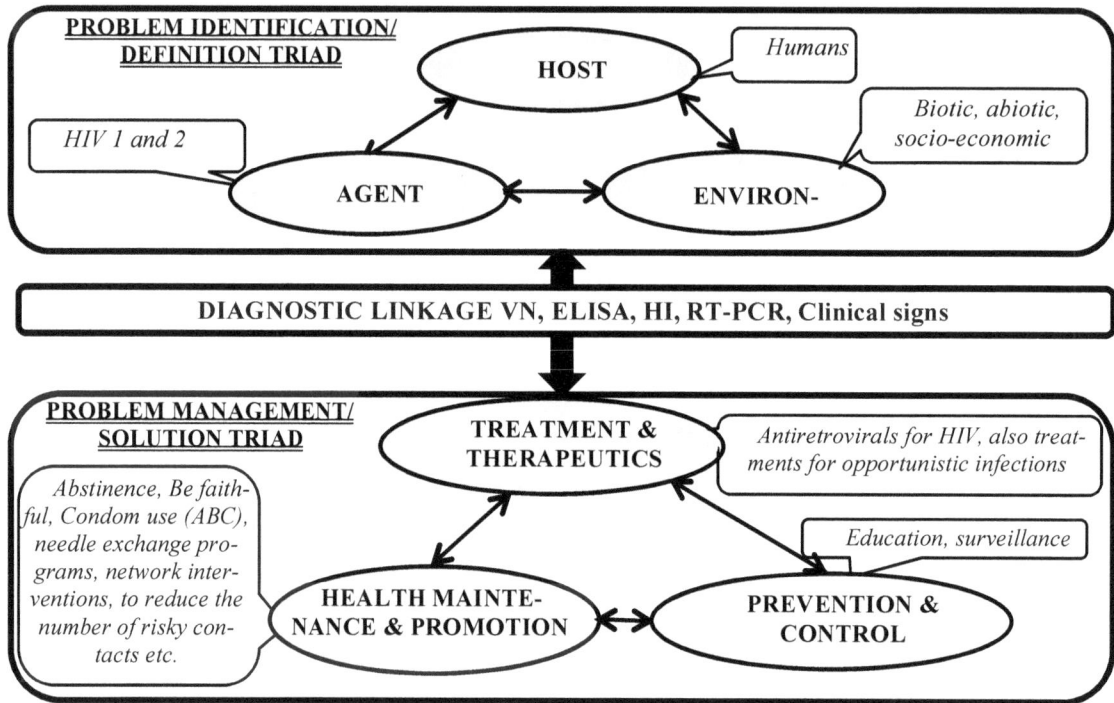

Figure 1:The Epidemiologic Problem Oriented Approach.

Data collection is crucial and central for development of the knowledge base, a lot of information and data have to be gathered depending on disease under study in this case HIV/AIDS. Sources and types of organizations that can provide or direct you to the key information include: academic and research institutions, ministries of health, other government agencies, hospitals and clinics, nongovernmental and community-based organizations, international organizations and partners involved in HIV/AIDS work, such as USAID, CDC, UNAIDS, WHO, national and/or regional associations of People Living With HIV/AIDS (PLWHA), private companies, media and the internet. Comprehensive program reviews produced by governments, donor agencies, and others, National HIV/AIDS program updates, including reports from behavioral and biological surveys, and from sentinel surveillance, Web-accessible libraries, meeting and conference reports, books, journals, and medical databases generated by research endeavors. The EPOA organizes this data collected into a well-structured format that is easily retrievable in the process of identifying variables and estimating parameters used in model development.

3.2   Conceptual Systems Dynamics Model Diagram

Once the knowledge base is developed based on the EPOA methodology a conceptual systems dynamics model diagram needs to be developed. The systems dynamic modelling (SDM) is an iterative process of scope selection, hypothesis generation, causal diagramming, and quantification; it consists of an interlocking set of differential and algebraic equations developed from a broad spectrum of relevant data. A completed SDM model may contain scores or even hundreds of equations along with the appropriate numerical inputs. Importantly, epidemiologic SDM models are designed to reproduce historical patterns and capable of generating useful insights. The data extrapolated from these epidemiological models are useful not only to study the past, but are reliable also to explore predictive and intervention possibilities (Forrester, 1960, 1985). With this in mind, a SDM model incorporating various HIV/AIDS-risky behaviors has been developed to model HIV/AIDS.

3.2.1   A Macro-epidemiologic Model of HIV Transmission

The dynamic epidemiologic model developed in the macro level of the transmission of HIV and its progression to AIDS relies on a set of multiple determinants that affect the epidemiology of HIV/AIDS in populations. At the macro level, the population is divided into three sub-populations based on their health status. These include those who are susceptible (S), infected with HIV (I), and advanced state of HIV infection or full blown AIDS (A). The transitions between the states of health are regulated by the respective rates such as birth rate, infection rate, progression rate to AIDS and death rate respectively see Figure 2. The macro model considers five ethnic populations: Whites (not Hispanic), African Americans, Hispanics, Asian/Pacific Islanders, and American Indian/Alaska Natives. Within each ethnic group, each individual has the demographic characteristics (age, gender, etc.) and HIV/AIDS risky behaviors: male to male sexual contact (MSM), injection drug use (IDU), male to male sexual contact and injection drug use (MSM/IDU), high risk heterosexual contact, and others (include hemophilia, blood transfusion, perinatal exposure, and risk factor not reported or not identified). The HIV/AIDS infection rate in a given susceptible population directly depends on the proportion of MSM, IDU, MSM/IDU, high-risk heterosexual contact, and other risk factors. Manipulation of one or several of these variables changes the behavior of the system dynamics and result in an increase or decrease of the incidence of HIV/AIDS; thus allowing critical evaluation of alternative disease control strategies.

3.2.2   Micro-epidemiologic Modelling

Cellular level modeling (CD4+ lymphocyte/HIV viral population dynamics): The host populations are CD4+ lymphocytes, the agent is HIV viral population and the environment is the cellular and intracellular/molecular ecosystems. The new state that represents infected CD4+ lymphocytes, referred to as "HIV infected CD4+ cell subpopulation", is further subdivided into four sub-states (Coffin 1995, Fauci 2014): *Productively infected, Latently infected, Defectively infected, and Chronically infected. Molecular level modeling: The CD4+ lymphocyte cell is assumed as infected as soon as the virion enters the host cell.* Ordinary differential equations were used to mathematically represent the viral kinetics as they move from reverse transcription through progeny formation and maturation.

4   Mathematical Epidemiology and Risk Assessment Model Applied in HIV/AIDS

Based on the conceptual model developed, a mathematical model which consists of several sub-models is developed. A mathematical model is more detailed, and is more based on data, than the conceptual model. If developed carefully, mathematical and statistical models can serve as tools to better understand the epidemiology of HIV/AIDS. Mathematical models of HIV/AIDS transmission dynamics also play an important role in understanding the epidemiological patterns and methods for disease control as they provide short and long term predictions of HIV and AIDS incidence and prevalence trends, and its dependence on various factors.

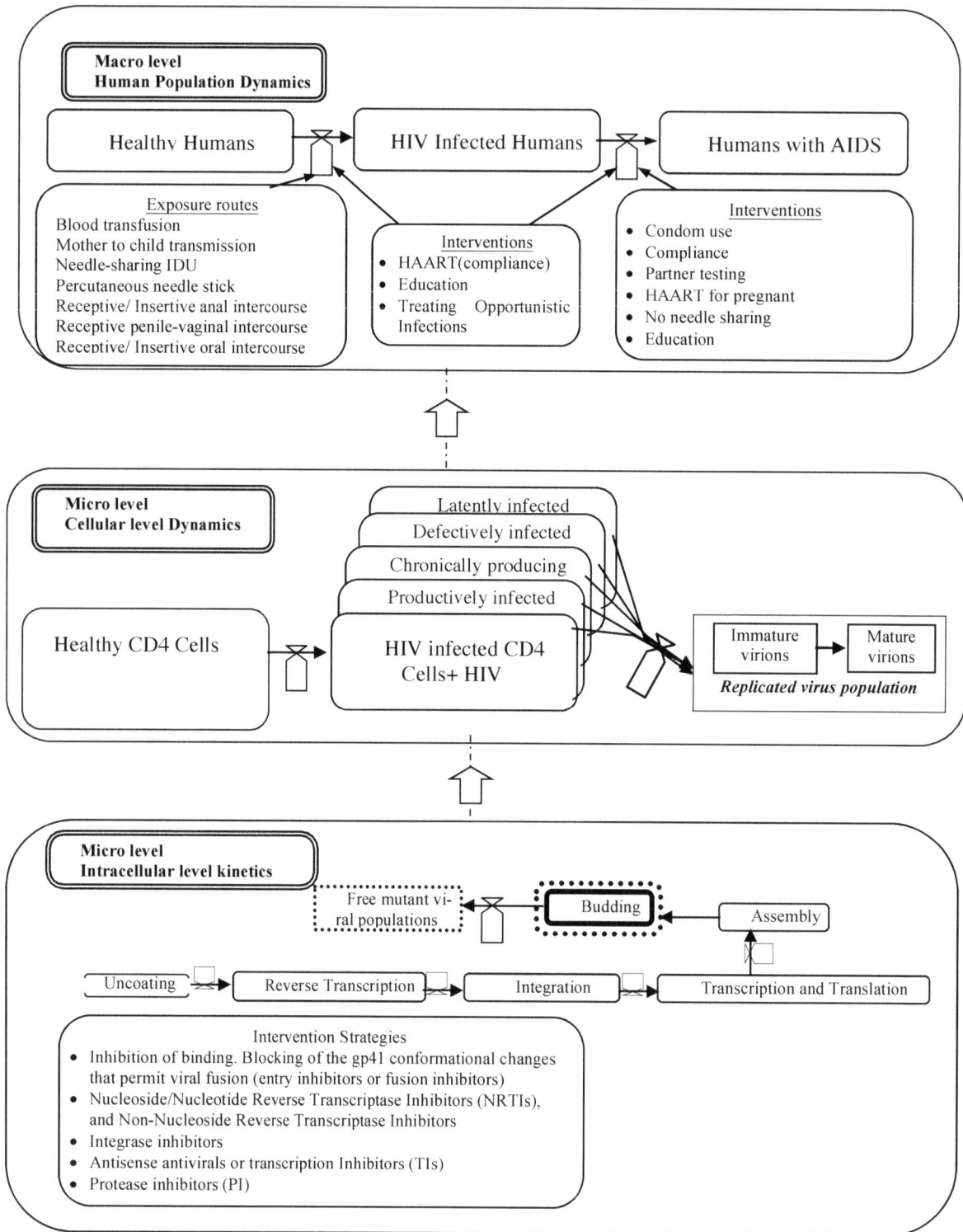

Figure 2: An epidemiologic systems model of macro-micro (human-Cellular) Population dynamics.

4.1   Mathematical Epidemiology

The framework for representing the integrated components of the HIV/AIDS epidemiologic model including macro level population dynamics as well as micro level population cellular/molecular level biological dynamics is shown in Figure 2. The dynamics of the model is described using a system of partial differential equations (Tameru *et al.*, 2010).

$$\frac{\partial \overline{S}\left(S_{ijk}(a,t,\overline{u})\right)}{\partial t} + \frac{\partial \overline{S}\left(S_{ijk}(a,t,\overline{u})\right)}{\partial a} = \left\{\sigma_{ijk}(\overline{u}(t),a)\left[1-\gamma_{ijk}(\overline{u}(t),a)\right]-1\right\}\overline{S}\left(S_{ijk}(a,t,\overline{u})\right) \quad (1)$$

where S_{ijk} denotes the number of susceptible individuals of drug use status k, sex related status j, ethnic group i, age a at time t; $\sigma_{ijk}(\overline{u}(t),a)$ is the age-group specific survival rate of individuals of drug use status k, sex related status j in ethnic group i; $\gamma_{ijk}(\overline{u}(t),a)$ is the HIV infection rate of individuals of age a at time t, drug use status k, sex related status j in ethnic group i, which depends on time of infection and the number of CD4+ count and the viral load at time t and cellular level dynamics of CD4+, $(\overline{u}(t),\tau)$, with $\overline{u}=(C_i(t,\tau),V_i(t,\tau))$ (C_i's are infected cells and V_i is the viral population), and age a of the individual.

$$\frac{\partial C_i(t,a,[dNTP])}{\partial t} + \frac{\partial C_i(t,a,[dNTP])}{\partial a} = -d_i C_i(t,a,[dNTP]), \quad (2)$$

with

$$C_i(t,0,[dNTP]) = \beta C_i(t,[dNTP])V(t,[RNA_{cor}]) \text{ for } i \in \{L,P,C,D\},$$

and

$$\frac{\partial V(t,[RNA_{cor}])}{\partial t} = \sum_{i\in\{L,P,C\}} \int_{a_{iP}}^{a_{max}} \gamma_i(a)C_i(t,a,[dNTP])da - uV(t,[RNA_{cor}]),$$

where for $i = D$, defectively infected CD4+ cells, for $i = L$, latently infected CD4+ cells, for $i = P$, productively infected CD4+ cells, and for $i = C$, chronically infected CD4+ cells and a is the age of the CD4 cell. A selected equation representing the molecular kinetic level interactions is shown below.

$$\frac{d[RNA_{cor}]}{dt} = -\frac{V_m[RNA_{cor}]}{K_{m(RNA_{cor})}+[RNA_{cor}]} \cdot \frac{[dNTP]}{K_{m(dNTP)}+[dNTP]} - (k_{RNA_{cor}}+\phi_{RT})[RNA_{cor}], \quad (3)$$

where $[RNA_{cor}]$ is the concentration of genomic RNA present in the viral core and $[dNTP]$ is the concentration of the dNTP pool of the host cell. $K_{m(RNA_{cor})}$ and $K_{m(dNTP)}$ are the Michaelis constants for reverse transcriptase with the substrates RNA_{cor} ($= 2*[V_F]$) and the dNTP (Deoxyribonucleoside triphosphate) pool, respectively. $k_{RNA_{cor}}$ is the degradation rate constant of the genomic RNA and φ_{RT} is the efficacy of the drug for reverse transcription inhibitor.

Other equations representing the various other states were developed in a similar fashion. The equations that describe the dynamics in HIV infected populations of drug use status k, ethnic group i, age a at time t are defined as follows:

$$\frac{\partial \overline{I}(I_{ijk}(a,t,\overline{u}))}{\partial t} + \frac{\partial \overline{I}(I_{ijk}(a,t,\overline{u}))}{\partial a} + \frac{\partial \overline{I}(I_{ijk}(a,t,\overline{u}))}{\partial \overline{u}} = \left\{\sigma_{ijk}(\overline{u}(t),a)\left[1-tr(\overline{u})\right]-1\right\}I_{ijk}(a,t,\overline{u}), \quad (4)$$

where $tr\left(\left(\overline{u}(t),\tau\right)\right)$ is the probability that an individual infected by HIV at time t-τ becomes an AIDS patient at time t, which is assumed to be the same for all ethnic groups. A similar equation can be given for the dynamics of AIDS patients populations.

$$\frac{\partial \overline{A}(A_{ijk}(a,t,\overline{u}))}{\partial t}+\frac{\partial \overline{A}(A_{ijk}(a,t,\overline{u}))}{\partial a}+\frac{\partial \overline{A}(A_{ijk}(a,t,\overline{u}))}{\partial \overline{u}}=\left\{\mu(\overline{u}(t),a)-1\right\}A_{ijg}(a,t,\overline{u}). \quad (5)$$

The role of individual characteristics from macro (age, gender and race), socioeconomic status (level of education, level of income and employment status), and psychosocial factors to the cellular level CD4+ count, HIV viral load, and the kinetics inside the cell are also incorporated in this model. We let $F_{ijk}(t)$ denote the events that an individual of drug use status k, sex related status j, in ethnic group i is infected by HIV during $[t, t+dt)$ due to sexual contact. An individual may have sexual contacts with partners from different ethnic groups. The probability of HIV transmission due to sexual contacts is formulated in terms of the number of partners, number of sexual contacts with each partner, the probability that a partner is infected, the HIV viral load of the infected and the probability that one contact with an infected partner will result in infection. In this study, since we consider six ethnic groups, each consisting of five risky behaviors related sub groups, the HIV prevalence differs from group to group. The probability that an individual of drug use status k, risky behaviors related status j in ethnic group i is infected by HIV at time t due to sexual contacts is given by:

$$P\left[F_{ijk}(a,t,\overline{u})\right]=1-\prod_{e=1}^{3}\left\{1-q_e(t)\right\}, \quad (6)$$

where

$$q_e(t)=1-\left\{1-p_e(t)\left[1-(1-r)^{m_{ijk,e}}\right]\right\}^{n_{ijk,e}}$$

is the probability that an individual of drug use status k, risky behaviors related status j in ethnic group i is infected by HIV during $[t, t+dt]$ due to sexual contacts with partners from ethnic group e, r is the probability of HIV transmission associated with a single sexual contact, $n_{ijk,e}$ is the number of sexual partners from ethnic group e, $m_{ijk,e}$ is the number of sexual contacts with a partner from ethnic group e, and $p_e(t)$ is the probability that a partner from ethnic group e is infected at time t.

4.2   Risk Assessment

Quantitative risk assessment (QRA) was performed after developing the risk pathway scenario tree based on a comprehensive review of published literature that have examined psychological, social and interpersonal variables as correlates of sexual risk behaviors in people who know they are HIV positive (Gerbi, et al., 2012). The main focus in this chapter is on individual level factors influencing HIV/AIDS risky behaviors. QRA provides the methods of measuring risks and provides decision makers with the information needed to make decisions which are scientifically based. The QRA process involves: (a) identification of the hazard, (b) developing a scenario tree outlining the pathway of expected events and all the failures that are likely to occur, (c) gathering and documenting evidence, (d) developing equations or functions, (e) performing calculations to summarize the likelihood of the hazard occurring, (f) considering risk management options and (g) preparing a written report.

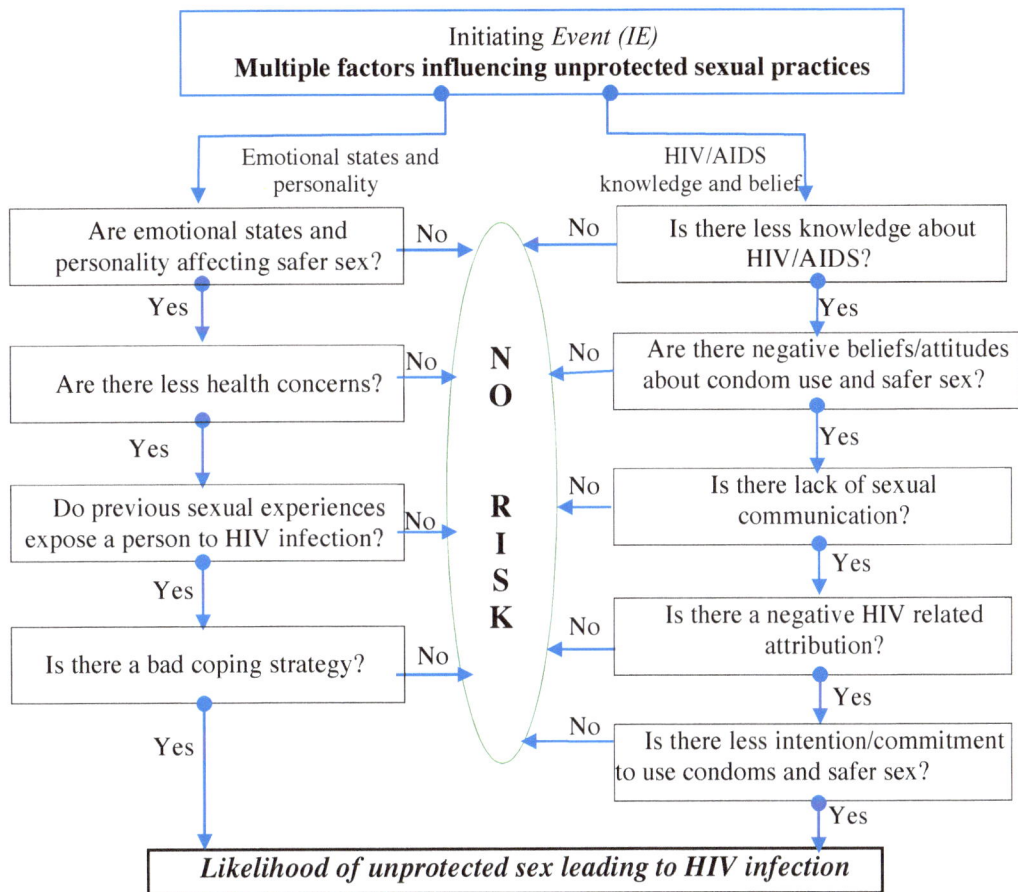

Figure 3: Risk scenario pathway for the likelihood of unprotected sex *leading to HIV infection.*

The risk pathway presented in Figure 3 consists of a sequence of specific events. For each node or event, a specific question related to the risk of unprotected sex is asked. The product of the probabilities of these answers to these questions determined the final risk related to HIV transmission through unprotected sex. In constructing the risk pathway, the epidemiology and determinants of HIV/AIDS transmissions provided the framework from which the risk assessment was conducted. Quantitative Risk Assessment requires that each parameter should be described and scientific evidence should be presented to justify the parameter estimates. This risk assessment relied on studies that have examined psychological, social, interpersonal, and medical variables as correlates of sexual risk behavior in people who know they are HIV positive. The quantified parameter values of the model were presented in terms of beta distributions which are used to determine the likelihood of HIV infection in men through unprotected sex. The beta distribution is seen as a suitable model in risk analysis and it is widely used to model probability distributions of variables in many areas of research (Soumyo, 1990).

5   Experimentation using the Computational Models

Once the development and integration of the computer modeling methodologies are completed, several simulations need to be conducted with varying initial and boundary conditions to test the validity of the model. The next step is the enhancements adjustments and modifications that need to be made until the model exhibit outputs which are biologically and mathematically reasonable and plausible. Sensitivity analysis must be performed to examine model stability too.

5.1   Macro Level

The macro level computational model developed integrated three stochastic and dynamic sub-models; one to represent AIDS at the human level, the second to represent CD4+ population dynamics at the cellular level, and the third to represent the kinetics at the intracellular viral kinetics level. Using the integrated model as the experimental medium, computer simulations were conducted to examine and answer specific scientific questions. The results of computational experiments showed that the prevalence of infection will be decreased if: a) the number of sexual partners per person is minimized; b) injecting drug use is decreased; c) condom use is increased; d) the number of sexual contacts per partner is decreased; and, e) if injecting drug needles are not shared. As a case example below is given for part c) effect of condom use (Habtemariam *et al.*, 2001).

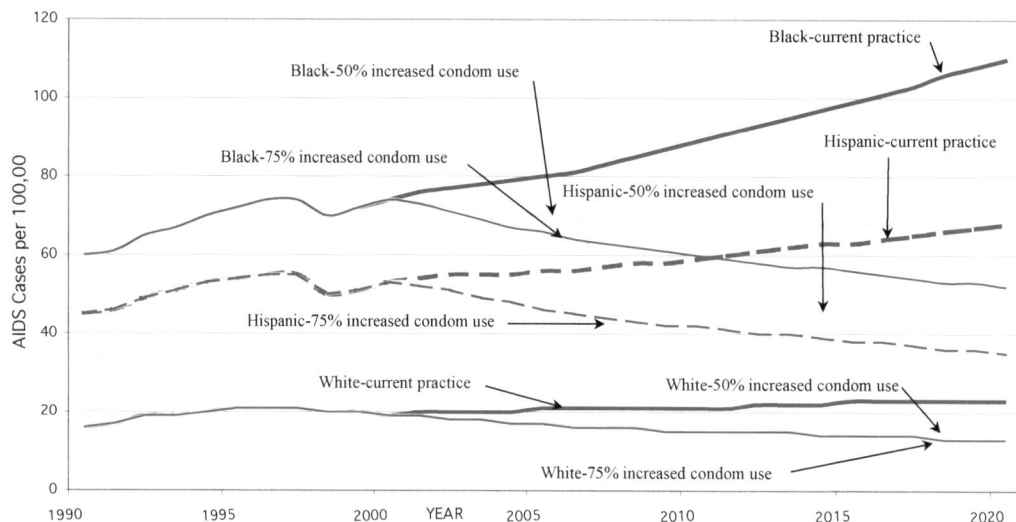

Figure 4: Projections of AIDS Cases in Blacks, Hispanics and Whites (under various levels of condom use).

In this predictive model, the focus was on the use of condoms and its impact on reducing the incidence of HIV in sexually active adults in the USA. The model (Figure 4) shows that if active HIV/AIDS prevention and control interventions are not pursued, the HIV/AIDS incidence in the black population would increase from 60 per 100,000 in 1990 to 110 per 100,000 in 2020. In the Hispanic population, it would increase from 40 per 100,000 to 68 per 100,000. In the white population, it would increase from around 16 per 100,000 to 23 per 100,000. These predictions show that there are significant increases for all populations but much more devastating for the Black subpopulation. Condom use in 25% (the status quo up to 1995 or so), 50% and 75% of sexually active adult populations was evaluated. The baseline of 25% was used in our model although the rates of condom use varied from low levels (5 to 10%) to 50% or more in surveys (CDC 1996, Douglas *et al.*, 1997; Peipert *et al.*, 1997). Figure 4 shows that increased condom use in 50% - 75% of the sexually active population, can decrease the rates to the pre 1991 levels, which were 47.9% for Blacks, 27.5% for Hispanics, and 11.6% for Whites. By the year 2020, the percentage reduction of AIDS will be 53% in Blacks, 49% in Hispanics and 43% in Whites. Our simulation only examined the proportion of condom use up to 75%, but if higher levels are evaluated, the rate of reduction will be higher and more consistent with the reported findings in the meta-analysis.

5.2   Micro level

The simulations of micro level model describe and quantitatively represent the cellular level dynamics between HIV virus and CD4+ lymphocytes (Figure 5 a) and b) (Habtemariam *et al.*, 2002). Several assumptions are relied upon and some of the parameter estimates that undoubtedly will improve over time. Of greater interest also is the intracellular dynamics that represent the molecular level dynamics and interactions between HIV and the biochemical and RNA kinetics. There is a need for and to see the importance of using computational models to represent complex biomedical systems. Consequently these systems can best be studied cohesively and rationally using integrative systems dynamics modeling.

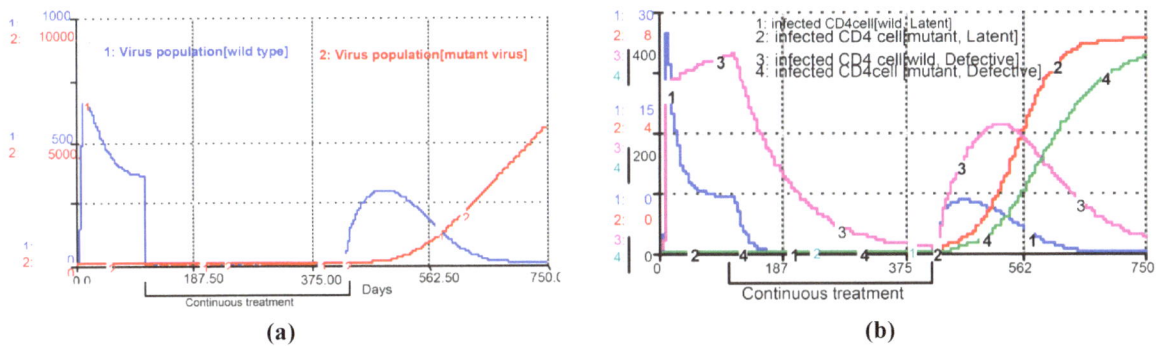

Figure 5 (a): Computer simulation of the model with drug intervention. **(b):** Computer simulation of the model for the virus without drug intervention).

5.3   Risk Assessments

After the risk pathway (scenario tree) culminating in the likelihood of unprotected sex leading to HIV infection is presented, parameters for each node were estimated using a review that included 17 English language published articles contributing tests of association for 23 variables associated with sexual risk behaviors. The majority of the studies 82% were conducted in the United States and about 18% of the studies were conducted in Europe. Participants were recruited from HIV outpatient clinics, sexually transmitted disease (STD) clinics, local or state health departments, or other community locations. A Monte Carlo Simulation with the software @Risk (Palisade Corporation) for excel was used for analysis. A total of 20,000 iterations were done for the simulation. The risk pathway consists of a sequence of specific events. For each node or event, a specific question related to the risk of unprotected sex is asked (Figure 3). The product of the answers to these questions determined the final risk related to unprotected sex leading to infection with HIV. There were 23 inputs and three outputs for the simulations. To see the effect of various inputs on the output, likelihood of HIV infection in men through unprotected sex, a sensitivity analysis was performed using regression tornado graphs (Figure 6). Sensitivity analysis identifies what is "driving" the risk estimates and provides a way to show how the results of the likelihood of unprotected sex due to: 1) less knowledge about HIV/AIDS and beliefs, 2) emotional states and personality would be affected and how sensitive those results would be to changes in the values of specific input variable.

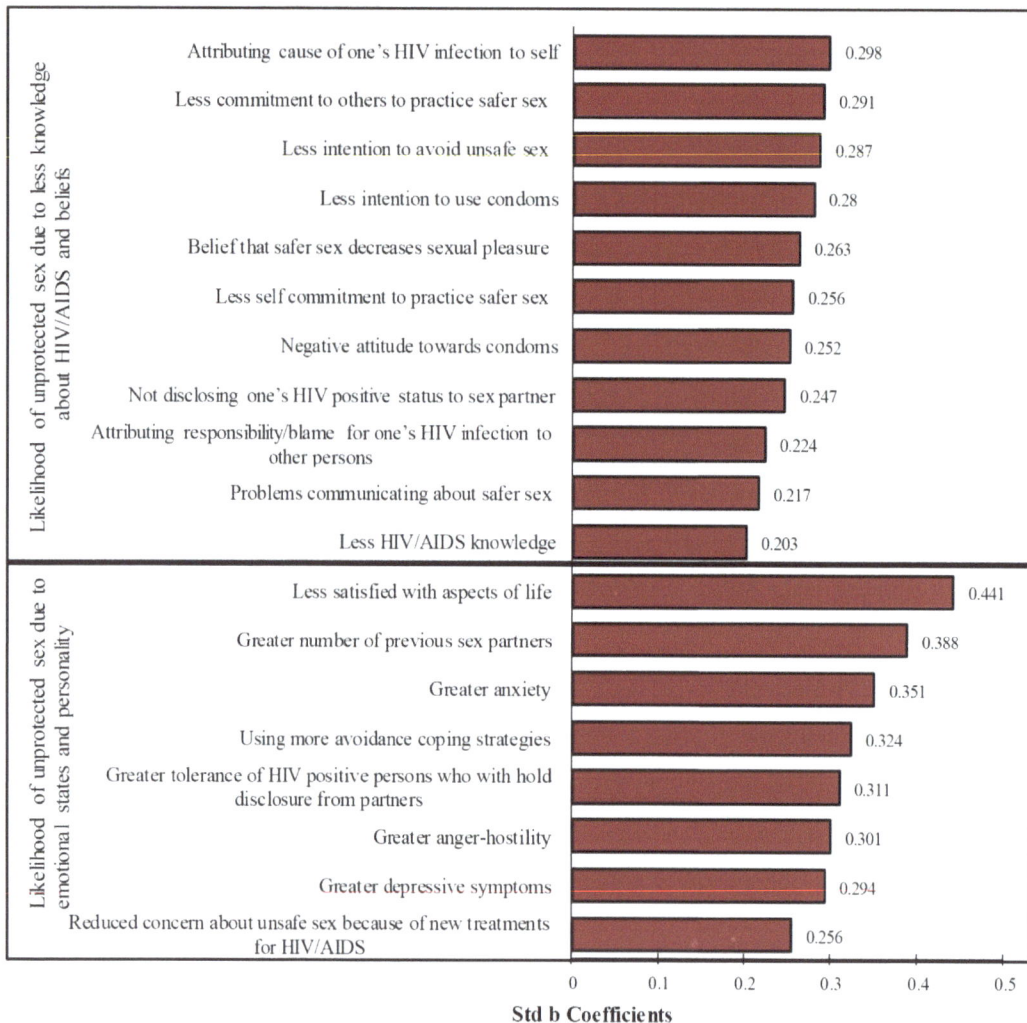

Figure 6: Tornado graph showing the likelihood of unprotected sex due to: 1) less knowledge about HIV/AIDS and beliefs, 2) emotional states and personality

6   Discussion

Models for HIV/AIDS could be conceptual, in-vivo or in-vitro, systems analysis, mathematical, or computational just to name a few. The knowledgebase developed using the EPOA methodology provides a well-organized structured source of information, which is used in the variable and parameter estimations and analysis (biological, mathematical, statistical and computer simulations) that are crucial in epidemiologic modeling of HIV/AIDS. These models are cost effective in that they are less time consuming, easily manipulated for different scenarios and not dangerous in comparison to human experimentations especially invasive ones for such a disease like HIV/AIDS. This ethical approach has enabled great strides to be achieved in the area of HIV/AIDS research which would have otherwise taken a long time especially due to the limited availability of suitable animal models. A model is evaluated first and foremost by its consistency to empirical data; any model inconsistent with reproducible observations must be modified or rejected. However, a fit to empirical data alone is not sufficient for a model to be accepted as valid. Other factors important in evaluating a model include; Ability to explain past observations; Ability to predict future observations; Cost of use, especially in combination with other models; Refutability, enabling estimation of the degree of confidence in the model and; Simplicity. Epidemiologic Problem Oriented Approach has become a crucial tool in the development of HIV/AIDS models that are important for decision making in public health as it relates to prevention, control and treatment strategies. As more knowledge becomes available, the knowledge bases can be updated and used to improve on the models thus enhancing better decisions to be considered as pertains to this HIV/AIDS pandemic. Furthermore, the results from this study may be extrapolated to assist in public health policy planning, decision-making, and in education to prevent and/or reduce the HIV/AIDS pandemic burden. In addition, the integration of the macro and micro modeling will help to see the effect of mitigation measures from individual level to the population level and ultimately to the national and international levels.

7   Conclusion

The rationale behind relying upon computational epidemiology and risk analysis modeling is that "Epidemiology has its tentacles in literally all disciplines, such as in mathematics and statistics, molecular epidemiology, socioepidemiology, computational epidemiology etc. In its simplicity, it focuses upon the study of population dynamics, whatever the population may be (biotic, *i.e.*, living or biological entities, as well as abiotic or non-living population entities)." Key to its breadth of application is epidemiology's extension into computational and risk analysis models, which can be used to examine and communicate a diversity of epidemiological concerns and scenarios. Excitingly, the role that computational and risk analysis models could play in the advancement of the theoretical understanding of disease processes and the identification of specific intervention strategies and scenarios holds the potential to impact and save human life.

Computational epidemiologic models provide insights in examining a variety of computational experimentations. Complimented with computational tools under the frame work of sound epidemiology, risk analysis can help the current and future problems in tackling the problem of HIV/AIDS by considering multiple scenarios and sensitivity analyses. Such experimentations can be of profound help in evaluating scientific questions related to effective strategies in HIV drug therapy interventions and risky behaviors.

Acknowledgement

This work is supported by a Research Centers in Minority Institutions (RCMI) Award, 2G12RR03059-16, from the National Center for Research Resources.

References

Anderson RM, May RM. (1992). Infectious Diseases of Humans: Dynamics and Control. Oxford University Press, Oxford.

Coffin JM. (1995). HIV population dynamics in vivo: Implications for genetic variation, pathogenesis, and therapy. Science 267:483-489.

Diaz T, Chu SY, Buehler JW, Boyd D, Checko PJ, Conti L, Davidson AJ, Hermann P, Herr M, Levy A, et al. (1994). Socio-economic differences among people with AIDS: results from a Multistate Surveillance Project. American Journal of Preventive Medicine 10(4):217–222.

Eubank S, Guclu H, Kumar VS, Marathe MV, Srinivasan A, et al. (2004). Modelling disease outbreaks in realistic urban social networks. Nature, (429):180-184.

Fauci AS. (2014). A Mississippi infant's case opens a new door on studying a cure for HIV. Opinions: The Washing Post June 2014

Forrester, J.W. (1961). Industrial dynamics. Cambridge, Mass.: The MIT Press.

Forrester, J.W. (1985). Future development of the system dynamic paradigm. Department Memo, SD group MIT, D-3715.

Gerbi GB, Habtemariam T, Robnett V, Nganwa D, Tameru B. (2012). Psychosocial factors as predictors of HIV/AIDS risky behaviors among people living with HIV/AIDS. Journal of AIDS HIV Research. 4(1):8-16.

Gerbi GB, Habtemariam T, Tameru B, Nganwa D, Robnett V.(2012) A quantitative risk assessment of multiple factors influencing HIV/AIDS transmission through unprotected sex among HIV-seropositive men. AIDS Care. 24(3):331-9.

Habtemariam T, Ghartey-Tagoe A, Robnett V, Trammel G (1988) Computational Epidemiology - New Research Avenues. Proceedings of the 5th International Symposium on Veterinary Epidemiology and Economics, Published in ActaVeterinaria Scandinavia, Supplementum 84:439-441.

Habtemariam T, Oryang D, Robnett V, Obasa M (1991). Computational epidemiology: integrating systems analysis and expert systems. Proceedings of the 6th International Symposium on Veterinary Epidemiology and Economics, Ottawa, Canada, Modelling & systems analysis session (pp. 538-540).

Habtemariam T, Yu P, Oryang D, Nganwa D, Ayanwale O, Tameru B, Abdelrahman H, Ahmad A, Robnett V (2001). Modelling Viral and CD4 cellular Population Dynamics in HIV:Aproaches to Evaluate Intervention Strategies. Cellular and Molecular Biology, 47(7), 1201-1208.

Habtemariam, T., Tameru, B. Nganwa, D. Ayanwale, L. Ahmed, A. Oryang, D. AbdelRahman, H. (2002) Epidemiologic modelling of HIV and CD4 cellular/molecular population dynamics. Kybernetes, 31 (9/10):1369–1379.

Ho DD, Neumann AU, Perelson AS, Chen W, Leonard JM, Markowitz M. (1995). Rapid turnover of plasma virions and CD4 lymphocytes in HIV-1 infection. Nature (373):123-126.

National Research Council (1983). Risk Assessment in the Federal Government: Managing the Process. Washington, DC: National Academy Press.

Nganwa D, Habtemariam T, Tameru B, Gerbi B, Bogale A, Robnett VWilson W. (2010). Applying the Epidemiologic Problem Oriented Approach (EPOA) Methodology in Developing a Knowledge Base for the Modeling of HIV/AIDS. Ethnicity and Disease 20(1) S1:173-177

Perelson AS, Nelson PW (1999). Mathematical analysis of HIV-1 dynamics in vivo. SIAM Revew, (41), 3-44.

Pool R. 1992. "The Third Branch of Science Debuts". Science. (256):44-47.

Risk Newsletter. Society for Risk Analysis Editorial, First Quarter 2000, 20(1):3-5.

Rvachev LA, Longini IM Jr(1985). A mathematical model for the global spread of influenza. Mathematical Biosciences (75):3-22.

Sattenspiel L, Simon CP (1988). The spread and persistence of infectious diseases in structured populations. Mathematical Biosciences, (90):341-366.

Tameru B, Gerbi G, Nganwa D, Bogale A, Robnett V, Habtemariam T. (2012). The Association between Interrelationships and Linkages of Knowledge about HIV/AIDS and its Related Risky Behaviors in People Living with HIV/AIDS. Journal of AIDS and Clinical Research 1:3(7):1-7.

Tameru B, Habtemariam T, Nganwa D, Ayanwale L, Beyene G, et al. (2008). Computational Modelling of Intracellular Viral Kinetics and CD4+ Cellular Population Dynamics of HIV/AIDS. Advances in Systems Science and Applications (l 8):40-45.

Tameru B, Habtemariam T, Nganwa D, Gerbi G, Bogale A, Robnett V, Wilson W.(2010). Assessing HIV/AIDS intervention strategies using an integrative macro-micro level computational epidemiologic modeling approach. Ethnicity & Disease 2010;20:S1-207-10.

Tameru B, Nganwa D, Bogale A, Robnett V, and Habtemariam T. (2012). The Role of Computational Epidemiology and Risk Analysis in the Fight against HIV/AIDS. Journal of AIDS and Clinical Research. 3(6), http://dx.doi.org/10.4172/2155-6113.1000e107.

Tan Wai-Yuan and Wu Hulin Eds. (2008). Deterministic and Stochastic Models of AIDS Epidemics and HIV Infections with Intervention. Hackensack, NJ: World Scientific Publishing Company.

Wei X, Ghosh SK, Taylor ME, Johnson VA, Emini EA, et al. (1995) Viral dynamics in human immunodeficiency virus type 1 infection. Nature, (373):117-122.

Decreasing Maternal Mortality in Africa: Integrating HIV Care and Maternal Care

Sara Gorman

Department of Health Policy and Management
Columbia University Mailman School of Public Health, USA

1   Introduction

As 2015 quickly approaches, we have been made increasingly aware of our progress toward Millennium Development Goals (MDGs). Some remarkable progress has indeed been made. For example, the proportion of underweight children younger than age five in developing countries has declined from 28% to 17% between 1990 and 2011(WHO Millennium Development Goals, 2012). Significant progress has also been made in reducing mortality among children under the age of five. In 1990, 12 million such children under five died, compared with 6.9 million children in 2011 (WHO Millennium Development Goals, 2012). In 2011, 2.5 million people were newly infected with HIV, representing a 24% decrease from the 3.1 million people newly infected in 2001 (WHO Millennium Development Goals, 2012). However, one millennium development goal has been particularly recalcitrant to progress: MDG 5, namely, improving maternal health. Improving maternal health involves not only reducing the maternal mortality ratio by 75% but also increasing the proportion of births attended by skilled health personnel and achieving universal access to reproductive health. Indicators for monitoring progress of universal access to reproductive health include contraceptive prevalence rate, adolescent birth rate, antenatal care coverage, and unmet need for family planning. Few countries are on track to achieve the first part of MDG 5's goals, reducing maternal mortality by 75% (WHO Trends in Maternal Mortality, 2010). Sub-Saharan Africa is in the most dire position, with a regional maternal mortality rate of 640 maternal deaths out of 100,000 live births, and a decline rate of merely 0.1% per year (WHO Trends in Maternal Mortality, 2010). In 2012, there were a total number of 25 million people living with HIV in sub-Saharan Africa, representing 71% of the global total, with 1.6 million newly infected over the course of the year (Kaiser Family Foundation, 2013). In the summer of 2012, the University of Cambridge hosted a conference on the topic of "New Approaches to Maternal Mortality," recognizing the crucial need to address the problem of global maternal mortality rates and to address potential solutions (University of Cambridge New Approaches to Maternal Mortality, 2012). There are some signs of global improvement in PMTCT and ART coverage, especially among women, which have led to reductions in maternal mortality (WHO and UNICEF, 2013). Yet many countries, especially in Africa, are nonetheless still not on track to meet MDG 5.

2   HIV in Pregnancy is Contributing to High Maternal Mortality Rates

What is contributing to such high maternal mortality rates and what can we do to help reduce them? In 2010, experts from WHO, UNICEF, United Nations Population Fund, and the World Bank came together to produce a report on global trends in maternal mortality (WHO Trends in Maternal Mortality, 2010). A relatively buried and subsequently unpublicized portion of the report revealed the key connection between maternal mortality and HIV infection. This key link has received little attention in both research and popular media, but the contribution of HIV infection to maternal morality is undoubtedly significant. The authors of the joint report estimated that in 2008 alone there were 42,000 deaths due to HIV/AIDS among pregnant women (WHO Trends in Maternal Mortality, 2010). 9% of all maternal deaths in sub-Saharan Africa were due to HIV in the period between 1990 and 2008 (WHO Trends in Maternal Mortality, 2010). One report in 2008 estimated that there would have been 61,400 fewer maternal deaths that year in the absence of HIV-related mortality (Rosen *et al.,* 2010). Zaba and colleagues estimate that roughly a quarter of pregnancy-related deaths in Africa are due to HIV (Myer, 2013). One study in Mulago Hospital Complex in Kampala Uganda ascertained that HIV-positive women were at five times the risk of dying from pregnancy-related complications compared with HIV-negative women (Wandabwa *et al.*, 2011). In another study in Benin City, Nigeria, about 25% of maternal deaths in a university teaching hospital were due to HIV/AIDS. The majority of these women (86.5%) did not have antiretroviral therapy initiated prior to presentation at the hospital, and two-thirds (64.6%) presented with stage III or IV HIV disease (Onakwhor *et al.*, 2011).

In countries with high HIV prevalence, such as eastern and southern Africa, HIV has become the leading cause of death among women during pregnancy and the postpartum period (WHO Trends in Maternal Mortality, 2010). The problem may only become worse as increasing numbers of HIV-positive pregnant women enter later stages of the disease (Le Coeur *et al.*, 2005). Goals of reducing worldwide maternal mortality cannot be realized without simultaneously addressing the HIV/AIDS epidemic among women, especially in resource-poor settings and especially in the southern regions of Africa.

A recent study emphasized the clear and considerable contribution of HIV/AIDS to global maternal mortality rates (Calvert & Ronsmans, 2013). The authors of this meta-analysis found that a very high proportion of pregnancy-related deaths are attributable to HIV at the population level. They estimate that 5% of pregnancy-related deaths worldwide are attributable to HIV. There are numerous single facility-based studies, especially in South Africa and sub-Saharan Africa, that further demonstrate this link. One study at a major tertiary hospital in KwaZulu-Natal in 2001 indicated a 32-fold increased risk of death among TB-HIV co-infected women, compared with non-infected women (Moodley *et al.*, 2010). Another study done in another major tertiary hospital in South Africa in 2007 showed that the majority of deaths among HIV-infected pregnant women were associated with co-infection with tuberculosis (22%), pneumonia (19.9%), and meningitis (Moodley *et al.*, 2010). A more recent 5-year review of maternal deaths at a tertiary health facility in Johannesburg found that maternal mortality ratios in HIV-infected women were 776/100,000, which was 62-fold higher than in HIV-negative women (Moodley *et al.*, 2010). Another study in Pointe Noire, Congo found that the maternal mortality ratios were 1842 and 478 per 100,000 births respectively in HIV-positive and negative women, demonstrating that HIV increased the maternal mortality ratio in the population as a whole by 18% (Le Coeur *et al.*, 2005). In other parts of Africa, the maternal mortality ratio is also higher for HIV-infected women than for non-infected women, and this threat sometimes extends for years beyond pregnancy and delivery. Studies done in Uganda and Zimbabwe demonstrated that HIV-infected women were more likely than non-infected women to be admitted to the hospital or die during the two years after delivery (Moodley *et al.*, 2010). In one study of 378 maternal deaths over a 7-year period in a hospital in Durban, South Africa, pregnancy-related sepsis occurred more frequently in HIV-infected than non-infected women (Ramogale *et al.*, 2004). At the same time, rates of TB-associated maternal deaths and TB in pregnancy are certainly on the rise in Africa. TB was the third leading infectious cause of maternal death in Durban (14.9%) and Lusaka (25%) (Grange *et al.*, 2010).

There is even reason to believe that these estimates of HIV-related maternal mortality might be underestimates. Maternal deaths often go undetected in the first place. Most of the research and data collection on maternal deaths focuses on facility-based deliveries, while many women in developing countries still give birth at home or in other non-traditional settings (Myer, 2013). WHO defines maternal death as the death of a woman while pregnant or within 42 days of termination of pregnancy, irrespective of the duration and site of the pregnancy, from any cause related to or aggravated by the pregnancy or its management but not from accidental or incidental causes. Maternal deaths must therefore be direct obstetric deaths from complications or misinformed treatment or indirect deaths resulting from previous existing disease or a disease developing during pregnancy that was made worse by the effects of pregnancy (Rosen *et al.*, 2012).

Classifying deaths as either HIV or pregnancy-related is difficult in developing countries, where accounts of death often rely upon verbal autopsies and where HIV status is often unknown (Le Coeur *et al.*, 2005). In some cases, the distinction between incidental and indirect causes of death is difficult to determine, especially in the case of HIV, in which the effects of pregnancy on disease progression are largely unknown. Because of this, many HIV-related deaths in pregnancy do not get recorded as "maternal deaths," even though it is very likely that pregnancy contributes negatively to disease progression (Rosen *et al.*, 2012). The need for more information on the contribution of HIV to maternal mortality is particularly urgent in places like sub-Saharan Africa, where the burden of the epidemic is large.

Interestingly, the epidemiological landscape of maternal mortality is starting to shift, in large part due to the HIV epidemic among women of reproductive age in areas of the world in which maternal mortality ratios tend to be high. In these regions, causes of maternal deaths are shifting from obstetric to non-obstetric causes. These nonobstetric causes are largely HIV-related opportunistic infections. One study done over a five-year period from 1995 to 2001 at the Johannesburg Hospital in South Africa found a change in the etiology of maternal mortality even over this short period. In 1995, most pregnant women died from complications associated with hypertension. By 2001, the HIV/AIDS epidemic had advanced and, as a result, pneumonia was the leading cause of death. The authors of this particular study note that this trend is similar to a national trend and not limited to Johannesburg and that this trend is also in keeping with an international increase in HIV/AIDS (Kruger *et al.*, 2002). This shift demands a similarly adaptive response to maternal mortality, and the global health community should be actively searching for ways to maximize the message that treatment of HIV/AIDS is an essential part of maternal health. For example, health workers should be trained to be on the lookout for respiratory symptoms among pregnant women in particular and should attend to respiratory symptoms as a matter of urgency, especially in pregnant patients with HIV or in patients whose HIV status is unknown.

3   We need to Better Understand the Link Between HIV and Maternal Death

Some have proposed that pregnancy might accelerate HIV progression or that the risk of obstetric complications may be increased in HIV-infected women (Calvert & Ronsmans, 2013). Recent evidence suggests that pregnancy appears to have no significant effect on the progression of HIV in asymptomatic pregnant women with the disease. However, symptomatic HIV-positive pregnant women are at greater risk of dying from opportunistic infections than non-infected pregnant women. This probably means that women who are either in the early stages of the disease or are using antiretrovirals to control their virus are protected from the risks presented by pregnancy to women with either advanced HIV infection or who are not able to control their illness with the appropriate medications. In resource-poor settings, opportunistic infections are usually bronchopneumonia, *Pneumocystis carinii* pneumonia, meningitis, tuberculosis, and malaria. The effects of pregnancy on respiratory diseases associated with HIV infection, the most common form of opportunistic infection that causes death among HIV-infected pregnant women, is not well known (Ramogale *et al.*, 2004). At the same time as opportunistic infections are emerging as an important cause of maternal death among HIV-infected women, one study that found a maternal mortality ratio 10 times higher in HIV-infected pregnant women than in uninfected women in South Africa discovered that HIV-infected pregnant women were also at higher risk of dying from pregnancy-related sepsis and complications of abortion (Moran *et al.*, 2012). These particular findings indicate a potential double burden for HIV-infected mothers: both improper treatment of and attention to their HIV infection as well as the possibility of HIV infection's direct contribution to pregnancy-related maternal deaths leave HIV-infected mothers much more vulnerable to postpartum complications than their uninfected counterparts.

Much more research is still needed on the biological basis of HIV-related maternal mortality (Abdool-Karim *et al.*, 2010). We know that the link exists, but we are still not entirely sure why it exists (Landes *et al.*, 2012). Evidence suggests that immune marker status of HIV infection itself is not worsened during pregnancy (Brettle *et al.*, 1995). One possibility lies in the changes in the maternal immune system that occur during pregnancy. Technically, a fetus is a semi-allograph because one-half of its antigens are paternal and therefore foreign proteins to the mother. The exact mechanisms by which the fetus avoids rejection by the mother have never been fully elucidated. Traditionally, it has been thought that tolerance of the fetus is accomplished by a maternal shift from Th1 to Th2 immunity during pregnancy. This notion, however, has recently been challenged (Mor & Cardenas, 2010). Investigators have searched for other, more subtle shifts in immune system function during pregnancy to explain why the fetus is not rejected and these may have some relevance to explaining why HIV-positive pregnant women are prone to increased morbidity and mortality.

Shifts in immunity might render the HIV-positive women more susceptible to the effects of opportunistic infections during pregnancy. It is known that women are more susceptible to malaria infection during the first half of pregnancy (Okoko *et al.*, 2003). During pregnancy there is a greater increase in regulatory T cells (Treg) in HIV-positive compared to HIV-negative women (Richardson & Weinberg, 2011; Kolte *et al.*, 2011). As Treg cells generally serve an anti-inflammatory function, this may help explain maternal tolerance of the fetus but also make the mother more susceptible to opportunistic infections like malaria. Hygino *et al.* (2012) found a lower immunoproliferative response and higher production of the anti-inflammatory cytokine interleukin-10 (IL-10) in HIV-positive pregnant women, which also may make them at risk for greater morbidity and mortality from opportunistic infections (Hygino *et al.*, 2012).

In order to understand the possible role of normal or exaggerated immune systems shifts during pregnancy in HIV-positive women in increasing susceptibility to opportunistic infections and increased mortality it will be necessary to investigate several aspects of this problem. First, more exact data on the cause of death of HIV-positive pregnant women is necessary to confirm that the underlying pathology involves opportunistic infection. Second, a more detailed and trimester-specific understanding of immune system changes that distinguish HIV-positive pregnant women from HIV-positive non-pregnant women and HIV-negative pregnant women is required. Finally, studies must investigate whether such immune system changes are proximally related (e.g. occur in the same trimester of pregnancy) to excess morbidity and mortality from opportunistic infections.

On a more psychosocial level, qualitative research in Kenya has shown that fear of HIV testing and unwanted disclosure of HIV status to spouse and family can cause some HIV-positive pregnant women to specifically avoid giving birth in a health facility (Medema-Wijnveen *et al.*, 2012). In another study of 1,777 HIV-positive pregnant women in Kenya, 20% of women agreed that women who give birth at health facilities can be tested for diseases without giving consent. In the same study, 57% of women agreed with the statement "HIV-positive women who give birth at health facilities are likely to have their HIV status revealed to their husband/partner or others in the community" (Medema-Wijnveen *et al.*,

2012). This variable was significantly associated with intention to give birth at home, with women agreeing with this statement being far more likely to choose to give birth at home rather than at a health facility. Women with HIV may be particularly afraid to give birth at a health facility because of the perception that giving birth at a facility will automatically entail testing without their consent and automatic disclosure of their test results to family members. In this way, HIV may contribute to maternal mortality, since giving birth in a health facility dramatically reduces the risk of death from immediate birth-related complications.

4   Prenatal Care and HIV Treatment must be Better Integrated

What would wider recognition of the crucial link between HIV and maternal mortality mean for interventions to reduce the maternal mortality ratio? For one thing, there should be an integrated approach to HIV and maternal health service delivery. Pregnant women with HIV worldwide should be given earlier access to antiretroviral treatment and access to family planning services (Abdool-Karim et al., 2012). Current funding schemes often award money for programs and treatments to address a particular illness. This has certainly been the case for HIV funding, where vertical programming has become the norm. Yet, more recently, concerns have been raised about the effects of vertical programs on the use and outcomes of reproductive health services. Some of these negative effects include: the diversion of funding away from reproductive health and the general health system toward HIV-specific services and increased demands on an already depleted health workforce (Van den Akker *et al.*, 2012). The perception that vertical HIV services increase stigma is also common among patients and may represent a barrier to seeking care (Topp *et al.*, 2010). In response to these hypotheses, some researchers have implemented interventions in developing countries to integrate reproductive health, PMTCT care, and maternal HIV treatment. These interventions have often demonstrated that integration of ART and reproductive health services result in an increase in the use of both HIV care and reproductive health care among HIV-positive pregnant women (Van den Akker *et al.,* 2012). Now is an opportune time to integrate HIV care and maternal care, since new testing approaches and technologies, including CD4 point-of-care testing assays, have become more widely available in low- and middle-income countries and make integration much more feasible (Hirnschall *et al.*, 2013). New WHO guidelines for the treatment and prevention of HIV released in 2013 demonstrate a growing international focus on improving retention in care and adherence to ART, decentralizing delivery of ART to primary health care, and integrating HIV care with maternal and child health, TB, and drug dependency programs (Hirnschall *et al.*, 2013).

Although it is clear that better integration of HIV treatment and prenatal care is crucial, much work remains to be done to pinpoint exactly how this integration should be achieved. Cost-effectiveness of integrated services and health outcomes such as HIV and STI incidence and mortality must continue to be investigated in order to inform the development of integrated programs and policies (Lindegren *et al.*, 2012). Prevention of mother-to-child transmission (PMTCT) has been enormously important in helping reduce the number of neonatal HIV infections worldwide. However, the focus on PMTCT might sometimes occlude the health needs of HIV-positive pregnant women (Mataka, 2007). The field of HIV prevention and treatment must pay more adequate attention to the health risks of pregnancy for the HIV-positive mother.

Some strategies for integration of these services include lifelong ART for HIV-positive pregnant women, which can help prevent mother-to-child transmission as well as maternal mortality due to complications related to HIV in subsequent pregnancies and send a message to communities that antiretroviral therapy should be continued for life (Suthar *et al.*, 2013). In 2013, the WHO came out with the *consolidated guidelines on the use of antiretroviral drugs for treating and preventing HIV infection* (Hirnschall *et al.*, 2013). The most important new clinical recommendations include: treating adults, adolescents, and older children earlier by initiating ART in all individuals with a CD4 count of 500 cells/mm^3 or less, giving priority to those with advanced clinical disease or a CD4 count less than 350 cells/mm^3; starting ART at any CD4 level in certain populations, including those with active TB, Hepatitis B and severe chronic liver disease, HIV-positive partners in serodiscordant couples, pregnant and breastfeeding women, and children younger than 5 years of age; a preferred first-line ART regimen of Tenofovir + 3TC or FTC + Efavirenz as a once-daily fixed dose combination for adults, pregnant women, and children 3 years and older; and the use of viral load testing as the preferred approach to monitoring response to treatment and detecting treatment failure (Hirnschall *et al.*, 2013). In 2010 WHO guidelines recommended lifelong ART for pregnant women with CD4 counts of 300 cells/mm^3 or less, and two prophylaxis options for those not eligible for ART. Option A provided twice-daily zidovudine from 14 weeks to the onset of labor and single-dose nevirapine and twice-daily zidovudine and lamivudine for several days post-partum. Option B provided triple ARV therapy to the mother until delivery or, if the mother was breastfeeding, until one week after all infant exposure to breast milk had completed (Hirnschall *et al.*, 2013). In 2013, WHO revised these recommendations, indicating international recognition of a dire need for better prevention of PMTCT and better protection of pregnant women against HIV-related maternal mortality. WHO now recommends ART in one simplified regimen to all pregnant and breastfeeding women regardless of CD4 count in the period of risk of mother-to-child transmission. Life-long ART for pregnant women regardless of CD4 count or clinical stage is also recommended, especially in areas of high fertility and limited access to CD4 testing (Hirnschall *et al.*, 2013). The recommendation for life-long ART for pregnant women is, however, provisional, with the caveat that the benefits of universal ART have not been entirely confirmed in the literature. WHO recommends that individual countries weigh the costs and benefits of life-long ART for pregnant women (Hirnschall *et al.*, 2013). The treatment entailed in Option A is no longer recommended. Of course, implementing life-long ART treatment in Africa carries its own potential drawbacks, including overburdening an already overstretched health system and increasing the threat of ART stock-outs in resource-poor settings.

There have been some concerns about the safety and toxicity of EFV and TDF during pregnancy, with some evidence that both drugs may contribute to certain types of birth defects. Isolated case reports of neural tube defects have produced some concern about using EFV in the first trimester of pregnancy (WHO consolidated guidelines, 2013). Results from an updated systematic review suggest that this risk is relatively low, however. The estimated prevalence of neural tube defect among women taking EFV during the first trimester of pregnancy was 7 per 10,000 population (0.07%) in the systematic review, compared with estimates of 0.02%-0.2% prevalence of neural tube defects in the general population (WHO consolidated guidelines, 2013). This potential low risk should be balanced against the benefits and importance of providing ART to HIV-positive pregnant women to maternal and child health and prevention of vertical transmission. Concerns about the safety of TDF in pregnancy include renal toxicity, adverse birth outcomes, and effects on bone density. In one important study, the prevalence of overall birth defects with exposure to TDF in the first trimester was 2.4%, which did not differ significantly from the overall birth defect rate (WHO consolidated guidelines, 2013). Studies also show no significant difference in fetal growth between infants exposed to TDF and infants not exposed to TDF. More extensive research is certainly needed, but the evidence suggests that EVF and TDF exposure in pregnancy is safe for both mother and child.

In countries with generalized HIV epidemics and antenatal HIV prevalence > 1%, ART should be offered to eligible pregnant women in maternal health clinics, rather than in separate specialized HIV clinics, to reduce transportation costs, lower risk of attrition and remove potentially stigmatizing obstacles (Suthar *et al.*, 2013). Lifelong use of ART among HIV-positive pregnant women also has the benefits of preventing HIV transmission during subsequent pregnancies (Suthar *et al.*, 2013). Preliminary investigations indicate that ART retention and treatment levels are higher among pregnant women attending maternal health services clinics that also provide HIV treatment services (Suthar *et al.*, 2013). Because many antenatal clinics lack the ability to perform CD4+ T-lymphocyte counts, antenatal clinics in some countries, such as Malawi, have begun initiating all HIV-positive pregnant women on ART regardless of CD4 count (Suthar *et al.*, 2013). The results of this strategy have not yet been fully ascertained, but preliminary evidence suggests that this tactic might be effective. One meta-analysis of studies of integrated HIV and ANC clinics in Mozambique, Rwanda, and Zambia found that the proportion of eligible pregnant women taking ART was consistently higher in integrated clinics than in non-integrated ANC clinics (Suthar *et al.*, 2013). In addition, integrated HIV and maternal care has in some cases also increased uptake of STI testing and treatment as well as family planning consultations (Van den Akker *et al.*, 2012).

Reaching women who deliver at home, common phenomenon especially in rural areas, is a particular challenge in preventing maternal deaths from HIV-related complications. One option is to scale up services provided by community health workers. One study in South Africa implemented and evaluated a comprehensive care package of antenatal care and HIV services in the home. The care packages were implemented by groups of community health workers. The authors note that interventions that better link the household and community level to health care through community health workers have the capacity not only to make a significant contribution to reducing maternal mortality but also to empowering the community. In addition, many countries are now showing an active interest in strengthening community-based care, and some evidence has suggested that home counseling is more effective than health facility counseling in changing and directing health-related behaviors (Tomlinson *et al.*, 2011). Integration of HIV and prenatal counseling at the household level could be another important step in reducing HIV-related maternal mortality.

Studies have also shown that integrated maternal/child health care (MCH) and HIV prevention and treatment programs are well-received by both health care workers and patients. One intervention in Mozambique that randomly assigned three existing health care facilities to the integrated intervention and three to the control group found that all personnel involved evaluated the integrated service delivery model positively (Geelhoed *et al.*, 2013). To personnel, it made more sense to attend to a mother with her child in a single, one-stop consultation than to treat the child first and have the mother return later in the day for evaluation and treatment. Participating staff felt well-equipped with appropriate technical knowledge to provide both MCH and HIV care. Staff noted increased efficiency in integrated care centers, partly due to the integration of routine data collection tools in addition to integrated service delivery. In general, when interviewed about integrated care, providers often cite increased efficiency, decreased time spent by patients in clinics, improved provider-patient relationships, and improved ART adherence (Suthar *et al.*, 2013). Nonetheless, several limiting factors were nearly unanimously noted by involved personnel in the Mozambique study. Frequent staff absences and irregular supply of essential drugs were noted as the most important among these factors. Indeed, months in which one or more staff had been absent resulted in a significantly lower number of HIV tests performed in children and a significantly lower number of HIV-exposed infants initiating follow-up care (Geelhoed *et al.*, 2013). These findings indicate a need for broader systemic changes and health systems strengthening, even in the presence of integrated care. Increasing psychosocial support for health care workers dealing with increased workloads and severe clinical cases would also be important (Mutemwa *et al.*, 2013). In another study of integrated HIV and reproductive health care in Kenya, providers reported that integration enhanced job satisfaction by providing a better quality service, which led to better feedback from clients (Mutemwa *et al.*, 2013). In addition, providers reported greater professional stimulation due to constantly changing clientele and confronting new and different health problems. Increased job satisfaction may help reduce rates of absenteeism, which presents a major barrier to the provision of appropriate care in developing countries.

Lower ART coverage among pregnant women is usually attributed to several specific factors, including: complex treatment regimens; complex referral systems; HIV test stock-outs; antiretroviral stockouts; HIV staff shortages; and slow processing of CD4+ T-lymphocyte test results (Suthar *et al.*, 2013). Integrated HIV and ANC clinics would take care of a number of these problems, including complex referral systems, staff shortages, and complex treatment regimens. In qualitative studies conducted in Malawi, Uganda, and Zimbabwe, several key reasons for loss to follow-up were identified, including: long lines at HIV clinics; cost of transport from home to clinics; fear of disclosure of HIV status; lack of support from partners who did not want to be tested for HIV; and staff suggestions not to breastfeed babies (Suthar *et al.*, 2013). Again, integrated HIV and ANC clinics could alleviate several of these problems, including cost of transport and problems related to fear of disclosure or stigma. In general, the process for delivering ART to a pregnant woman generally involves: attendance at an ANC clinic; provider-initiated HIV testing and counseling; referral to an HIV clinic; enrollment in care at the HIV clinic; assessment of eligibility for ART (based on CD4+ T-lymphocyte counts); initiation of ART if eligible; maintaining high adherence to ART (Suthar *et al.*, 2013). The chances that an HIV-positive pregnant woman will default from care increases with every additional clinic she must visit. In studies from four different African countries, 30 to 83% of HIV-positive pregnant women were lost from care during referral from ANC to HIV clinics (Suthar *et al.*, 2013).

Integrating ART and other HIV services into antenatal clinics will require training nurses, midwives, and OB/GYNs to provide HIV care and ART as well as HIV testing and counseling. Other health workers, including community health workers, might be needed in these integrated clinics to avoid overburdening nurses and midwives. Studies have shown no difference in mortality or loss to follow up when nurses or non-physician clinicians or community health workers initiate people on ART as compared to physicians (WHO consolidated guidelines, 2013). This kind of task shifting is also likely to reduce overall costs by lowering overhead expenses for delivering quality care and decreasing facility and utility costs (WHO consolidated guidelines, 2013). Training of non-physicians and community health workers may include developing standardized manuals for educating maternal health care providers about delivering HIV services.

Clinics should be jointly owned by existing maternal and child health programs and HIV programs, integrating staff from both antenatal clinics and HIV clinics into one location. Ideally, electronic monitoring of ART should be available and patient registers used in reproductive health and antenatal services should include information about HIV status and treatment (Suthar *et al.*, 2013). Health workers should be better trained in information collection practices, and, where available, should be trained to record patient information electronically. In one South African study, health workers recorded only a portion of information about PMTCT and ART activity, making it difficult to improve current practices and systems. This poor data organization and incomplete information collection is likely representative of a lot of facilities in resource-poor areas (Sprague *et al.*, 2011). Organizational problems in HIV clinics have historically led to delayed payment of lay HIV counselors, which often results in low morale and absenteeism, further resulting in serious delays in pregnant women's HIV care. Measures must be taken to improve the organization of integrated ANC and HIV clinics to ensure that all staff is paid on time in full and that staff is held accountable for absences and tardiness (Sprague *et al.*, 2011). Integrated clinics would also have to better monitor and treat opportunistic infections, since these now represent a major cause of pregnancy-related mortality among HIV-positive women in African countries. More intensive medical inputs for cardiac, respiratory, and metabolic disorders which are often HIV-related would be essential (Madzimbamuto *et al.*, 2013). Health workers at these integrated clinics would thus also need to be trained to recognize the signs of HIV-related opportunistic infections. All HIV-positive pregnant women should be screened for opportunistic infections at these clinics.

Preventing unwanted pregnancies is another key strategy in reducing maternal deaths as a result of HIV, as well as teaching women to space births out, since health status decreases with each pregnancy. Family planning programs to avert unwanted pregnancies among HIV-positive women has been determined to be cost-effective in studies in sub-Saharan African populations. For the same cost, contraceptive strategies could avert 28.6% more HIV-positive births than the nevirapine intervention currently used for PMTCT. Reducing rates of these unwanted pregnancies would also reduce rates of neonatal HIV infection. There are many opportunities to provide better family planning for HIV-positive women, including at the time of discharge from maternity units, in postnatal clinics, when mothers bring children in for immunizations, and the post-abortion and post-partum periods (Moodley *et al.*, 2011). Providing family planning to women in developing countries would prevent 54 million unintended pregnancies, including 21 million unplanned births, 26 million induced abortions, and seven million miscarriages. It would also prevent 79,000 maternal deaths and 1.1 million infant deaths (Warren *et al.,* 2013). In settings of low contraceptive prevalence and high HIV prevalence, women living with HIV have shorter birth spacing intervals than HIV-negative women; suggested limited access to family planning services following childbirth for this population in particular (Warren *et al.*, 2013). In an intervention in Swaziland providing integrated reproductive and family planning services for postpartum HIV-positive and HIV-negative women, HIV-positive women were much more likely to have discussed family planning with the provider during their visit than HIV-negative women, suggesting a need for these kinds of services for this population (Warren *et al.*, 2013).

At the policy level, strategic planning and budgeting with relevant stakeholders for maternal health and HIV services will be necessary to help provide and sustain funds for integration of services, training of employees, and monitoring and evaluation. International aid agencies will need to be encouraged to provide funds specifically for integrated services, rather than focusing on one disease or health issue at a time. Some international donors are already taking notice of the need for funds directed specifically at integrated services of this kind. For example, at the 2010 Women Deliver conference, Melinda Gates pledged $1.5 billion over the next five years to stimulate investment in integrated women's health programs, including programs that combine maternal health and HIV services (PLoS Medicine Editors, 2010). Communication and coordination across departments dealing with HIV and maternal health within local ministries of health must be strengthened, a process that is already under way in many countries. In order to avoid duplication and to maximize the use of available resources, national interagency coordination committees addressing the integration of these services should be formed, and continuous planning and management is essential (WHO, Technical consultation, 2008).

To aid pregnant women with disclosure of HIV status to their partners, clinics should offer couples testing and counseling at the first antenatal visit. Evidence has suggested that integrating couples counseling into antenatal care greatly increases pregnant women's uptake of efforts to prevent HIV transmission, including good ART retention (Farquar et al., 2004). Since lack of partner support is associated with decreased use of ART, incorporating couples counseling into antenatal care for HIV-positive pregnant women might encourage usage of life-saving therapies that may also help reduce maternal mortality rates. Couples counseling sessions may also be an ideal time to introduce the importance and effectiveness of ART in preventing transmission of HIV infection to the newborn child. Other possible interventions include integration of HIV services in general primary care or having HIV service providers visit antenatal clinics on specified days. However, fully integrated HIV and antenatal services at antenatal clinics probably have the greatest potential to control HIV infection among pregnant women, thereby reducing the chances of obstetric complications and maternal death (Turan et al., 2012).

5   Conclusion

Greater attention to and greater provisions for HIV-specific services in young women of reproductive age could have a major impact on the global maternal mortality rate, especially in places like sub-Saharan Africa, where both HIV rates and the maternal mortality ratio are high. Moreover, progress on four main sub-goals across two of the Millennium Development Goals (5 and 6) will be enhanced by closer attention to treating, managing, and preventing HIV infection in pregnant women: reducing the maternal mortality ratio by 75%; achieving universal access to reproductive health; halting and reversing the spread of HIV/AIDS; and achieving universal access to treatment for HIV/AIDS for all those who need it. Integrated maternal health and HIV services would help reduce rates of maternal death due to obstetric complications associated with HIV; would connect more women at risk with reproductive health services, including prevention and treatment of STI's other than HIV; would control HIV infection among a vulnerable population of sexually active women and prevent transmission to HIV-negative partners and mother-to-child transmission; and would help connect a large population of HIV-positive women to treatment.

Maternal deaths often represent problems with the broader health system in general, and there is evidence that improvements in maternal and child health have been associated with improvements in health systems overall (Madzimbamuto et al., 2013). In Mozambique, integration of HIV services and antenatal services even strengthened health infrastructure, leading to system efficiency through reduced workforce gaps, improved supervision, improved patient flows, and coordination between laboratories, pharmacies, and clinics (Madzimbamuto et al., 2013). Thus it seems that integrated care in general can result in increased efficiency and benefit the entire system.

In broader terms, it may be wise to take a more integrated approach to the Millennium Development Goals, recognizing that they may not be as isolated from each other as they might seem. Millennium Development Goal 6, combatting HIV/AIDS, malaria and other diseases, should be integrated with MDG 5, improving maternal health and reducing maternal mortality. Part of the goals of MDG 6 would directly influence efforts to reduce maternal mortality, including reducing HIV prevalence in people aged 15-24 years and increasing the proportion of the population with advanced HIV infection with access to antiretroviral drugs. The MDGs cannot be achieved in isolation from each other; in fact, MDGs 3 (eliminate gender disparities in education), 4 (reduce the under-five mortality rate by two-thirds), 5, and 6 are all connected in vital ways. Promoting gender equality and empowering women through better education and higher wages is directly related to women's ability to seek and obtain better antenatal care, to prevent and treat HIV infection that contributes to maternal mortality, and to reduce the incidence of obstetric complications that contribute to both maternal and child mortality. To be sure, goals of reducing incidence of HIV and reducing maternal mortality rates are inextricably linked.

References

Abdool-Karim Q., AbouZhar C., Dehne K., et al. (2010). HIV and maternal mortality: turning the tide. The Lancet, 375, 1948-1949.

Brettle RP., Raab GM., Ross A., Fielding KL., Gore SM. et al. (1995). HIV infection in women: immunological markers and the influence of pregnancy. Aids, 9, 177-1184.

Calvert C. & Ronsmans C. (2013). The contribution of HIV to pregnancy-related mortality: a systematic review and meta-analysis [published online ahead of print 25 February 2013]. AIDS. Available: http://journals.lww .com/aidsonline/pages/articleviewer.aspx?year=9000&issue=00000&article=98660&type=abstract. Accessed 20 March 2013.

El-Sadr WM., Lundgren JD., Neaton JD., Gordin F., Abrams D., Arduino RC. et al. (2006). Strategies for management of antiretroviral therapy (SMART) study group CD4+ count-guided interruption of antiretroviral treatment. N Eng J Med, 355, 2283-96.

Farquhar C., Kiarie JN., Richardson BA., et al. (2004). Antenatal couple counseling increases uptake of interventions to prevent HIV-1 transmission. J Acquir Immune Defic Syndr., 37(5), 1620-1626.

Geelhoed D., Lafort Y., Chissale É., Candrinho B. & Degomme O. 2013. Integrated maternal and child health services in Mozambique: structural health system limitations overshadow its effect on follow-up of HIV-exposed infants. BMC Health Serv Res., 13, 207.

Grange J., Adhikari M., Ahmed Y., Mwaba P., Dheda K., Hoelscher M. & Zurnla A. (2010). Tuberculosis in association with HIV/AIDS emerges as a major nonobstetric cause of maternal mortality in sub-Saharan Africa. Int J Gynaecol Obstet., 108(3), 181-183.

Hirnschall G., Harries A.D., Easterbrook P.J., Doherty M.C., & Ball A. (2013). The next generation of the World Health Organization's global antiretroviral guidance. Journal of the International AIDS Society, 16, 18757.

Hygino J., Vieira MM., Kasahara TM. et al. (2012). The impact of pregnancy on the HIV-1-specific T cell function in infected pregnant women. Clinial Immunology, 145, 177-188.

Kaiser Family Foundation (2013). The global HIV/AIDS epidemic. Available: http://kff.org/global-health-policy/factsheet/the-global-hivaids-epidemic/. Accessed 1 December 2013.

Kolte L., Gaardbo JC., Karlsson K. et al. (2011). Dysregulation of CD4+CD25+CD127^{low}FOXP3+regulatory T cells in HGIV-infected pregnant women. Blood, 117, 1861-1866.

Kruger A.M. & Bhagwanjee S. (2003). HIV/AIDS: Impact on maternal mortality at the Johannesburg Hospital, South Africa, 1995-2001. International Journal of Obstetric Anesthesia, 12, 164-168.

Landes M., van Lettow M., Bedell R., et al. (2012). Mortality and health outcomes in HIV-infected and HIV-uninfected mothers at 18-20 months postpartum in Zomba District, Malawi. PLoS One, 7(9), e44396.

Le Coeur S., Khlat M., Halembokaka G., Augereau-Vacher C., Batala-M'Pondo G., Baty G. & Ronsmans C. (2005). HIV and the magnitude of pregnancy-related mortality in Pointe Noire, Congo. AIDS, 19(1), 69-75.

Lindegren ML., Kennedy CE., Bain-Brickley D., et al. (2012). Integration of HIV/AIDS services with maternal, neonatal and child health, nutrition, and family planning services. Cochrane Database Syst Rev., 12(9), CD010119.

Madzimbamuto FD., Ray S. & Mogobe KD. 2013. Integration of HIV care into maternal health services: a crucial change required in improving quality of obstetric care in countries with high HIV prevalence. BMC Int Health Hum Rights, 13, 27.

Mataka E. 2007. Maternal health and HIV: bridging the gap. Lancet, 370(9595), 1290-1291.

Medema-Wijnveen JS., Onono M., Bukusi EA., Miller S., Cohen CR. & Turan JM. (2012). How perceptions of HIV-related stigma affect decision-making regarding childbirth in rural Kenya. PLoS One, 7(12), e51492.

Moodley J., Pattison RC., Baxter C., Sibeko S. & Abdool-Karim Q. (2011). Strengthening HIV services for pregnant women: an opportunity to reduce maternal mortality rates in Southern Africa/sub-Saharan Africa. BJOG, 118(2), 219-225.

Moran NF. & Moodley J. (2012). The effect of HIV infection on maternal health and mortality. Int J Gynaecol Obstet., 119 Suppl 1, S26-29.

Mor G. & Cardenas I. (2010). The immune system in pregnancy: a unique complexity. Am J Reprod Immunol, 63, 425-433.

Mutemwa R., Mayhew S., Colombini M., Busza J., Kivunaga J. & Ndwiga C. 2013. Experiences of health care providers with integrated HIV and reproductive health services in Kenya: a qualitative study. BMC Health Serv Res., 13, 18.

Myer L. (2013). Maternal deaths and HIV treatment in sub-Saharan Africa. The Lancet, 381, 1699-1700.

Okoko BJ., Enwere G. & Ota MO. (2003). The epidemiology and consequences of maternal malaria: a review of immunological basis. Acta Trop., 87, 193–205.

Onakewhor JU., Olagbuji BN., Ande AB., Ezeanochie MC., Olokor OE. & Okonofua FE. (2011). HIV-AIDS related maternal mortality in Benin City, Nigeria. Niger J Clin Pract., 14(2), 140-145.

Oyugi JH., Byakika-Tusiime J., Ragland K., Laeyendecker O., Mugerwa R., Kityo C. et al. (2007). Treatment interruptions predict resistance in HIV-positive individuals purchasing fixed-dose combination antiretroviral therapy in Kampala, Uganda. AIDS, 21, 965-971.

Ramogale MR., Moodley J. & Sebiloane MH. (2004). HIV-associated maternal mortality—primary causes of death at King Edward VII Hospital, Durban. S Afr Med J., 97(5), 363-366.

Richardson K. & Weinberg A. (2011). Dynamics of regulatory T-cells during pregnancy: effect of HIV infection and correlations with other immune parameters. PLoS One, 6, e28172.

Rosen J.E., de Zoysa I., Dehne K., Mangiaterra V. & Abdool-Karim Q. (2012). Understanding methods for estimating HIV-associated maternal mortality. Journal of Pregnancy.

Sprague C., Chersich MF. & Black V. 2011. Health system weaknesses constrain access to PMTCT and maternal HIV services in South Africa: a qualitative enquiry. AIDS Res Ther., 8, 10.

Suthar AB., Hoos D., Beqiri A., Lorenz-Dehne K., McClure C. & Duncombe C. 2013. Integrating antiretroviral therapy into antenatal care and maternal and child health settings: a systematic review and meta-analysis. Bull World Health Organ., 91(1), 46-56.

The PLoS Medicine Editors. (2010). HIV in maternal and child health: concurrent crises demand cooperation. PLoS Med., 7(7), e1000311.

Tomlinson M., Doherty T., Jackson D., Lawn J.E., Ijumba P., Colvin M. (2011). An effectiveness study of an integrated, community-based package for maternal, newborn, child and HIV care in South Africa: study protocol for a randomized controlled trial. Trials, 12, 236.

Topp S.M., Chipukuma J.M., Giganti M., Mwango L.K., Chiko L.M., Tambatamba-Chapula B., et al. (2010). Strengthening health systems at facility-level: feasibility of integrating antiretroviral therapy into primary health care services in Lusaka, Zambia. PLoS One, 5(7), e11522.

Turan JM., Hatcher AH., Medema-Wijnveen J., et al. (2012). The role of HIV-related stigma in utilization of childbirth services in rural Kenya: A prospective mixed-methods study. PLoS Med, 9(8), e1001295.

University of Cambridge, Centre for Research in the Arts, Social Sciences and Humanities. (2012). New Approaches to Maternal Mortality in Africa. Available: http://www.crassh.cam.ac.uk/events/1977/. Accessed 20 March 2013.

Van den Akker T., Bemelmans M., Ford N., Jemu M., Diggle E., Scheffer S., Zulu I., Akkeson A. & Shea J. 2012. HIV care need not hamper maternity care: a descriptive analysis of integration of services in rural Malawi. BJOG, 119(4), 431-438.

Wandabwa JN., Doyle P., Longo-Mbenza B., Kiondo P., Khainza B., Othieno E. & Maconichie N. (2011). Human immunodeficiency virus and AIDS and other important predictors of maternal mortality in Mulago Hospital Complex Kampala Uganda. BMC Public Health, 11, 565.

Warren C.E., Abuya T., & Askew I. (2013). Family planning practices and pregnancy intentions among HIV-positive and HIV-negative postpartum women in Swaziland: a cross sectional survey. BMC Pregnancy and Childbirth, 13, 150.

World Health Organization and UNICEF (2013). Accountability for maternal, newborn and child survival: the 2013 update. Available: http://www.countdown2015mnch.org/documents/2013Report/Countdown_2013-Update_withprofiles.pdf. Accessed 30 November 2013.

World Health Organization. (2013). Consolidated guidelines on the use of antiretroviral drugs for treating and preventing HIV infection. Available: http://www.who.int/hiv/pub/guidelines/arv2013/download/en/index.html. Accessed 12 August 2013.

World Health Organization. (2012). Millennium Development Goals. Available: http://www.who.int/mediacentre/factsheets/fs290/en/index.html. Accessed 20 March 2013.

World Health Organization. (2008). Technical consultation on the integration of HIV interventions into maternal, newborn and child health services. Available: http://apps.who.int/iris/bitstream/10665/69767/1/WHO_MPS_08.05_eng.pdf. Accessed 23 April 2013.

World Health Organization. (2010). Trends in Maternal Mortality: 1990-2008. Available: http://whqlibdoc.who.int/publications/2010/9789241500265_eng.pdf. Accessed 24 April 2013.

Change in Cellular Gene Expression by Hepatitis B virus (HBV)

Keiji Ueda

Division of Virology, Department of Microbiology and Immunology
Osaka University Graduate School of Medicine, Osaka, Japan

1   Introduction

Hepatitis B virus (HBV) is a causative agent for acute, chronic hepatitis leading to liver cirrhosis and finally to hepatocellular carcinoma, which are serious problems where HBV is prevalent such as east and south-east Asia, middle east countries, Africa, the equator of south America, Alaska, the coast area of Greenland (Seeger *et al.*, 2007).

HBV was identified as an Australian antigen firstly by Blumberg about a half century ago (Blumberg *et al.*, 1965). It is obvious that HBV infection is involved in the several diseases mentioned above (Liang, 2009). The pathophysiology, however, that HBV causes, and the viral life cycle itself, have not been yet to be clarified, largely due to limited propagation system of this virus (Ueda, 2013). Even though there are several animal models similar to HBV such as avihepadnaviruses (duck hepatitis B virus [DHBV] and heron hepatitis B virus [HHBV] etc.,) and the other orthohepadnaviruses like grand squirrel hepatitis virus (GSHV) and woodchuck hepatitis virus (WHV), they are still inconvenient for daily research activity (Seeger *et al.*, 2007). Of course, orthohepadnaviruses have been identified in primates; wooly monkey hepatitis B virus (WMHBV), gibbon ape hepatitis B virus (GAHBV), orangutan hepatitis B virus (OHBV) and chimpanzee hepatitis B virus (CHBV) (Seeger *et al.*, 2007), but their usage in the species are beset with ethical issues.

Molecular studies of HBV clarified many functions of HBV related gene products. Such data, however, should be verified in the natural life cycle *in vitro* and/or *in vivo* and further more, there are a lot of mysteries about HBV including the covalently closed circular DNA (cccDNA) formation and its regulation, the entry and the egress (Glebe & Urban, 2007). HBV infects efficiently primary human hepatocytes (PHH) in vitro (Gripon *et al.*, 1988; Ochiya *et al.*, 1989) and tupaia primary human hepatocytes (Walter *et al.*, 1996). PHH is now commercially available from human liver-uPA-SCID mouse (Meuleman & Leroux-Roels, 2008), but too expensive for ordinary research. A hepatocellular carcinoma-originated cell line called HepaRG was reported to become permissive for HBV several weeks after differentiation induction with 2% dimethyl sulfoxide (DMSO) (Gripon *et al.*, 2002). Nonetheless, its infectivity is limited as much as twenty to thirty percent and the HepaRG is also commercially sold and restricted for its use and propagation. Therefore, more useful and convenient HBV infection system must be established.

Thus, it is very difficult to understand accurate HBV life cycle and we only test HBV amplification mechanism by transfecting cloned HBV genome into hepatocellular-originated cell lines such as HepG2, HuH6, HuH7 and so on. The limited transfection efficiency to these cell lines seems not to be appropriate how HBV affects the cellular gene expression profile. And there have been only two reports about cellular gene expression profiles under HBV producing and infecting models (Fletcher *et al.*, 2012; Hajjou *et al.*, 2005).

In this report, we analyzed cellular gene expression profiles comparing HBV producing cells to its parental HBV non-producing cells and recognized that considerable numbers of gene expression level was altered by HBV amplification. We also picked up several characteristic gene expression level involved in cell cycle and interferon system.

2   Materials and Methods

Cell. HuH6 and HB611 cells were grown in DMEM (low glucose; 1.0g/L) (Nakalai tesque®) supplemented with 10% fetal bovine serum, 10IU/ml penicillin G and 10μg/ml streptomycin (Nakalai tesque®).

In case of HB611 culture, G418 (Nakalai tesque®) was added in the media at 0.5mg/ml. HepaRG cells were purchased from Biopredic International and cultured in Williams E meidium supplemented with 10% fetal bovine serum, 10IU/ml penicillin G, 10μg/ml streptomycin (Nakalai tesque®), 50μM hydrocortisone and 5μg/ml insulin. For differentiation induction, 2% dimetylyl sulfoxide (DMSO) was added into the medium for HepaRG. HepG2 and HuH7 cultured as HuH6.

RNA purification. HuH6 and HB611 cells were grown on the 10 cm cell culture dish (Iwaki®) at almost confluent condition whose cell number was about 2~3 x 10^6/dish. The cells were washed with phosphate buffered saline (PBS) twice and then lysed directly in 3ml Trizol® (Invtrogen-Life Technologies). Each lysed solution was transferred into a 15ml centrifugation tube (BD™), respectively and total RNA was purified according to the manufacturer's protocol. The RNA was finally solved in TE solution (10mM Tris-HCl pH7.6, 1mM EDTA) and the concentration was measured with a UV Spectrophotometer (DU800™, Beckman). RNA from normal human liver was purchased from Takara Bio®. RNA from HepaRG, differentiated HepaRG, HepG2 and HuH7 was extracted as described above. Quality of the extracted RNA was checked with Agilent 2200 TapeStation®.

DNA microarray analysis. Each total RNA (250ng) was labeled with GeneChip® 3'IVT Express Kit aRNA amplification procedure according to the manufacturer's protocol (GeneChip® 3'IVT Kit User Manual, P/N 702646 Rev.1; Chapter 2 aRNA Amplification Protocol and Chapter 3 Evaluation and Fragmentation of aRNA). The probe was hybridized on a DNA microarray, Human Genome U133 Plus2.0® (Affymetrix™) with a hybridization oven (Hybridization Oven 640 110V®; Affymetrix 800138) and washed with Fluidics Station 450® (Affymetrix 00-0079). The microarray was scanned with GeneChip Scanner 3000® (Affymetrix 00-0074) and analyzed with GeneChip Operating Software ver1.4® (Affymetrix 690036).   The analysis protocol was GeneChip Expression Analysis Data Fundamentals® (Chapter 4 First-Order Data Analysis and Data Quality Assessment and Chapter 5 Statistical Algorithms Reference) with GeneChip Operating Software ver1.4®.

RT-PCR. 5μg RNA from each cell line was reverse-transcribed with random primers and Superscript III® reverse transcriptase (Invitrogen-Life Technologies) according to manufacturer's direction to generate their cDNA. Typical genes described in this report; fatty acid binding protein 7 (FABP7, gi: 4557584), alfa-fetoprotein (AFP, gi: 4501988), platelet-derived growth factor receptor alfa (PDGFRα, gi: 5453869) as well as glyceraldehyde-3-phosphate dehydrogenase (GAPDH, gi:19684109) as a control were tested. Primers were 5'-aagaattcatggtggaggctttctgtgcta-3' and 5'-aaggatccttatgccttctcatagtggcg-3' for FABP7, 5'-tcctactaaattttactgaatc-3' and 5'-gctgcagcagtctgaatgtccg-3' for AFP, 5'-tatggggacttcccatccg gcg-3' and 5'-tgtctgagtgtggttgtaatag-3' for PDGFRα. These primers generate about 400bp (FABP7), 320bp (AFP), 320bp (PDGFRα) and 210bp (GAPDH), respectively.   PCR was performed 96˚C for 30 sec, 54˚C for 30 sec and 72˚C 60 sec, 25 cycles with ExTag DNA polymerase (Takara Bio) and ProFlex® PCR System (Life Technologies®).

3   Results

HB611. This cell was established by transfecting three tandemly arranged HBV genomes (adr4) in a plasmid containing the G418 resistance gene into HuH6 cells (Figure 1) (Tsurimoto *et al.*, 1987; Ueda *et al.*, 1989). HB611 cells maintains one copy of three tandemly arranged HBV genomes and is supposed to reflect all pathways of the HBV life cycle except the attachment and the entry process and the covalently

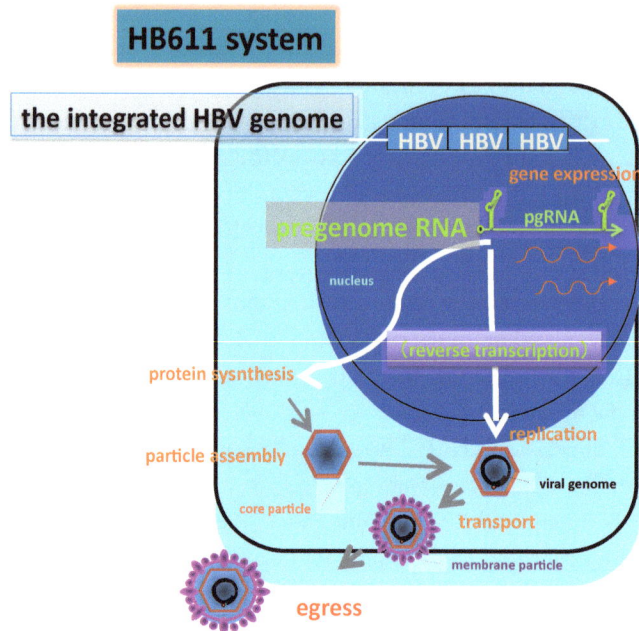

Figure 1: HB611 system. In HB611 cells three tandemly arranged HBV genomes are integrated in the host chromosome. Viral genes including pregenome RNA (pgRNA) are transcribed from the genome. The viral genome is synthesized through reverse transcription pathway while packaging into core particle.

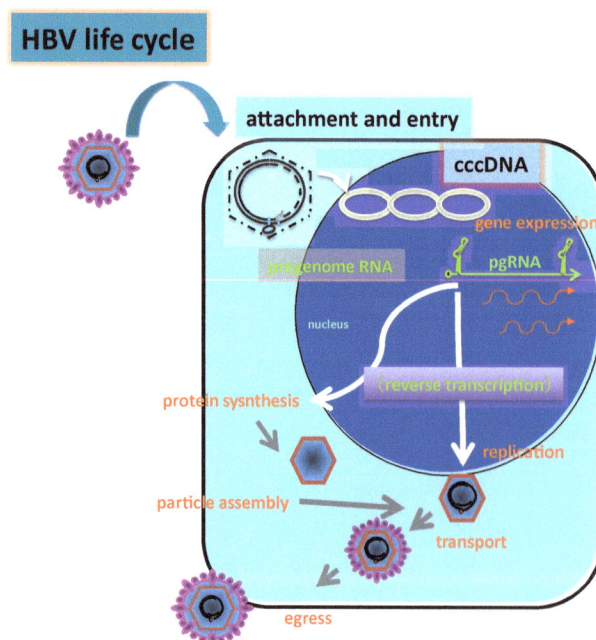

Figure 2: Natural HBV life cycle. In the natural infection course of HBV, the viral genome is not integrated into the host genome. The partially double stranded DNA genome is converted to covalently closed circular DNA, which is maintained in the infected cell nucleus and produces viral related transcripts including pgRNA. The pathway after this is the same as shown in Figure 1.

closed circular DNA (cccDNA) formation (Figure 1 and Figure 2). The integrated HBV genome functions as cccDNA and produces HBV-related transcripts. The difference between HB611 and HuH6 cells is that the HBV genome is integrated into a host chromosome with transcription competence and there is no other system affecting cell physiology such as an immune system and therefore it could be possible to compare gene expression profiles purely by HBV production.

Global differences of gene expression profiles between HB611 and HuH6. This time, we analyzed gene expression profiles of HB611 cells, an HBV amplifying cells and its parental counterpart, HuH6 cells to understand how HBV gene expression and replication affect the host cell gene expression newly and independently of previous analysis (Nakanishi *et al*, 2005) and utilized the newest version of the Affymetrix Human Genome U133 Plus2.0™. This microarray loaded more than 50,000 probes. The scatter plot shows that 95% genes are expressed at the same level within eight folds difference (Figure 3A, and 3B). Ten to twenty genes are drastically changed for their expression (arrows in the Figure 3, Table 1 and Table 2). Typical ones were picked up and drawn on the graph. Interestingly, some genes such as steroid sulfatace (microsomal) isozyme S, microsomal triglyceride transfer protein and fatty acid binding protein involved in fatty acids metabolism were highly expressed in HB611. And cell-growth related genes such as *CD24* (gi; 180167), platelet-derived growth factor receptor α (*PDGFRα*) and *myc* (*N-myc* related) were also highly expressed in HB611 (Table 2, Figure 7). Some of them were tested with semi-quantitative RT-PCR and verified the DNA array data (Figure 8). This analysis included human normal liver, and the hepatocellular carcinoma originated cell lines such as HepaRG and its differentiated one with 2% DMSO for two weeks, HepG2 and HuH7.

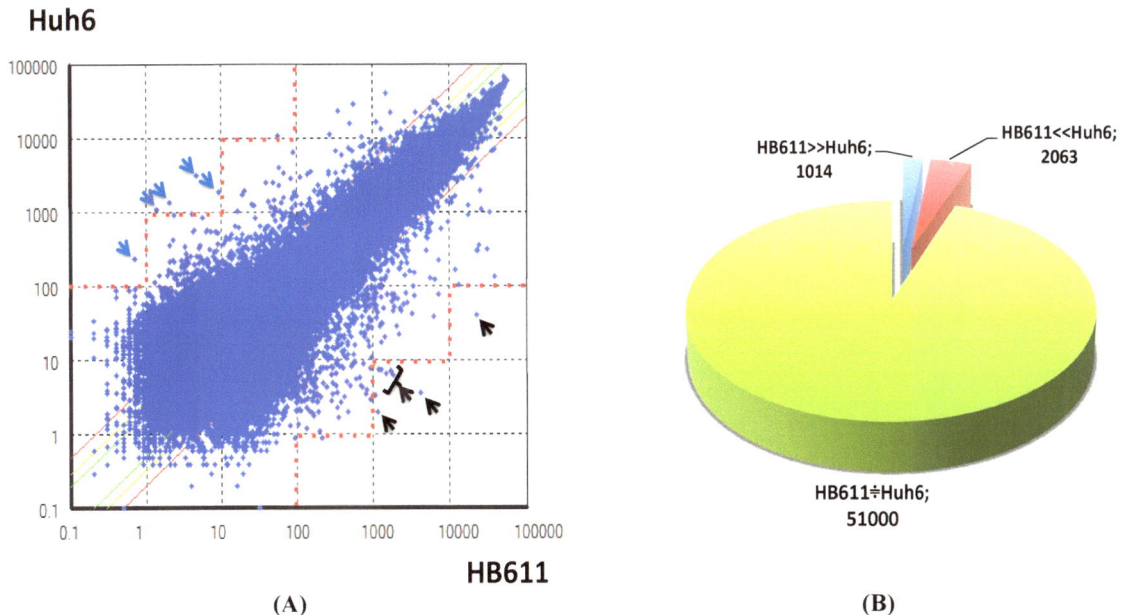

(A)   **(B)**

Figure 3: Gene expression profile of HB611 and its parental HuH6 cells. (A) Scatter plot analysis of expressed genes in HB611 and HuH6 cells. Orange dotted lines shows the boundary of extreme difference in expression level more than one hundred. Arrows represent picket-up genes that show extreme difference in expression. (B) Pie chart of the gene expression profile. The light blue zone represents highly expressed genes in HB611 more than eight times and light red section represents highly expressed genes in HuH6 more than eight times.

gene	gi No.	HuH6	HB611
hox transcript antisense RNA	10939596	235.7	0.7
EST*	5863388	1128.8	1.4
plastin 3	7549808	1398.5	2.1
transmembrane channel like 5	13417048	3166.5	4.8
kelch-like	9511250	1970.7	9.2
Wntless homolog	2835015	10967.0	55.9

* is a transcript identified as an expression sequence tag (EST).
Gene name and its gi number are shown on the left two columns.
The values represent signal intensity detected in this analysis.

Table 1: Genes extremely highly expressed in HuH6.

gene	gi No.	HuH6	HB611
CD24	180167	77.5	7083.8
gremlin-1	10863087	2.0	1136.2
steroid sulfatase (microsomal) isozyme S	3538520	3.7	4229.7
steroid sulfatase (microsomal) isozyme S*	13162281	7.7	1179.1
microsomal triglyceride transfer protein	4648246	6.3	1855.5
fatty acid binding protein	4557584	41.4	22460.8
lysyl oxidase	4505008	7.3	1696.3
PDGFR-α	5453869	7.7	1297.9
myc (N-myc related)	12803748	6.8	1495.5

* is another gene of steroid sulfatase (microsomal) isozyme S.
Gene name and its gi number are shown on the left two columns.
The values represent signal intensity detected in this analysis.

Table 2: Genes extremely highly expressed in HB611.

Not a few genes seem to be changed by HBV production for their expression. 1014 genes (~2.0%) were highly expressed in the HB611 cells more than eight times and 2063 genes (~4%) were highly expressed in the HuH6 cells more than eight times. These data suggest that HBV production should affect cellular gene expression program.

Cell cycle control genes. It is interesting how HBV production affects cell cycle since HBV is a major cause of liver cancer in the world. We mined the data related to cell cycle control; cyclins, cyclin dependent kinases (*CDKs*) and cyclin dependent kinase inhibitors (*CKIs*). In these cells, cyclin

D1(*CYCD1*, gi; 12652656), cyclin A2 (*CYCA2*. gi; 4502612), cyclin B1 (*CYCB1*, gi; 1443518) and cyclin B2 (*CYCB2*, gi; 1093801) were modestly expressed, but the expression level did not show much difference (Figure 4). Among *CDKs*, these cells expressed *CDK4* that functions in G0-G1 phase. *CDK1*, *CDK2* and anther G0-G1 cyclin, *CDK6* were modestly expressed and their expression level was not different between HB611 cells and HuH6 cells (Figure 5). As for *CKIs*, $p21^{Cip1}$ and $p27^{Kip1}$ were mainly expressed in these cells and suggest that they should probably work as major cell cycle controllers (Figure 5). We would better take into consideration that 80 ~90 % cells were in the G1 in the ordinary culture condition, since almost all cells attach dishes neither condensed chromatin nor dividing status (data not shown).   In this term, it is interesting that S phase and M phase cyclins were relatively highly expressed and *CDK4* was fairly highly expressed in these cells. This might represent that these cells were transformed cell lines.

Liver specific genes. The analysis was based on the hepatocellular carcinoma (HCC) originated cells with or without HBV production and therefore liver specific gene expression could be maintained modestly but fairly reduced. As expected, some liver specific transcription factors such as hepatocyte nuclear factor 1A (*HNF1A*, gi; 184264), 1B (*HNF1B*, gi; 4507396), 4A (*HNF4A*, gi; 3250320) and 4G (*HNF4G*, gi; 5636455) were at low expression (Figure 6). Albumin (*ALB*, gi; 7959790) is one of the typical liver specific genes (Knowles *et al.*, 1980) and its expression was a kind of repressed in these cell lines, which suggests that these HCC originated cell lines or otherwise, HCC itself were dedifferentiated in the course of transformation (Figure 6). Interestingly, alphafetoprotein (*AFP*, gi; 4501988) was extremely highly expressed in HB611 cells. This might suggest that HBV production should drastically changed the expression program of this gene. As shown in Table 2, a couple of genes were much highly expressed in the HB611 cells. It seems to be interesting how the gene expression was controlled, in a similar way or in a different way?

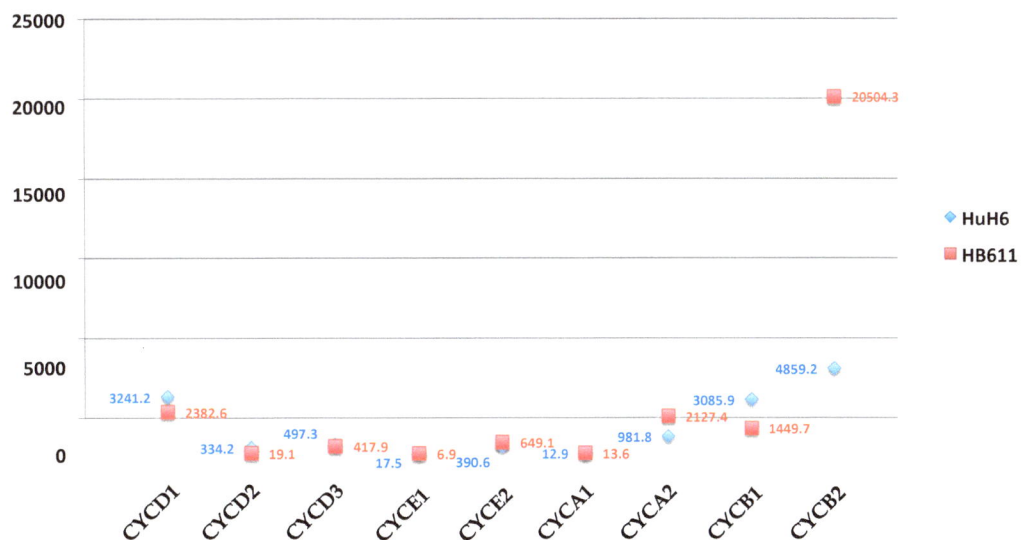

Figure 4: Expression level of cell cycle control genes. The value represents signal strength in the DNA microarray analysis. Orange figures shown on the right of the market represent the value for HB611 cells and the blue ones on the left for HuH6.

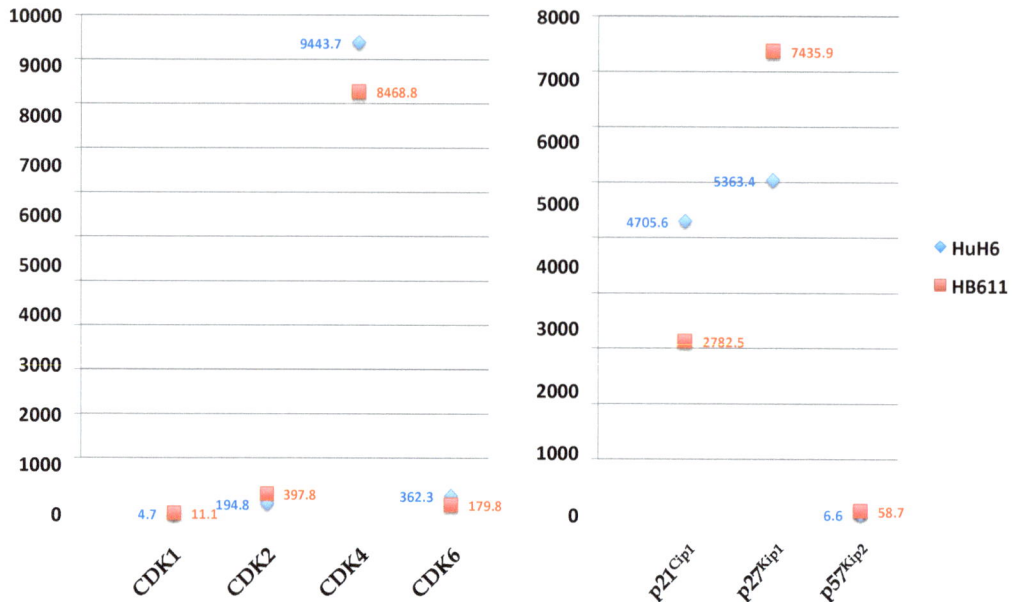

Figure 5: Expression level of cyclin dependent kinases (CDKs) (left) and cyclin dependent kinase inhibitors (CKIs) (right). Orange figures shown on the right of the market represent the value for HB611 cells and the blue ones on the left for HuH6.

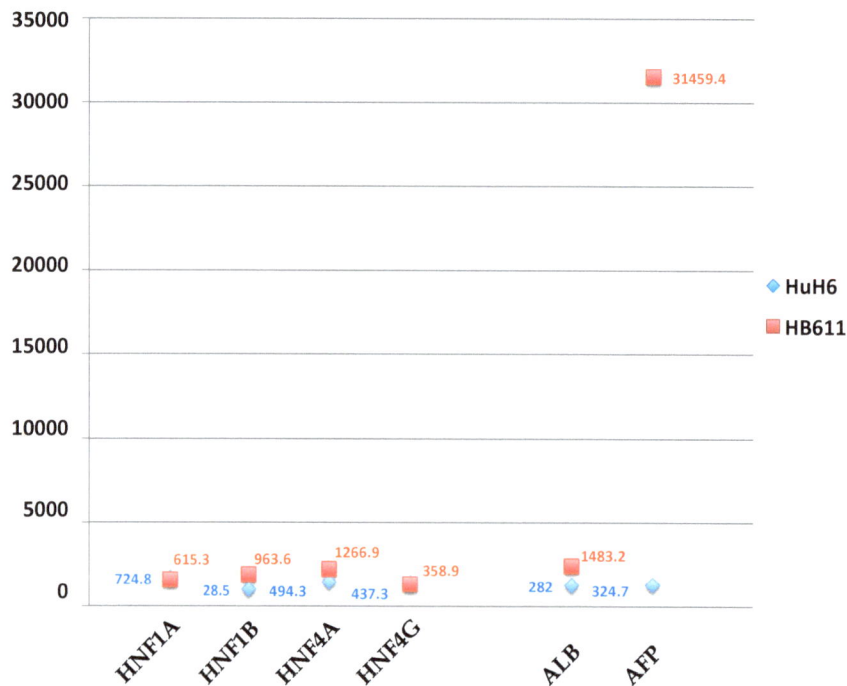

Figure 6: Expression level of liver specific genes. Orange figures shown on the right of the market represent the value for HB611 cells and the blue ones on the left for HuH6.

Other interesting genes. While we were mining data, we found interesting expression profiles of some genes. Sodium taurocholate co-transporting polypeptide (*NTCP* or *NTCP1*, gi; 4506970) was reported to be an HBV receptor last year (Yan *et al.*, 2012). The report pointed out that HCC originated cultured cell line such as HepG2 and HuH7 did not express this gene and correction of this gene expression by transfection endowed these cell lines with HBV infectivity and viral amplification. We checked the gene expression in this study. Beyond my expectations, HB611 cells expressed moderately NTCP (Fig. 7), which suggests that HBV produced from the HB611 cells could reinfect the cells. But so far, cccDNA was not observed in the HB611 (Tsurimoto *et al.*, 1987; Ueda *et al.*, 1989), which suggests that there was some obstruction to HBV infection in this system. HBV membrane protein, large S (LS), middle S (MS) and small S (SS or simply HBs) produced from the cells might interfere the HBV reinfection. On the other hand, another similar gene, *NTCP2* (gi; 456972) was at no expression level.

We checked about hundreds interferon related genes including INFs, IFN receptors and IFN regulatory factors (IRFs) but there was almost no difference between HB611 cells and HuH6 cell, expressed or not expressed (data not shown). Likewise, Janus kinase (JAK)/ signal transduction and transcription factors) STATs related genes were not changed (data not shown), although it was reported that HBV polymerase (HBVpol) inhibited the activities of the STAT proteins (Wu *et al.*, 2007).

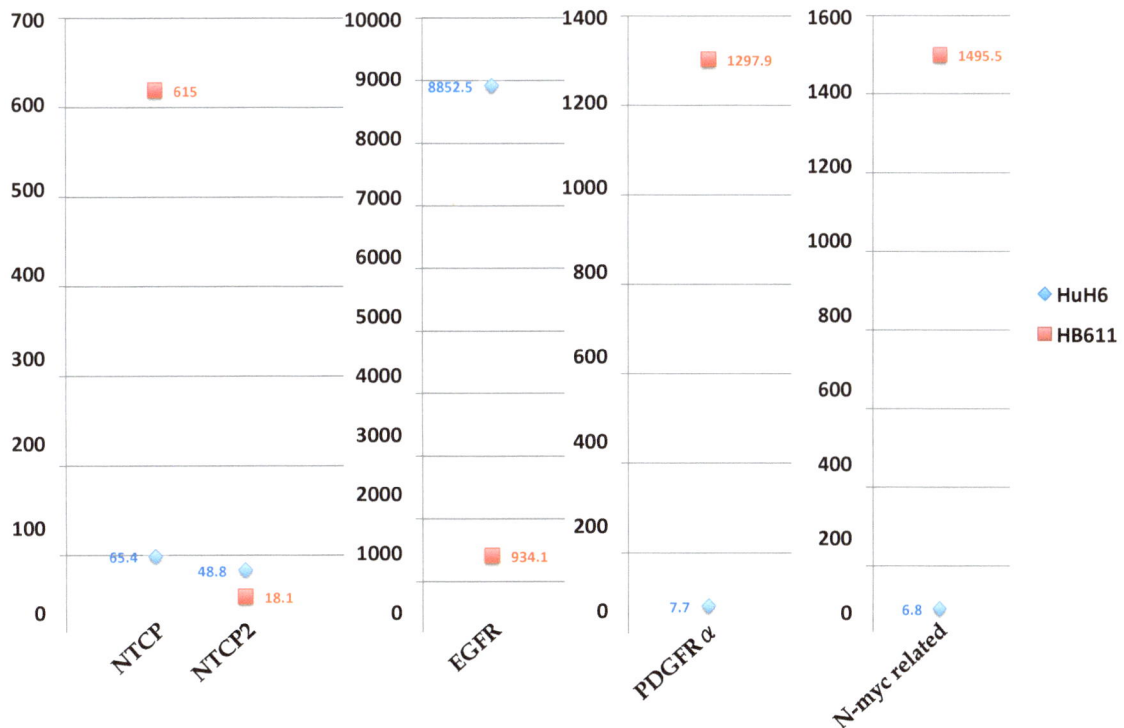

Figure 7: Expression level of NTCP's and typical growth related genes. Orange figures shown on the right of the market represent the value for HB611 cells and the blue ones on the left for HuH6.

4   Discussion

In this report, we analyzed how HBV production affected cellular gene expression profiles using an artificially HBV producing system based on an HCC-originated cultured cell line. HBV never infects cultured cell lines and experimental animals. Needless to say, this kind of analysis should be done in natural infection system. HBV, however, has strict species specificity and there is no very convenient and useful infection system for HBV. HepaRG, a HCC derived cell line, and PHH separated from SCID-hu hepatocytes are commercially available. Even though PHH shows high competency for HBV infection, both cell lines are very expensive and inconvenient for daily HBV study. Therefore, more convenient and useful systems for HBV infection must be explored and currently we can utilize an HBV production system designed artificially in HCC derived cultured cell lines (Sells *et al.*, 1987; Tsurimoto *et al.*, 1987). Nevertheless, it was clear that such analysis was very informative and HBV production affected remarkably the cellular gene expression profiles and expression level of some genes appeared to be drastically changed by HBV production.

Considerable numbers of gene seemed to be affected for their gene expression. Since it was reported that hepatitis C virus infection affected lipid metabolism (Moradpour *et al.*, 1996), it is very interesting that the expression level of some genes such as fatty acid binding protein (gi; 4557584) involved in lipid metabolism was remarkably changed in the presence of HBV related products in the cells. Change in lipid metabolism might lead to cellular phenotypic change.

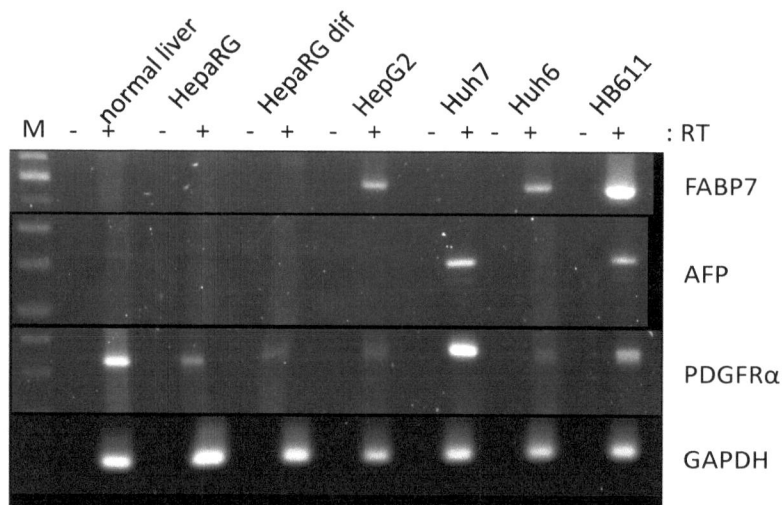

Figure 8: RT-PCR of RNA extracted from several hepatocellular carcinoma cells. Typical genes which showed much difference in the expression level were tested with RT-PCR, including GAPDH as a control for RNA preparation and expression.

Some genes related to cell growth such as PDGFRα and myc (N-myc related in this case, gi; 33877057) were extremely overexpressed in the HB611 cells. N-myc overexpression was observed in woodchuck hepatitis virus (WHV) involved hepatocarcinogenesis (Hansen *et al.*, 1993; Ueda *et al.*, 1996). WHV genome was found near or in the N-myc locus, which resulted in overexpression of N-myc gene

(Ueda *et al*., 1996). In our case or human HCC, there has been no evidence that the HBV genome integrated in or near the N-myc locus. Therefore, N-myc overexpression in our system is not the case and maybe there could be different mechanism.   HBV infection might increase the gene expression and facilitate hepatocyte growth.

Cell cycle engine is accelerated by cyclins (*CYCs*) and cyclin dependent kinase (*CDKs*) which are checked and controlled by CKI. Although *CYCs* and *CDKs* should be activated in immortalized and transformed cells, *CYCD1* (gi; 12652656) as a G1 phase cyclin, *CYCA2* (gi; 4502612) as a S phase cyclin and *CYCB2* (gi; 1093801) and less *CYCB1* (gi; 1443518) as an M phase cyclin were relatively activated in both HB611 and HuH6 cells. *CDK4* rather than *CDK6* was favored in these cell lines. $p57^{Kip2}$ (gi; 854949) is thought to be a CKI unique for stem cells and $p21^{Cip1}$ (gi; 11386202) and $p27^{Kip1}$ (gi; 12805034) were main CKIs in this case as expected.

Liver specific gene expression could be important to show how much such cell lines maintained well-differentiated hepatocyte characters. Although normal liver gene expression profiles were not investigated, liver specific transcription factors such as *HNF1A, 1B, 4A* and *4G* were expressed at low level but not absent. *ALB* (gi; 7959790) is one of the characteristic liver specific genes and was at low expression level. In contrast, *AFP* (gi; 4501988) was upregulated in HB611 cells, the mechanism of which could not be assessed in this report but HBV production might cause blastic change in hepatic cells.   *NTCP* (gi; 4506970) is a notable factor as an HBV receptor (Yan *et al*., 2012). Considering that cultured HCC derived cell lines never permit HBV infection, NTCP expression had not been expected. HB611 cells, however, showed moderate expression of *NTCP*. This fact lets us expect that HB611 cells should competent for HBV infection and reinfection circuit could go around. So far, we have not observed cccDNA formation in the HB611 cells and this is not the case perhaps because S related membrane proteins secreted from HB611 cells should block the receptor and the ligand interaction.

We found a big difference of three genes influencing cell growth. EGF as well as hepatocyte growth factor (HGF) is a hepatocyte growth factor (McGowan *et al*., 1981; Michalopoulos, 1990) and therefore its receptor, *EGFR* (gi; 6228471) expression should be important for tumor growth dependent on EGF. HBV production, however, could change drastically growth factor usage to platelet derived growth factor (PDGF) by increasing PDGFRα (gi; 5453869).

It is fascinating how gene expression profiles are altered by HBV production, though functional analyses of grossly changed genes for their expression should be further investigation. Some gene expression profiles including the other HCC derived cell lines were verified by RT-PCR and their gene expression profiles were different each other. Still, core protein, polymerase and X protein could be good candidates that change the gene expression and these phenomenon have to be assessed in a natural HBV infection system using PHH. Furthermore, we should pay attention to non-coding short RNA (ncsRNA) expression status in presence or absence of HBV. ncsRNA including miRNA basically have a negative effect on the target gene (Gebauer & Hentze, 2004). Such RNA molecules should have remarkable effects on cellular and viral gene expression program and might be expressed from HBV genome as well as host genome (Figure 9), though ten or more miRNAs have been reported to regulate HBV gene expression (Liu *et al*., 2011; Zhang *et al*., 2012).

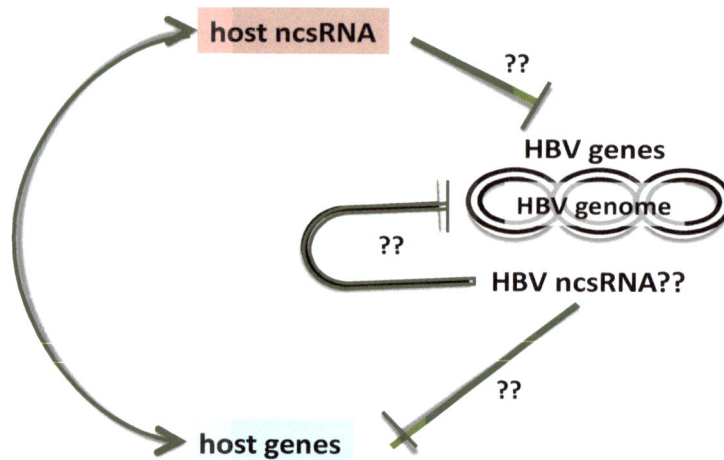

Figure 9: Non-coding viral RNA could be expressed from the HBV genome and affects cellular gene expression program as well as the viral one.

References

Blumberg, B. S., Alter, H. J., and Visnich, S. (1965) A "New" Antigen in Leukemia Sera, JAMA 191, 541-546.

Fletcher, S. P., Chin, D. J., Ji, Y., Iniguez, A. L., Taillon, B., Swinney, D. C., Ravindran, P., Cheng, D. T., Bitter, H., Lopatin, U., Ma, H., Klumpp, K., and Menne, S. (2012) Transcriptomic analysis of the woodchuck model of chronic hepatitis B, Hepatology.

Gebauer, F., and Hentze, M. W. (2004) Molecular mechanisms of translational control, Nature reviews. Molecular cell biology 5, 827-835.

Glebe, D., and Urban, S. (2007) Viral and cellular determinants involved in hepadnaviral entry, World J Gastroenterol 13, 22-38.

Gripon, P., Diot, C., Theze, N., Fourel, I., Loreal, O., Brechot, C., and Guguen-Guillouzo, C. (1988) Hepatitis B virus infection of adult human hepatocytes cultured in the presence of dimethyl sulfoxide, J Virol 62, 4136-4143.

Gripon, P., Rumin, S., Urban, S., Le Seyec, J., Glaise, D., Cannie, I., Guyomard, C., Lucas, J., Trepo, C., and Guguen-Guillouzo, C. (2002) Infection of a human hepatoma cell line by hepatitis B virus, Proc Natl Acad Sci U S A 99, 15655-15660.

Hajjou, M., Norel, R., Carver, R., Marion, P., Cullen, J., Rogler, L. E., and Rogler, C. E. (2005) cDNA microarray analysis of HBV transgenic mouse liver identifies genes in lipid biosynthetic and growth control pathways affected by HBV, J Med Virol 77, 57-65.

Hansen, L. J., Tennant, B. C., Seeger, C., and Ganem, D. (1993) Differential activation of myc gene family members in hepatic carcinogenesis by closely related hepatitis B viruses, Mol Cell Biol 13, 659-667.

Knowles, B. B., Howe, C. C., and Aden, D. P. (1980) Human hepatocellular carcinoma cell lines secrete the major plasma proteins and hepatitis B surface antigen, Science 209, 497-499.

Liang, T. J. (2009) Hepatitis B: the virus and disease, Hepatology 49, S13-21.

Liu, W. H., Yeh, S. H., and Chen, P. J. (2011) Role of microRNAs in hepatitis B virus replication and pathogenesis, Biochim Biophys Acta.

McGowan, J. A., Strain, A. J., and Bucher, N. L. (1981) DNA synthesis in primary cultures of adult rat hepatocytes in a defined medium: effects of epidermal growth factor, insulin, glucagon, and cyclic-AMP, Journal of cellular physiology 108, 353-363.

Meuleman, P., and Leroux-Roels, G. (2008) *The human liver-uPA-SCID mouse: a model for the evaluation of antiviral compounds against HBV and HCV, Antiviral Res 80, 231-238.*

Michalopoulos, G. K. (1990) *Liver regeneration: molecular mechanisms of growth control, FASEB journal : official publication of the Federation of American Societies for Experimental Biology 4, 176-187.*

Moradpour, D., Englert, C., Wakita, T., and Wands, J. R. (1996) *Characterization of cell lines allowing tightly regulated expression of hepatitis C virus core protein, Virology 222, 51-63.*

Nakanishi, F., Ohkawa, K., Ishida, H., Hosui, A., Sato, A., Hiramatsu, N., Ueda, K., Takehara, T., Kasahara, A., Sasaki, Y., Hori, M., and Hayashi, N. (2005) *Alteration in gene expression profile by full-length hepatitis B virus genome, Intervirology 48, 77-83.*

Ochiya, T., Tsurimoto, T., Ueda, K., Okubo, K., Shiozawa, M., and Matsubara, K. (1989) *An in vitro system for infection with hepatitis B virus that uses primary human fetal hepatocytes, Proc Natl Acad Sci U S A 86, 1875-1879.*

Seeger, C., Zoulim, F., and MASON, W. S. (2007) *Hepadnaviruses, Vol. II, 5 ed., Lippincott Williams and Wilkins, Philadelphia.*

Sells, M. A., Chen, M. L., and Acs, G. (1987) *Production of hepatitis B virus particles in Hep G2 cells transfected with cloned hepatitis B virus DNA, Proc Natl Acad Sci U S A 84, 1005-1009.*

Tsurimoto, T., Fujiyama, A., and Matsubara, K. (1987) *Stable expression and replication of hepatitis B virus genome in an integrated state in a human hepatoma cell line transfected with the cloned viral DNA, Proc Natl Acad Sci U S A 84, 444-448.*

Ueda, K. (2013) *Start or End? One of the biggest Mysteries is Finally Solved, J Infect Dis Ther 1, 1.*

Ueda, K., Tsurimoto, T., Nagahata, T., Chisaka, O., and Matsubara, K. (1989) *An in vitro system for screening anti-hepatitis B virus drugs, Virology 169, 213-216.*

Ueda, K., Wei, Y., and Ganem, D. (1996) *Activation of N-myc2 gene expression by cis-acting elements of oncogenic hepadnaviral genomes: key role of enhancer II, Virology 217, 413-417.*

Walter, E., Keist, R., Niederost, B., Pult, I., and Blum, H. E. (1996) *Hepatitis B virus infection of tupaia hepatocytes in vitro and in vivo, Hepatology 24, 1-5.*

Wu, M., Xu, Y., Lin, S., Zhang, X., Xiang, L., and Yuan, Z. (2007) *Hepatitis B virus polymerase inhibits the interferon-inducible MyD88 promoter by blocking nuclear translocation of Stat1, J Gen Virol 88, 3260-3269.*

Yan, H., Zhong, G., Xu, G., He, W., Jing, Z., Gao, Z., Huang, Y., Qi, Y., Peng, B., Wang, H., Fu, L., Song, M., Chen, P., Gao, W., Ren, B., Sun, Y., Cai, T., Feng, X., Sui, J., and Li, W. (2012) *Sodium taurocholate cotransporting polypeptide is a functional receptor for human hepatitis B and D virus, eLife 1, e00049.*

Zhang, Q., Pu, R., Du, Y., Han, Y., Su, T., Wang, H., and Cao, G. (2012) *Non-coding RNAs in hepatitis B or C-associated hepatocellular carcinoma: potential diagnostic and prognostic markers and therapeutic targets, Cancer letters 321, 1-12.*

Theoretical Approach to the Deposition of Variably Shaped Particles in the Lungs of Children and Adults

Robert Sturm

Department of Physics and Biophysics, Faculty of Natural Sciences
University of Salzburg, Austria

1   Introduction

According to a largely accepted paradigm, the shape of aerosol particles acts as a determinant affecting well-known phenomena such as dry deposition, cloud scavenging, and deposition in the human respiratory tract. Most aerosol particles occurring in the ambient air deviate remarkably from spherical shape. This class of nonspherical particles among other consists of fibers, disk- or platelet-shaped particulate structures, and various kinds of agglomerates. In general, fibers are elongated particles with an aspect ratio (*i.e.*, the ratio of the length to the diameter) greater than 3 (IARC, 2002; Su & Cheng, 2006; Figure 1). In the past, fibrous substances were categorized as notorious occupational hazards, whereby especially the exposure to airborne asbestos fibers was proven to increase the incidence of lung cancer (Lippmann, 1990; Heesterberg & Hart, 2001; Kamstrup *et al.*, 2002; IARC, 2002). These finds resulted in an enhanced scientific interest in all kinds of fibrous particles and, as a consequence of that, in a better understanding of fibrous particle behavior in the human respiratory tract (Myojo, 1987; Cai & Yu, 1988; Chen & Yu, 1991; Dai & Yu, 1998; Arsenijevic *et al.*, 1999; DeCarlo *et al.*, 2004; Slowik *et al.*, 2004). From the 1990s on, asbestos fibers had to be substituted by particulate materials with similar properties, among which man-made vitreous fibers (MMVF) turned out to be most appropriate (Heesterberg & Hart, 2001). However, it could be detected by experiments with laboratory animals that MMVFs have similar effects on the lungs as asbestos (IARC, 2002). Disks or platelets are the preferential particle shapes of dust aerosols that are produced by mechanical processes such as friction, grinding, burnishing, etc. Aspect ratios of these particulate structures are commonly smaller than 1 (Figure 1). Any studies concerning the behavior of dust particles in the human respiratory tract are still hard to find, although this knowledge would undisputedly mean an enormous progress in aerosol sciences and pneumology. Agglomerated particulate substances or aggregates are usually formed by combustion processes. High significance with regards to atmospherical and hygienic effects has to be attributed to soot which is currently produced in large amounts by all kinds of diesel engines (Yu & Xu, 1987; Bayram *et al.*, 2006). Shape of these particles is currently approximated by (a) the use of spherical components (Kasper, 1982a, 1982b; Sturm, 2010) or (b) the application of fractional geometry, with the help of which individual agglomerate populations may be characterized (Virtanen *et al.*, 2002).

During the past 40 years, the number of scientific articles and books dealing with aerosol particle uptake by adults has been exponentially increased (Gilbert *et al.*, 1972; Stahlhofen *et al.*, 1981; Heyder *et al.*, 1982; Bennett, 1988; Heyder *et al.*, 1988; Stahlhofen *et al.*, 1989; Schiller-Scotland *et al.*, 1994; ICRP, 1994). On the other hand, detailed studies on the inhalation of different aerosol particles by children and the consequences of this respiratory uptake for the child's lungs have been conducted for about two decades (Pope & Dockery, 1992; Chua *et al.*, 1994; Bennett & Zeman, 1998; Conceicao *et al.*, 2001; Bennett & Zeman, 2004; Schüepp *et al.*, 2004). In the meantime, it is a verified fundamental in pediatric science that children especially living in urban environments may be exposed to higher aerosol doses (*e.g.*, CO, CO_2, diverse dusts produced and raised by traffic, soot; Conceicao *et al.*, 2001). Contrary, in rural environments children may be increasingly confronted with biogenic aerosols, among which some types could be identified as triggers of infectious or allergic diseases (Burge, 1990; Vedal *et al.*, 1998; Schüepp *et al.*, 2004). Regarding the carcinogenicity of airborne particulate substances, especially four categories of aerosols have to be considered in conjunction with children and adults (Figure 2): Besides all kinds of dusts, which are characterized by a peculiarity regarding their deposition and clearance in the human respiratory tract (Lippmann, 1990; Pope & Dockery, 1992), some types of bioaerosols as well as smokes /soot and ultrafine particles, among which nanomaterials have continuously gained importance, may act as triggers of malignant transformations of various lung tissues (Yu & Xu, 1987; Burge, 1990; Bennett & Zeman, 1998, 2004). In environmental aerosols, the four particle categories may occur in very different amounts: Whilst in urban areas with extensive industry dusts, soot, and ultrafine particles may be most prominent constituents of the ambient air, in rural regions bioaerosols may be of enhanced importance. Particulate composition of aerosols also depends upon the season, with *e.g.*, bioaerosols occurring in higher amounts during spring and summer. Statistics concerning the distribution of particle shapes in the specific aerosols are not available yet, but few electronmicroscopic studies on sampled aerosol particles yield evidence that the ratio of nonspherical particles to spherical particles is greater than 9:1.

Deposition experiments carried out with children of different age and gender could demonstrate that tidal volume positively correlates with age, whereas breathing frequency continuously decreases from younger to older subjects (Gilbert *et al.*, 1972; Tabachnik *et al.*, 1981; Bennett & Zeman, 2004). As a result of this physiological development, deposition fractions among children as well as between children and adults may be characterized by significant differences (Schiller-Scotland *et al.*, 1994; Chua *et al.*, 1994; Bennett & Zeman, 1998). Despite these preliminary results lots of questions regarding the deposition behavior of inhaled particles in children's lungs have to be studied more in detail in order to be brought to a largely accepted solution.

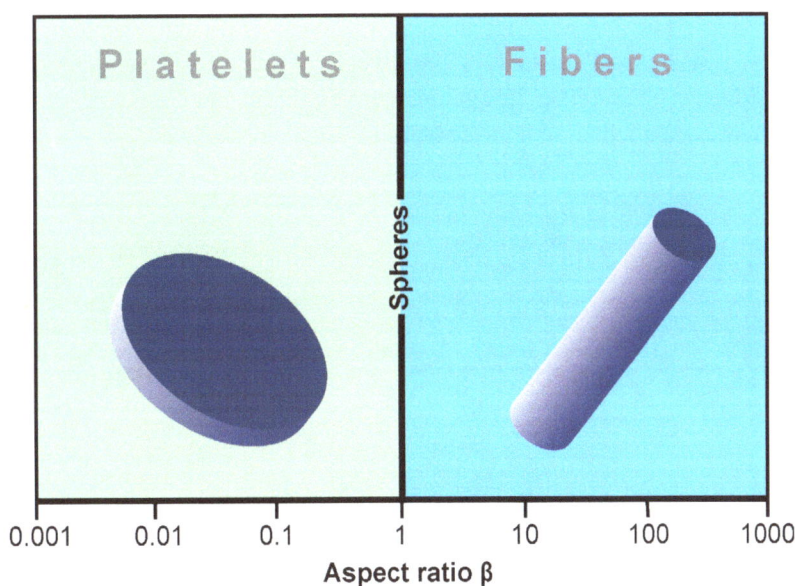

Figure 1: Diagram illustrating particle categorization based on the aspect ratio. Whilst for fibers with cylindrical or rod-like shapes aspect ratio β takes values > 1 (by convention even values > 3), for oblate disks β is characterized by values < 1.

Theoretical approaches to the deposition of nonspherical particles in the human respiratory tract are mainly based on the concept of the aerodynamic diameter which represents the diameter of a unit-density sphere with identical settling velocity as the particle of interest. For μm-sized and sub-micron aerosol particles the effect of shape on particle kinetics is commonly expressed by the dynamic shape factor taking values greater than 1 in the case of non-sphericity (Stöber, 1972; Davies, 1979; Kasper, 1982a, 1982b; DeCarlo *et al.*, 2004; Slowik *et al.*, 2004; Sturm & Hofmann, 2006, 2009; Sturm, 2010a).

In the past, theoretical determination of this factor succeeded in several ways, e. g. by the definition of individual particle mobilities parallel and perpendicular to the airflow (Dai & Yu, 1998) or by the calculation of fractal dimensions (Virtanen *et al.*, 2002). Computer models solely working on the basis of the aerodynamic diameter could demonstrate that for sitting breathing conditions (tidal volume: 750 ml, breathing frequency: 12 min⁻¹) alveolar deposition of fibers with aspect ratios smaller than 10 is similar to that of spheres, but also remains appreciable for longer fibers (Sturm & Hofmann, 2006, 2009). Comparable results for the deposition of oblate disks and agglomerates are not available at the moment. An alternative mathematical approach described the behavior of single nonspherical particles in the flow field of airway bifurcations by the application of numerical concepts such as computational fluid dynamics (CFD). As a main result of these theoretical models particle deposition was represented as a function of the Stokes number (St) which itself is directly proportional to particle size, particle density, and flow velocity. Computer simulations which founded upon CFD and were carried out during the past decades clearly demonstrated that bronchial deposition of fibers among other depends upon their orientation relative to the airflow (Balásházy *et al.*, 1990; Sommerfeld, 1990; Asgharian & Anjilvel, 1995; Shams *et al.*, 2001; Hölzer & Sommerfeld, 2009). Therefore, particles oriented perpendicular to the flow vector are characterized by a significantly increased deposition in the most proximal airway bifurcations due to the additional occurrence of interception as an essential deposition mechanism. Fibers oriented parallel to the flow vector are deposited in the bronchi to a lower extent, but are preferentially transported to distal lung regions, where they may be accumulated in the alveoli. Similar CFD simulations dealing with the transport and deposition of oblate disks or agglomerates in the tracheobronchial tree are missing at the moment, but might represent a remarkable research field in aerosol science.

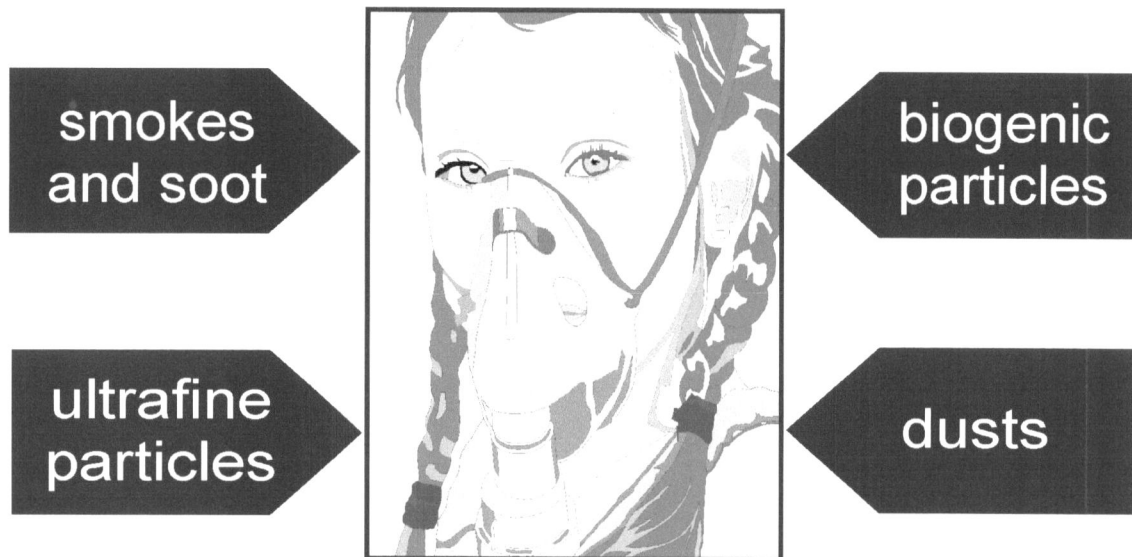

Figure 2: Sketch illustrating those aerosol particle categories which are commonly known to have a hazardous effect on children and adults. Besides the particles acting as triggers for infections and allergic reactions, some of these particulate substances are also discussed to possess carcinogenic properties.

The purpose of this contribution was to extend our knowledge on particle deposition in the lungs of infants (1 year), children (5 years), adolescents (15 years) and adults. Particle shape is approximated by using the aerodynamic diameter concept and dynamic shape factors, which are based upon the aspect ratios of the particles. In order to come to satisfactory results, a theoretical model that has been continuously extended and improved over the past ten years was applied. This mathematical approach is based on stochastic descriptions of lung architecture and particle transport and additionally enables the variation of a high number of morphometric and physiological parameters. Based on the modeling computations it is hypothesized that particle behavior may be indeed categorized according to the age of the studied subjects.

2 Description of the Model

2.1 Mathematical Approach to Lung Morphometry

In general, lung morphometry was modeled by application of the stochastic approach originally introduced by Koblinger and Hofmann (1985). This mathematical model is characterized by extensive statistical evaluations of morphometric data obtained from interferometric measurements of the tracheobronchial tree (Raabe *et al.*, 1976) and the acinar compartment of the human lung (Haefeli-Bleuer & Weibel, 1988). This procedure resulted in the definition of generation-specific probability density functions for the distributions of airway diameters, airway lengths, branching angles, and gravity angles (*i.e.*, the angles of single airway tubes relative to the direction of gravity). For generation of a nearly-realistic lung architecture airway parameters were selected from the related probability density functions with the help of a pseudo-random number generator. During this step of the mathematical process also potential correlations between the morphometric parameters themselves were considered. The procedure resulted in the construction of random airway paths and the junction of a pre-selected number of these paths (*e.g.*, 10,000) to the stochastic lung.

	1 year	5 years	15 years	adult
SF	0.353	0.517	0.780	0.840
T (s)	1.39	2.00	3.24	4.17
BH (s)	0.00	0.00	0.50	1.00
BF (min⁻¹)	43.2	30.0	18.5	14.4
FRC (ml)	244	767	2,650	3,300
TV (ml)	102	213	625	750

Table 1: Scaling and breathing parameters (no physical activity) of the age groups investigated in the present paper (Abbreviations: BF = breathing frequency, BH = breath-hold, FRC = functional residual capacity, SF = scaling factor, T = breath-cycle time, TV = tidal volume).

In the original model, stochastic lung size was normalized to a functional residual capacity (FRC) of 3,300 ml, which represents the mean value for a male Caucasian adult (ICRP, 1994). In order to model lung morphometry of subjects with various ages in an appropriate way, respective dimensions of the tracheobronchial tree were re-calibrated by application of scaling factors. As found by Phalen *et al.* (1985), the dimensions of the trachea and bronchi may be related to body height according to the simple mathematical equation:

$$SF = a \cdot (H_S - 1.76) + 1. \tag{1}$$

In equation (1) the scaling factor, SF, denotes the ratio of airway diameter or length in the subject compared to that in reference man, whilst H_S is the height of the subject in meters and a an airway-generation-specific constant (Phalen *et al.*, 1985; ICRP, 1994). Alternatively, scaling factors for the diameters and lengths of the tracheobronchial airways were calculated according to the expression:

$$SF = \left(\frac{FRC_S}{FRC_R} \right)^{1/3}, \tag{2}$$

where FRC_S denotes the functional residual capacity of the subject of interest and FRC_R represents the functional residual capacity of a reference subject (ICRP, 1994). Respective values for airway calibration derived from equation (2) are summarized together with age-specific physiological parameters necessary for modeling computations in Table 1.

2.2   Modeling Particle Geometry and Deposition

Simulation of nonspherical particle deposition in the lung is based on the concept of aerodynamic diameters (Stöber, 1972; Davies, 1979; Kasper, 1982a, 1982b; Sturm & Hofmann, 2006, 2009). For a particle with arbitrary shape and/or density, the aerodynamic diameter, d_{ae}, is defined by the equation:

$$d_{ae} = d_{ev} \cdot \sqrt{\frac{1}{\chi} \cdot \frac{\rho_p}{\rho_0} \cdot \frac{C_C(d_{ev})}{C_C(d_{ae})}}. \tag{3}$$

In Equation (3), d_{ev} denotes the so-called equivalent volume diameter, whereas χ, ρ_p, ρ_0, $C_c(d_{ev})$ and $C_c(d_{ae})$, respectively, represent the dynamic shape factor, the density (g·cm^{-3}) of the particle, unit density (= 1 g·cm^{-3}), the Cunningham slip correction factor for a particle with diameter d_{ev} as well as the correction factor for a particle with diameter d_{ae}. By definition, the equivalent volume diameter is equal to the diameter of a sphere with exactly the same volume as the particle of interest (Sturm, 2012b). Mathematically, d_{ev} can be defined as follows:

$$d_{ev} = \sqrt[3]{1.5 \cdot d_p \cdot \beta}, \tag{4}$$

where d_p denotes the cylindrical diameter of the nonspherical particle and β the aspect ratio. The dynamic shape factor, χ, of a particle with irregular shape and random orientation within the flow field of a bronchial airway is given by the mathematical equation:

$$\frac{1}{\chi} = \frac{1}{3\chi_{//}} + \frac{2}{3\chi_\perp}, \tag{5}$$

with $\chi_{//}$ denoting the dynamic shape factor of the particle oriented and moving parallel to the flow vector and $\chi_\perp$ denoting the dynamic shape factor for the particle oriented perpendicular to the flow vector

(Kasper, 1982b; Su & Cheng, 2006). Generally, the dynamic shape factor of a fiber (prolate shape) or platelet (oblate shape) may be determined according to the following approximation (Kasper, 1982a):

$$\chi = \frac{\dfrac{a_1}{3} \cdot \left(\beta^2 - 1\right) \cdot \beta^{-\frac{1}{3}}}{\left(\dfrac{2\beta^2 - a_2}{\sqrt{a_3}}\right) \cdot F\left(a_4\right) + a_5} .$$

(6)

In Equation (6), $a_1 - a_5$ represents specific numerical coefficients, whereas F is assumed as a mathematical function, being different for fibers and disks (Table 2). Whilst for fibers the approximation is valid for values of β greater than 1, for platelets β has to be smaller than 1. For $\beta = 1$, particle shape is commonly supposed to be spherical with $\chi = 1$ (Sturm, 2012b; Figure 3). The Cunningham slip correction factor C_c of Equation (3) may be determined according to the equation:

$$C_c = 1 + \frac{\lambda}{d_{ev}} \cdot \left[2.514 + 0.800 \cdot \exp\left(-0.55 \cdot \frac{d_{ev}}{\lambda}\right)\right],$$

(7)

where λ denotes the mean free path of air molecules, which adopts a value of 0.066 μm at standard conditions (20 °C and 1.013 atm). In order to adapt λ to the temperature and pressure conditions in the human respiratory system, it has to be re-calculated with the help of the formula:

$$\lambda = \frac{R_g \cdot T}{\sqrt{2} \cdot \pi \cdot d_{air}^2 \cdot N_A \cdot P} .$$

(8)

In Eq. (8), R_g is the gas constant (8.344 Pa·m^3·mol^{-1}·K^{-1}), d_{air} the mean diameter of the air molecules, N_A the Avogadro number (6.022·10^{23}), T the air temperature and P the related pressure (Sturm, 2012b). While air temperature in the lung takes an average value of 36 °C, pressure in single airway tubes is calculated according to the Hagen-Poiseuille-law:

$$\frac{V}{\Delta t} = \frac{\pi \cdot \Delta P \cdot R^4}{8 \cdot \eta \cdot L} .$$

(9)

In the equation noted above, R and L denote the radius and length of a selected airway, whilst η is the dynamic viscosity of the fluid passing through the tube system. For air it adopts a value of 1.8·10^{-4} Pa·s or 0.18 cP (Centipoise). The factor Δt, corresponding to $t_i - t_{i-1}$, describes the difference of time for a given air volume to pass the airway tube $i - 1$ and the following tube i. ΔP, which can be written as $P_i - P_{i-1}$, describes the air pressure difference between airway tube $i - 1$ and the following tube i.

In the stochastic deposition approach three basic drag forces exerting on a particle are distinguished: inertial impaction, gravitational settling, and Brownian diffusion. Aerodynamic diameters for nonspherical particles introduced in Equation (3) are commonly applied to all empirical deposition formulae. For each airway tube an individual deposition probability is computed which in the case of inertial impaction results from the equation (Ingham, 1975; Yeh & Schum, 1980; Koblinger & Hofmann, 1990; Cohen & Asgharian, 1990; Sturm, 2012b):

$$p_I = 1 - \frac{2}{\pi} \cdot \cos^{-1}\left(\theta \cdot St\right) + \frac{1}{\pi} \cdot \sin\left[2 \cdot \cos^{-1}\left(\theta \cdot St\right)\right].$$

(10)

		fibers		oblate disks	
		$\chi_{/\!/}$	$\chi_\perp$	$\chi_{/\!/}$	$\chi_\perp$
a_1		8	8	4	4
a_2		3	1	3	1
a_3		$\beta^2 - 1$	$\beta^2 - 1$	$1 - \beta^2$	$1 - \beta^2$
a_4		$\beta + (\beta^2 - 1)^{0.5}$	$\beta + (\beta^2 - 1)^{0.5}$	β	β
a_5		β	$-\beta$	β	$-\beta$
F		ln	ln	arccos	arccos

Table 2: Dynamic shape factors of nonspherical particles, using the definition of the coefficients outlined in Eq. (4).

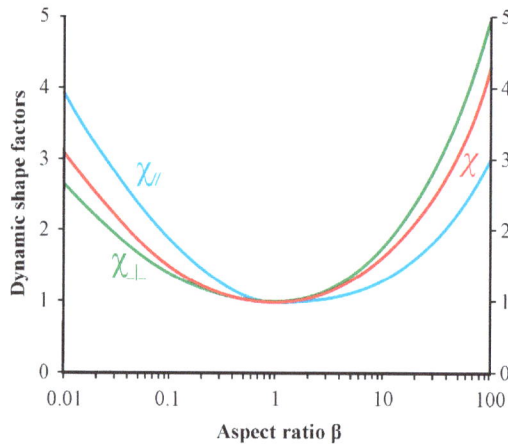

Figure 3: Dynamic shape factors for particles with aspect ratios ranging from 0.01 (thin platelets) to 100 (long fibers). For spherical particles ($\beta = 1$) dynamic shape factors commonly adopt the value 1.

In Equation (10), θ denotes the half branching angle between the two daughter airways in an airway bifurcation and St the Stokes number. The formula is only valid for $St < 1$, while for $St \geq 1$ p_I commonly adopts the value 1. Deposition probability based upon gravitational settling is determined by:

$$p_S = 1 - \exp\left(\frac{4 \cdot g \cdot C_c \cdot \rho_p \cdot d_{ae} \cdot L \cdot \cos\Phi}{18 \cdot \pi \cdot \eta \cdot R \cdot v} \right), \tag{11}$$

where g, d_{ae}, Φ, and v, respectively, represent the gravitational constant (9.81 m·s^{-2}), the aerodynamic diameter of the particle of interest, the angle of a given airway tube axis relative to the direction of gravity, and the flow velocity in the airway tube. Deposition probability based upon Brownian diffusion is determined according to the formula:

$$p_D = 1 - \sum_{i=1}^{3} a_i \cdot \exp(-b_i \cdot x) - a_4 \cdot \exp\left(-b_4 \cdot x^{\frac{2}{3}} \right). \tag{12}$$

In Eq. (12) a_i and b_i are empirical coefficients (Koblinger & Hofmann, 1990), whereas x is defined as follows:

$$x = \frac{L \cdot D}{2 \cdot R^2 \cdot v} \cdot \qquad (13)$$

D denotes the diffusion coefficient of the particle with aerodynamic diameter. It is calculated for the fluid and temperature of interest according to the well known Einstein equation. Assuming a total number of 100,000 particles, whose trajectories are simulated by the model, the amount of particles deposited in the bronchial airway j is obtained according to the following considerations:

$$N_j = \left[100,000 \cdot \prod_{i=1}^{j-1} (1 - p_i) \right] \cdot p_j \cdot \qquad (14)$$

In the formula noted above p_i and p_j include the deposition probabilities for inertial impaction, gravitational settling, and Brownian diffusion which were introduced in Eq. (10)-(14).

3   Modeling Results

3.1   Normalized Particle Mobilities and Calculated Diameters

As already illustrated in the preceding section, the aerodynamic diameter d_{ae} of nonspherical particles is mainly determined by the equivalent volume diameter d_{ev} of those particles. Additionally, the aerodynamic diameter is also affected to a certain extent by the dynamic shape factor χ, which consists of the two components $\chi_{//}$ and $\chi_{\perp}$, but, on the other hand, does not depend on particle size. In order to express dependence of aerodynamic diameter calculations on particle size, normalized mobilities $b_{//}$ and $b_{\perp}$ were computed, thereby using the simple relationship $b = \chi \cdot C_c$ (Figure 4). Normalized particle mobilities of selected oblate disks ($\beta = 0.1$) are commonly marked by an exponential decrease with increasing cylindrical diameter d_p. Whilst particles with $d_p < 0.1$ µm show high mobilities due to high Cunningham correction factors, large particles with $d_p > 1$ µm are characterized by almost negligible values for $b_{//}$ and $b_{\perp}$. For d_p ranging from 0.001 to 0.1 µm $b_{\perp}$ commonly exceeds $b_{//}$ by a factor of 1.1 to 1.2. Selected fibers ($\beta = 10$) show rather similar trends concerning their normalized particle mobilities as oblate disks. The graph of Figure 4 clearly demonstrates that values for $b_{//}$ and $b_{\perp}$ are significantly lower than those for oblate disks.

Figure 5 illustrates computed values for d_{ev} and d_{ae}, whereby unit-density particles ($\rho_p = \rho_0$) were supposed for the calculations. As clearly recognizable from the graph, d_{ev} exceeds d_{ae} for fibrous as well as disk-like particles due to χ taking values >1 within both particle categories. Based on the respective geometry, calculated diameters of oblate disks are commonly lower than related values for d_p, while calculated diameters of fibers show a contrary behavior. These results bear a significant consequence concerning the transport and deposition behavior of nonspherical particles in the human respiratory tract.

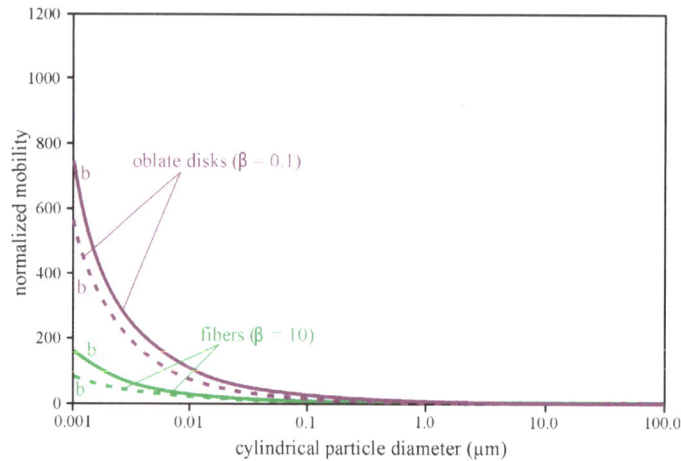

Figure 4: Normalized mobilities $b_{//}$ and $b_{\perp}$ of fibers and oblate disks with aspect ratios β of 10 and 0.1, respectively. Cylindrical particle diameters d_p range from 0.001 μm to 100 μm.

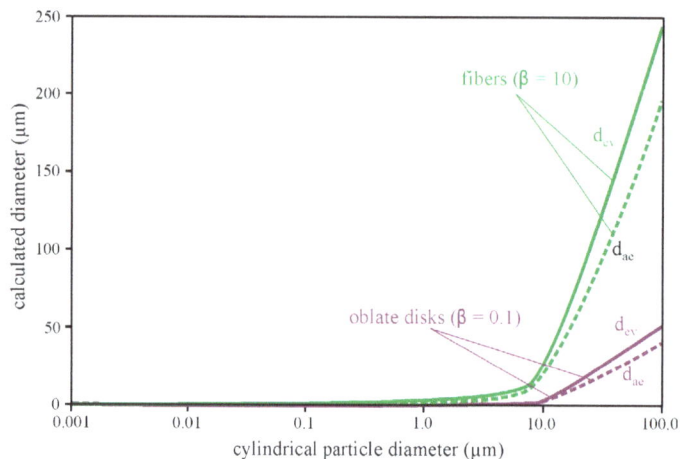

Figure 5: Computed equivalent volume diameters d_{ev} and aerodynamic diameters d_{ae} of fibers and oblate disks with aspect ratios β of 10 and 0.1, respectively. Cylindrical particle diameters d_p range from 0.001 μm to 100 μm.

3.2   Particle Deposition in Lungs of Subjects with Different Age

The graphs of Figure 6 underline the largely accepted paradigm, according to which deposition of particulate matter in the human respiratory tract is dependent on the inhaled particle size expressed by the aerodynamic diameter (see above). Within all subject age groups, total and regional (that is tubular and alveolar) lung deposition present as functions of the aerodynamic diameter: Very small (ultrafine) particles (< 100 nm) and large particles (> 1 μm) are characterized by deposition behaviours that are quite different from those of intermediately sized particles (100 nm–1 μm). With regards to total deposition this observation results in the development of U-shaped or V-shaped functions. Tubular deposition, where inhaled particulate matter is accumulated in all kinds of bronchial structures, differs from total deposition insofar as deposition maxima are slightly displaced towards intermediate aerodynamic diameters (Figure 6). Smallest (1 nm) and largest particles (10 µm) of the scale are again characterized by a more or less dramatic decline of deposition. In the case of 10-µm particles deposition is significantly decreased with respect to 3-µm particles. Alveolar deposition, where particle accumulation takes place in the zone of gas exchange, is marked by a further displacement of deposition maxima intermediate aerodynamic diameters. It commonly amounts to 2 – 20 % of the whole particulate mass inhaled during a breathing cycle (Figure 6). Particles of molecular size as well as largest particles are practically not deposited in the alveolar structures, lowering their significance in the case of microdosimetric considerations.

Whilst total deposition of variably sized particles is rather similar among the subjects' age classes, there may be noticed partly significant differences regarding particle deposition in the tubular and alveolar structures (Figure 6). In general, total deposition positively correlates with age, with respective values for adult lungs exceeding those for infants by a factor of 1.5 – 3 and those of children by a factor of 1.3 – 2.5. Total deposition functions change from broad U-shape in infants to nearly V-shape in adults. Lower values of total deposition in infants' and children's lungs have consequences with regards to regional deposition: whilst tubular accumulation of particulate matter amounts to about 20 % (infants) and 50 % (children) with respect to that in adolescents and adults, alveolar deposition commonly reaches values of 10 % (infants) and 40 % (children) compared to that in adolescents and adults.

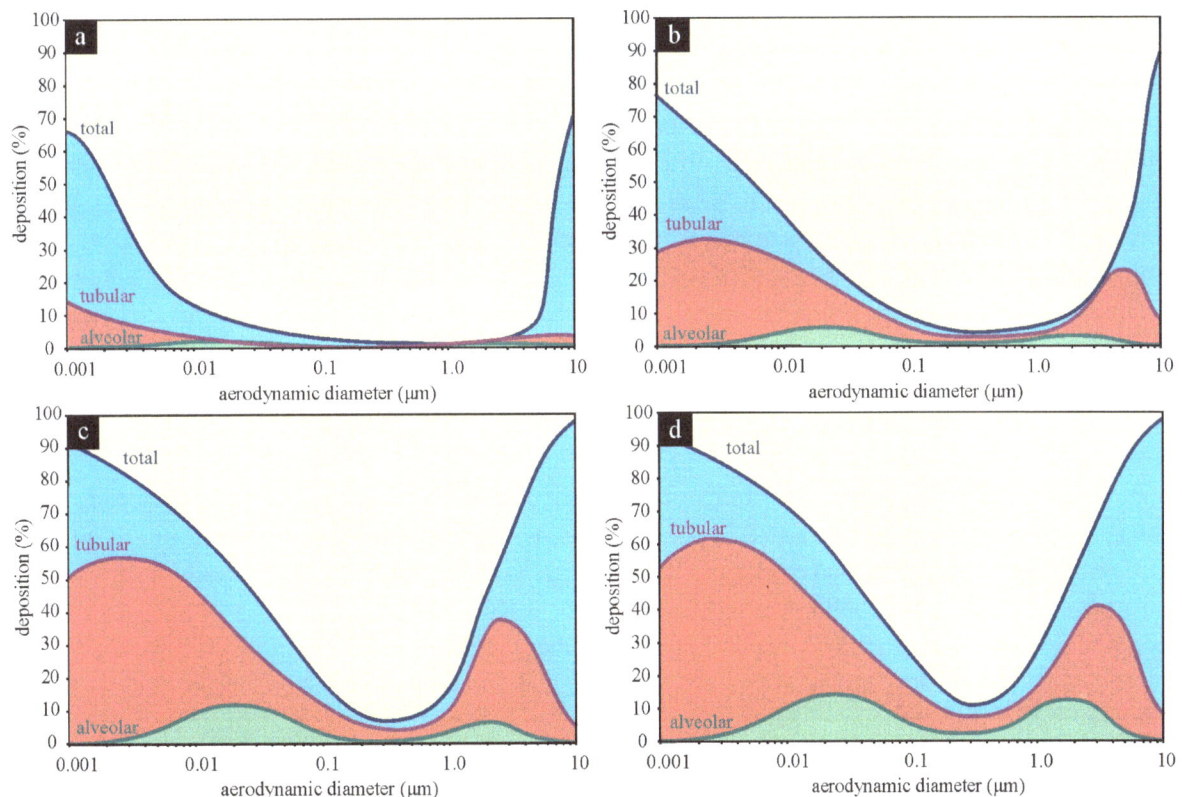

Figure 6: Total, tubular (*i.e.*, bronchial and bronchiolar), and alveolar deposition of particles and their dependence on the aerodynamic particle diameter: a) infants (1 y), b) children (5 y), c) adolescents (15 y), and d) adults. Note: The fraction of exhaled particles is marked in yellow colour.

4   Discussion

Environmental aerosols commonly consist of particles that deviate from spherical shape. Detailed knowledge regarding the deposition of such airborne particulate matter in the human respiratory tract may be regarded as basal knowledge in modern pneumology. However, mathematical approaches to the transport and deposition of nonspherical particles in the lungs are mostly founded upon the aerodynamic diameter concept (Stöber, 1972; Davies, 1979; Kasper, 1982a, 1982b; DeCarlo et al., 2004; Slowik et al., 2004; Sturm & Hofmann, 2006, 2009; Sturm, 2010a) and, in rare cases, upon numerical algorithms (Balásházy et al., 1990; Sommerfeld, 1990; Asgharian & Anjilvel, 1995; Shams et al., 2001; Hölzer & Sommerfeld, 2009). In the meantime, the aerodynamic diameter concept has been subjected to numerous experimental validations, resulting among other in its implementation in the stochastic particle transport and deposition code introduced by Koblinger and Hofmann (1990). The aerodynamic diameter of fibers and oblate disks depends on the so-called dynamic shape factor χ explaining the deviation of the particle shape from spherical geometry (Sturm & Hofmann, 2009). According to widely applied mathematical formulae, χ commonly takes values greater than 1 for both fibrous particles and oblate disks. These data correspond well with experimental and theoretical data provided by the pioneering works of the 1970s and 1980s (Stöber, 1972; Kasper, 1982a, 1982b). As an essential consequence of the calculated χ-values fibrous and disk-shaped particles yielding an identical equivalent volume diameter d_{ev} are marked by different aerodynamic diameters d_{ae} and, hence, by very individual deposition patterns in the human lungs (Figure 6).

The aerodynamic diameter concept may be also extended to particles with highly irregular shape (e.g., diesel soot) and, thus, has been established as mostly applied theoretical approach to particle geometry during the past decades. Despite its numerous advantages, the concept also bears a significant drawback insofar as particles with completely different aspect ratio and, therefore, with highly dissimilar geometry may have the same aerodynamic diameter, resulting in the same deposition behavior. As suggested by Fig. 3, platelets with an aspect ratio of 0.03 have almost identical values of χ, d_{ev}, and d_{ae} as fibers with an aspect ratio of 30. Plotting of deposition ratios against aspect ratios, however, would not account for overall particle size and, therefore, reveals as completely unusable for any interpretations. Percentual distributions of certain particle geometries in the ambient air are not considered at this stage of modeling, because deposition is generally represented as a function of d_{ae}. For the clarification of hygienic or microdosimetric problems, however, considerations concerning particle geometry distributions will have to be made.

Deposition of inhaled particulate matter depends on numerous factors, among which lung morphometry plays a superior role. As already proven by numerous inhalation experiments, the probability of particles being deposited in the respiratory tract increases with the length of the path, upon which these particles are transported (Koblinger & Hofmann, 1990; ICRP, 1994). A counterpart to the airway path length is commonly given by the medium airway caliber (sensu Horsfield et al., 1971) that exhibits a negative correlation with deposition probability. Since both morphometric factors do not fully compensate each other, discrepancies in particle deposition may be already observed between lungs of nearly identical size (note: breathing parameters are assumed to be constant) and principally between lungs of adult males and females belonging to the same age group. Highest relevance of this phenomenon may be observed by the comparison of infants, children, and adolescents, whereby gender-specific differences remain insignificant (ICRP, 1994; Chua et al., 1994; Bennett & Zeman, 1998).

Theoretical results summarized in Figure 6 clearly underline the fact that particle deposition is partly characterized by significant differences among the investigated age groups, with highest deposition fractions being commonly recognizable for adolescents (15 y) and adults and lowest deposition fractions being computed for infants (1 y). A physical reason for this phenomenon may be found in the complex interaction between deposition mechanisms and breathing parameters which both depend on lung morphometry (Gilbert *et al.*, 1972; Tabachnik *et al.*, 1981, ICRP, 1994). Low tidal volumes measured in infants (Table 1) cause a rather shallow breathing with the important consequence that residence times of inhaled particles are set to a minimum. The contrary case may be observed for the lungs of adolescents (high tidal volumes and higher particle residence times). On the other hand, lung architecture of infants increases the efficiency of single deposition forces (Brownian motion, inertial impaction, interception and gravitational settling) which all depend on airway diameter and, slightly less important, airway length (Koblinger & Hofmann, 1990). Brownian motion results in an enhanced deposition of ultrafine particles in the upper bronchi, whilst inertial impaction, interception and gravitational settling mainly affect larger particles (> 1 μm) to be accumulated in the proximal and distal lung. In adolescents and adults the increased efficiency of deposition forces due to lung morphometry is much less significant (Table 1) (Sturm, 2012a).

An important question concerns the filtering efficiency of the human respiratory tract and its dependence upon subject's age. As specifically computed for cylindrical particles with a diameter of 1 μm and aspect ratios ranging from 0.01 to 100 (Figure 7), the capability of filtering inhaled particles out of the air stream in the extrathoracic region is most highly developed in infants and children, where fibrous particles are mostly captured in the oral air passages. As an interesting phenomenon, filtering efficiency of thin platelets, representing *e.g.*, fine dust particles, is much lower than filtering efficiency of long fibers. These results, however, are in good correspondence with other studies (Sturm & Hofmann, 2009; Sturm, 2010b).

It has to be noted, however, that deposition of nonspherical particles was limited to a specific breathing scenario (*i.e.*, sitting breathing *sensu* ICRP (1994)). If breathing is combined with light or heavy physical activity, deposition patterns introduced above become modified in several aspects (Sturm & Hofmann, 2009). Hence, total deposition of most particles is significantly enhanced with increasing flow rate of the inhaled air. Further, ultrafine particles with $d_{ae} < 100$ nm are more frequently transported to distal lung regions and deposited in respiratory bronchioles and alveoli. Large particles with $d_{ae} > 1$ μm, on the other hand, are more preferably deposited in the extrathoracic airways and upper bronchi, where they may cause serious damages of the epithelium and, in the worst case, malignant transformations of certain epithelial cells (Sturm, 2010b).

Another factor, which has to be considered in the case of comprehensive particle deposition modeling, is the subject's gender. Among infants, children, and adolescents, differences between males and females with regards to lung morphometry and breathing behavior have to be evaluated is insignificant. Among adults, however, these discrepancies may reach valuable extents (ICRP, 1994). Under assumption of a mean functional residual capacity of 2,650 ml for Caucasian females, female lung dimensions are reduced by about 10% with respect to male lung dimensions (FRC = 3,300 ml; Table 1). This circumstance has measureable consequences for nonspherical particle deposition. Particle deposition behavior in adult females can be best compared with the deposition behavior of inhaled particulate matter determined for male adolescents (15 years), whose physiological parameters are very similar to those of women. In future models, gender-specific calculations will become more emphasized in order to clarify questions concerning a possible gender specificity of particle clearance or occurrence of certain lung diseases.

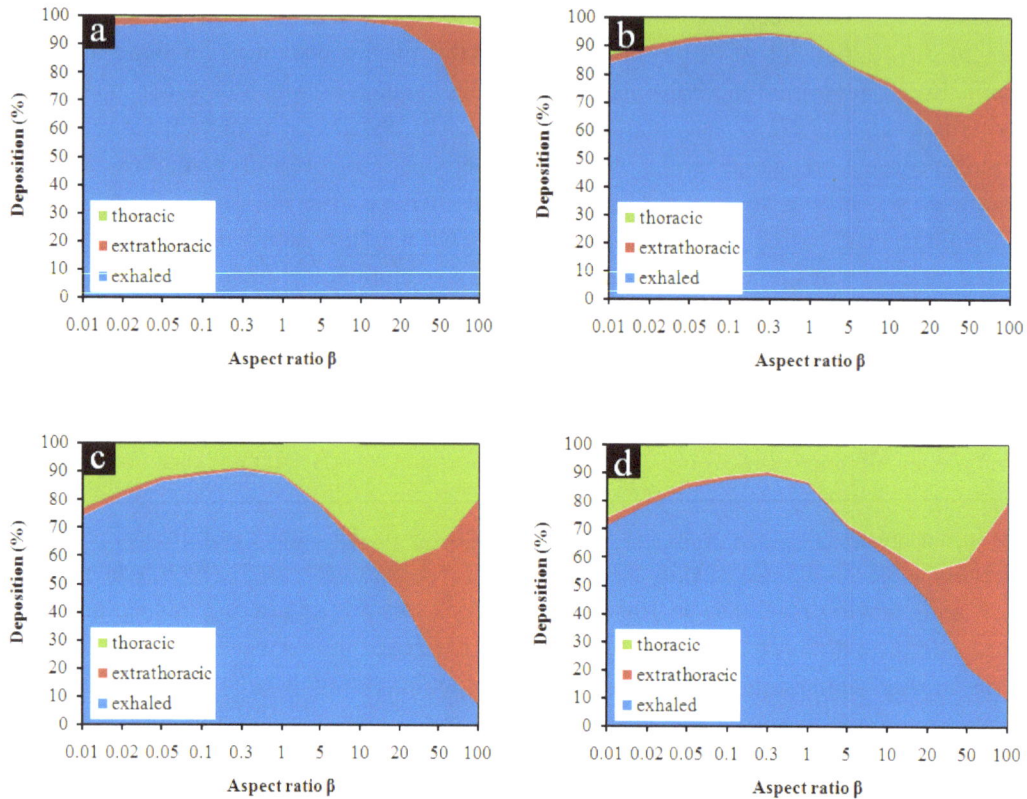

Figure 7: Particle fractions deposited in the extrathoracic region, thoracic region, and exhaled from the respiratory system as functions of the aspect ratio β (cylindrical diameter of the particles: 1 μm). The extrathoracic fraction (*i.e.*, the particle fraction deposited in the extrathoracic airways) may be assumed as an indicator for the filtering efficiency of the human respiratory tract; a) infants (1 y), b) children (5 y), c) adolescents (15 y), and d) adults.

5   Conclusions

According to the results presented here, deposition of hazardous particles has to be regarded as a phenomenon depending on subjects' ages. Nevertheless, it has to be further noted that also within a specific age group great discrepancies in particle deposition, commonly known as intersubject variability, may occur. This circumstance significantly influences the precise investigation of relationships between age and particle behavior in the human respiratory tract (Sturm, 2012a). Therefore, this contribution concerns mean values of deposition and clearance that have been derived from numerous inhalation experiments and related hypothetical computations.

Children develop protective mechanisms against carcinogens transported as aerosols in such a way that most particle sizes are already separated from the inhaled air in both the extrathoracic region and the main bronchi. The penetration of particulate matter into the alveoli is additionally limited by the shallow breathing behavior of infants and children. Nevertheless, the risk of malignant transformations in the extrathoracic and upper bronchial compartments should not be underestimated, especially in regions with enhanced exposure to hazardous aerosols.

Acknowledgement

The author is indebted to W. Hofmann, who has helped to realize most of the theoretical work.

References

Arsenijevic, Z. L., Grbavcic, Z. B., Garic-Grulovic, R. V., & Zdanski, F. K. (1999). Determination of non-spherical particle terminal velocity using particulate expansion data. Powder Technology, 103, 265–273.

Asgharian, B. & Anjilvel, S. (1995). Movement and Deposition of Fibers in an Airway with Steady Viscous Flow. Aerosol Science & Technology, 22, 261–270.

Balásházy, I., Martonen, T. B., & Hofmann, W. (1990). Fiber Deposition in Airway Bifurcations. Journal of Aerosol Medicine, 3, 243–260.

Bayram, H., Ito, K., Issa, R., Ito, M., Sukkar, M., & Chung, K. F. (2006). Regulation of human lung epithelial cell numbers by diesel exhaust particles. European Respiratory Journal, 27, 705–713.

Bennett, W. D. (1988). Human variation in spontaneous breathing deposition fraction: a review. Journal of Aerosol Medicine, 1, 67–80.

Bennett, W. D. & Zeman, K. L. (1998). Deposition of fine particles in children spontaneously breathing at rest. Inhalation Toxicology, 10, 831–842.

Bennett, W. D. & Zeman, K. L. (2004). Effect of body size on breathing pattern and fine-particle deposition in children. Journal of Applied Physiology, 97, 821–826.

Burge, H. (1990). Bioaerosols: prevalence and health effects in the indoor environment. Allergy & Clinical Immunology, 86, 686–701.

Cai, F. S. & Yu, C. P. (1988). Inertial and interceptional deposition of spherical particles and fibers in abifurcating airway. Journal of Aerosol Science, 19, 679–688.

Chen, Y. K. & Yu, C. P. (1991). Sedimentation of fibers from laminar flows in a horizontal circular duct. Aerosol Science & Technology, 14, 343–347.

Chua, H. L., Collis, G. G., Newbury, A. M., Chan, K., Bower, G. D., Sly, P. D., & Le Souef, P. N. (1994). The influence of age on aerosol deposition in children with cystic fibrosis. European Respiratory Journal, 7, 2185–2191.

Cohen, B. S. & Asgharian, B. (1990). Deposition of ultrafine particles in the upper airways. Journal of Aerosol Science, 21, 789–797.

Conceicao, G. M., Miraglia S. G., Kishi, H. S., Saldiva, P. H., & Singer, J. M. (2001). Air pollution and child mortality: a time-series study in Sao Paulo, Brazil. Environmental Health Perspectives, 109, 347–350.

Dai, Y. T. & Yu, C. P. (1998). Alveolar deposition of fibers in rodents and humans. Journal of Aerosol Medicine, 11, 247–258.

Davies, C. N. (1979). Particle-Fluid Interaction. Journal of Aerosol Science, 10, 477–513.

DeCarlo, P. F., Slowik, J. G., Worsnop, D. R., Davidovits, P., & Jimenez, I. L. (2004). Particle Morphology and Density Characterization by Combined Mobility and Aerodynamic Diameter Measurements. Part 1: Theory, Aerosol Science & Technology, 38, 1185–1205.

Gilbert, R., Auchincloss, J. H., Brodsky, J., & Boden, W. (1972). Changes in tidal volume, frequency, and ventilation induced by their measurement. Journal of Applied Physiology, 33, 252–254.

Haefeli-Bleuer, B. & Weibel, E. R. (1988). Morphology of the human pulmonary acinus. Anatomical Records, 220, 401–414.

Heesterberg, T. W. & Hart, G. A. (2001). Synthetic vitreous fibers: A review of toxicology research and its impact on hazard classification. Critical Reviews in Toxicology, 31, 1–53.

Heyder, J., Gebhart, J., Stahlhofen, W., & Stuck, B. (1982). Biological variability of particle deposition in the human respiratory tract during controlled and spontaneous mouth-breathing. Annals of Occupational Hygiene, 26, 137–147.

Heyder, J., Gebhart, J., & Scheuch, G. (1988). Influence of human lung morphology on particle deposition. Journal of Aerosol Medicine, 1, 81–88.

Hölzer, A. & Sommerfeld, M. (2009). Lattice Boltzmann simulations to determine drag, lift and torque acting on non-spherical particles. Computers and Fluids, 38, 572–589.

Horsfield, K., Dart, G., Olson, D. E., Filley, G. F., & Cumming G. (1971). Models of the human bronchial tree. Journal of Applied Physiology, 31, 207–217.

Ingham, D. B. (1975). Diffusion of aerosol from a stream flowing through a cylindrical tube. Journal of Aerosol Science, 6, 125–132.

International Agency for Research on Cancer (IARC) (2002). IARC monographs on the evaluation of carcinogenic risks to humans, Vol 81: Man-made vitreous fibers. Lyon: IARC Press.

International Commission on Radiological Protection (ICRP) (1994). Human respiratory tract model for radiological protection, Publication 66. Oxford: Pergamon Press.

Kamstrup, O., Ellehauge, A., Collier, C. G., & Davis, J. M. G. (2002). Carcinogenicity studies after intraperitoneal injection of two types of stone wool fibres in rats. Annals of Occupational Hygiene, 46, 135–142.

Kasper, G. (1982a). Dynamics and measurement of smokes. I Size characterization of nonspherical particles. Aerosol Science & Technology, 1, 187–199.

Kasper, G. (1982b). Dynamics and measurement of smokes. II The aerodynamic diameter of chain aggregates in the transition regime. Aerosol Science & Technology, 1, 201–215.

Koblinger, L. & Hofmann, W. (1985). Analysis of human lung morphometric data for stochastic aerosol deposition calculations. Physics in Medicine and Biology, 30, 541–556.

Koblinger, L. & Hofmann, W. (1990). Monte Carlo modeling of aerosol deposition in human lungs. Part I: Simulation of particle transport in a stochastic lung structure. Journal of Aerosol Science, 21, 661–674.

Lippmann, M. (1990). Effects of fiber characteristics on lung deposition, retention, and disease. Environmental Health Perspectives, 88, 311–317.

Myojo, T. (1987). Deposition of fibrous aerosol in model bifurcating tubes. Journal of Aerosol Science, 18, 337–347.

Phalen, R. F., Oldham, M. J., Beaucage, C. B., Crocker, T. T., & Mortensen, J. D. (1985). Postnatal enlargement of human tracheobronchial airways and implications for particle deposition. Anatomical Records, 212, 368–380.

Pope, C. A. & Dockery, D. W. (1992). Acute health effects of PM10 pollution on symptomatic and asymptomatic children. American Reviews of Respiratory Disease, 145, 1123–1128.

Raabe, O. G., Yeh, H. C., Schum, G. M., & Phalen, R. F. (1976). Tracheobronchial Geometry: Human, Dog, Rat, Hamster, LF-53. Albuquerque: Lovelace Foundation.

Schiller-Scotland, C. H. F., Hlawa, R., & Gebhart, J. (1994). Total deposition of monodisperse aerosol particles in the respiratory tract of children. Toxicologic Letters, 72, 127–144.

Schüepp, K. G., Straub, D., Möller, A., & Wildhaber, J. H. (2004). Deposition of aerosols in infants and children. Journal of Aerosol Medicine, 17, 153–156.

Shams, M., Ahmadi, G., & Rahimzadeh, H. (2001). Transport and deposition of flexible fibers in turbulent duct flows. Journal of Aerosol Science, 32, 525–547.

Slowik, J. G., Stainken, K., Davidovits, P., Williams, L. R., Jayne, J. T., Kolb, C. E. et al. (2004). *Particle Morphology and Density Characterization by Combined Mobility and Aerodynamic Diameter Measurements. Part 2: Application to Combustion-Generated Soot Aerosols as a Function of Fuel Equivalence Ratio. Aerosol Science & Technology, 38,* 1206–1222.

Sommerfeld, M. (1990). *Particle dispersion in turbulent flow: The effect of particle size distribution. Particle and Particle Systems Characterization, 7,* 209–220.

Stahlhofen, W., Gebhart, J., & Heyder, J. (1981). *Biological variability of regional deposition of aerosol particles in the human respiratory tract. American Industrial Hygiene Association Journal, 42,* 348–352.

Stahlhofen, W., Rudolf, G., & James, A. C. (1989). *Intercomparison of experimental regional aerosol deposition data. Journal of Aerosol Medicine, 2,* 285–308.

Stöber, W. (1972). *Dynamic shape factors of nonspherical aerosol particles. In T. Mercer (ed.), Assessment of airborne particles (pp. 247–289).*

Sturm, R. & Hofmann, W. (2006). *Computer model for the simulation of fiber deposition in the human respiratory tract. Computers in Biology & Medicine, 36,* 1252–1267.

Sturm, R. & Hofmann, W. (2009). *A theoretical approach to the deposition and clearance of fibers with variable size in the human respiratory tract. Journal of Hazardous Materials, 170,* 210–221.

Sturm, R. (2010a). *Theoretical models of dynamic shape factors and lung deposition of small particle aggregates originating from combustion processes. Zeitschrift für medizinische Physik, 20,* 226–234.

Sturm, R. (2010b). *Deposition and cellular interaction of cancer-inducing particles in the human respiratory tract: Theoretical approaches and experimental data. Thoracic Cancer, 1,* 141–152.

Sturm, R. (2012a). *Theoretical models of carcinogenic particle deposition and clearance in children's lungs. Journal of Thoracic Disease, 4,* 368–376.

Sturm, R. (2012b). *A computer model for the simulation of nonspherical particle dynamics in the human respiratory tract. Physics Research International, 2,* Article ID 142756, 11 pages.

Su, W. C & Cheng, Y. J. (2006). *Deposition of fiber in a human airway replica. Journal of Aerosol Science, 37,* 1429–1441, 2006.

Tabachnik, E., Muller, N., Toye, B., & Levison, H. (1981). *Measurement of ventilation in children using the respiratory inductive plethysmograph. Journal of Pediatry, 99,* 895–899.

Vedal, S., Petkau, J., White, R., & Blair, J. (1998). *Acute effects of ambient inhalable particles in asthmatic and nonasthmatic children. American Journal of Respiratory and Critical Care Medicine, 157,* 1034–1043.

Virtanen, A., Ristimäki, J., & Keskinen, J. (2004). *Method for Measuring Effective Density and Fractal Dimension of Aerosol Agglomerates, Aerosol Science & Technology, 38,* 437–446.

Yeh, H. C. & Schum, G. M. (1980). *Models of human lung airways and their application to inhaled particle deposition. Bulletin of Mathematical Biology, 42,* 461–480.

Yu, C. P. & Xu, G. B. (1987). *Predicted deposition of diesel particles in young humans. Journal of Aerosol Science, 18,* 419–429.

Epidemiology of *Streptococcus agalactiae* and Streptococcosis in Tilapia Fish

Carlos Iregui, Paola Barato, Alba Rey, Gersson Vasquez
Veterinary Pathobiology Group, Faculty of Veterinary Medicine
Universidad Nacional de Colombia

Noel Verjan
Veterinary Pathobiology Group, Faculty of Veterinary Medicine
Universidad Nacional de Colombia
Research Group in Immunobiology and Pathogenesis
Universidad del Tolima, Colombia

1   Introduction

Tilapia (*Oreochromis* sp.) are freshwater fish species belonging to the Cichlidae family, native to Africa and Middle East regions (Trewaves, 1983), and the third largest family of bony fish. Illustrations from Egyptian tombs suggest that Nile tilapia (*Oreochromis niloticus*) have been cultivated for over 4,000 years (Balarin & Hatton, 1979). However, it was not until the second half of the twentieth century that tilapia were introduced into many tropical, sub-tropical and temperate regions of the world (Pillay, 1990), and it is currently one of the most cultured fish species contributing to the food fish industry worldwide (FAO, 2004).

The estimated world production of tilapia by the year 2012 was 2.5 million metric tons (MT), that when compared to 28,260 MT in 1970 indicates a significant and steadily increased growth rate. Similarly, the market value of farmed tilapia increased from about 154 million USD in 1984 to 4,000 million USD in 2010 (FAO, 2012). Among the largest tilapia producers are China, with 706,585 MT and accounting for almost 50% of the total global production, followed by Egypt with 167,735 MT, and Philippines with 122,390 MT, whereas Colombia was located in the ninth place with 24,000 MT (FAO, 2004; El-Sayed, 2006), although latest report indicates the tilapia production in Colombia has almost doubled to 44,000 MT by 2012 (CCI - MADR, 2012).

Some of the features that have made tilapia an advantageous fish species for culture are: rapid growth rate, firm and white muscle, the ability to survive in poor water conditions, and high reproductive success with limited requirements during incubation (Nandlal & Pickering, 2004). Last but not least, tilapia belongs to the base of the food chain, which makes them suitable to consume low cost and wide range of food sources with reduced ecological impact (Beveridge & Baird, 1998).

Initially it was thought that tilapia were more resistant to bacterial, parasitic, fungal and viral diseases compared with other farmed fish species (Popma *et al.*, 1999; Klessius *et al.*, 2008; Amal *et al.*, 2011). More recently, it has been shown that tilapia is also susceptible to many bacterial, parasitic, nutritional and fungal diseases. The most common bacterial pathogens of tilapia include *Streptococcus* sp., *Flavobacterium columnare*, *Aeromonas hydrophila* and *Edwardsiella tarda*; and within parasitic infections are found *Ichthyophthirius multifiliis* and *Trichodina* sp., (Iregui *et al.*, 2004; Klessius *et al.*, 2008). Of note, infections by the genus *Streptococcus* sp., are perhaps the most important health problem in farmed tilapia, with serious economic losses that were estimated at 250 million USD in 2008 globally (Klesius *et al.*, 2008). The most significant *Streptococcus* species that cause disease in the tilapia industry worldwide are *S. iniae*, *S. agalactiae, S. dysgalactiae* and *Lactococcus garviae* (Evans *et al.*, 2006; Netto *et al.*, 2011), while in Colombia *Streptococcus agalactiae* is the most important bacterial pathogen of tilapia (Iregui *et al.*, 2004; Jimenez *et al.*, 2007), up to date we do not have any evidence for other Gram-positive cocci causing disease in this fish species. Thus, this chapter only deals with the infection and disease caused by *Streptococcus agalactiae*.

2   *Streptococcus*

The Genus *Streptococcus* contains Gram-positive spherical bacteria less than 2 microns diameters that typically grow in pairs and form chains when grown in liquid media. Most members are facultative anaerobes, meaning that they can grow in absent or limited oxygen conditions; they are catalase negative with varying nutritional requirements, which reflects adaptation as commensals or parasites. Commonly,

Streptococcus is grown in culture media supplemented with red blood cells that may allow a preliminary classification based on the production of hemolysis, which can be classified as β-hemolytic, α-hemolytic (approx. 1% of cases) or non-hemolytic strains (Edwards & Nizet, 2011). In Colombia, the entire *Streptococcus agalactiae* strains isolated from tilapia by the Veterinary Pathobiology Group at the Universidad Nacional de Colombia (VPG, UNC) have been found to be non-hemolytic and belonging to the serotype Ib. The identification scheme followed in our laboratory is based on colony characteristics, hemolytic properties, carbohydrate and protein antigen composition, sugar fermentation and other biochemical reactions. More recently, DNA sequencing of 16 and 23S rRNA genes, in addition to molecular typing at the species level has been carried out using multilocus enzyme electropherotype and multilocus sequence typing (MLST) (Unpublished data).

The majority of pathogenic streptococci have a serologically reactive carbohydrate sheath that is antigenically different from one species or group of species to another. These cell wall associated antigens are designated A-H and K-V, and are the basis of the Lancefield groups.

2.1 *Streptococcus agalactiae* and Streptococcosis

Before going further, it is important to clarify the difference between the terms *infection* and *infectious disease*. *Infection* refers to the presence of a microorganism in a host without disease manifestations, whereas *infectious disease* refers to the expression of clinical signs by the host as a result of the presence and growth of that microorganism within its tissues. Although this explanation seems very simple, it seems to be the cause of most serious mistakes in the livestock practices, daily medical care and research. In this text, Streptococcosis is a word that implies a disease caused by *S. agalactiae* infection.

2.1.1 Disease (Streptococcosis) by *S. agalactiae* in Humans, Bovines and Fish

S. agalactiae is the lone member of the Lancefield group B (GBS) and a pathogen that frequently affects three animal species: humans, cattle and fish, in which it is responsible for several pathologies such as neonatal meningitis and sepsis (early-onset and late-onset disease) that is is the primary outcome in human being, mastitis in cattle and meningoencephalitis, epicarditis and choroiditis in fish (Evans *et al.*, 2002; Mitchell, 2003; Oliveira *et al.*, 2006; Mian *et al.*, 2009). Sporadically, *S. agalactiae* is responsible for disease in many other hosts such as chickens, camels, dogs, horses, cats, bottlenose dolphins, frogs, hamsters, mice, monkeys and otters (Elliot *et al.*, 1990; Yildirim *et al.*, 2002a, b; Hetzel *et al.*, 2003; Johri *et al.*, 2006). *S. agalactiae* is also considered an obligate parasite of the ruminant mammary gland epithelium and tissues; in human *S. agalactiae* is primarily a commensal bacterium of the gastrointestinal and genitourinary tracts (Timoney, 2010), while the status of *S. agalactiae* in fish has not yet been elucidated.

There are substantial differences in biochemical, serological and molecular features among *S. agalactiae* strains isolated from human and bovine species, in which this pathogen has been most studied (Pattison *et al.*, 1955; Finch & Martin, 1984). For many years the relationships between GBS strains of human and bovine have been investigated, and so far there is no solid evidence to prove that cattle serve as a reservoir for GBS strains that cause human disease, which is corroborated by the low transmission of GBS from cattle to humans (Finch & Martin, 1984; Sukhanand *et al.*, 2005). Controversial results about if GBS belonging to the hypervirulent clonal complex 17 isolated from humans, are derived from a common bovine GBS ancestor, have been described based on molecular characterization with 15 housekeeping genes. Bovine CC67 and human CC17 differed in alleles of seven out of eight additional MLST housekeeping genes examined and they are more distantly related than predicted by analysis based on the seven MLST gene loci and do not support the conclusion that the highly virulent human CC17 emerged recently form bovine CC67 (Sorensen et al., 2010; Timoney, 2010).

The initial report of *Streptococcus* sp., in fish was made in rainbow trout (*Onchorynchus mykiss*) cultured in Japan in 1957 (Hoshina *et al.*, 1958). Subsequently, two outbreaks of disease in golden shiner (*Notemigonus crysoleucas*) were documented in USA (Robinson & Meyer, 1966). Plumb *et al.* (1974) isolated *Streptococcus* sp. in more than 50% of eight different fish species dying during an epidemic outbreak in estuarine beaches of Florida, Alabama and the Gulf of Mexico in the U.S. in 1972. In tilapia, the first report of streptococcosis was made by Al-Harbi (1994).

The group B streptococci and particularly *S. agalactiae* cause significant mortality and morbidity in a wide variety of freshwater and saltwater fish species worldwide (Robinson & Meyer, 1966; Plumb *et al.*, 1974; Evans *et al.*, 2002). There are reports of this pathogen in the U.S, Israel, Japan, Kuwait, Thailand, Honduras, Costa Rica, Brazil and Colombia. In addition, this microorganism has been isolated from 17 species of fish including rainbow trout, seabream, tilapia, yellowtail, catfish, croaker, killifish, menhaden, mullet, and silver pomfret (Wilkinson *et al.* 1973; Plumb *et al.* 1974; Rasheed & Plumb, 1984; Berry *et al.*, 1989; Elliot *et al.*, 1990; Eldar *et al.*, 1995; Vandamme *et al.*, 1997; Evans *et al.*, 2002; Duremdez *et al.*, 2004; Suanyuk *et al.*, 2005; Salvador *et al.*, 2005; Evans *et al.*, 2006; Kim *et al.*, 2007; Garcia *et al.*, 2008). *S. agalactiae* is so far the only species of *Streptococcus* isolated in tilapia farms with streptococcosis in Colombia (Jimenez *et al.*, 2007).

Conventional serotyping and molecular typing, including multiplex PCR and multilocus sequence typing (MLST), of various capsular strains isolated from fish, dolphins, human and bovine showed that *S. agalactiae* strains isolated from dolphins and fish in Kuwait, share the same sequence type ST-7 and serological type described for human strains that caused neonatal infection in Japan (Evans *et al.*, 2008; Pereira *et al.*, 2010). Although the ability of this pathogen to cross the species barrier, meaning that *S. agalactiae* of human origin could infect animals, or vice versa, is currently unknown, Pereira *et al.*, (2010) demonstrated that *S. agalactiae* of human and bovine origin can infect fish and that genetic similarity between strains (i.e. a clonal relationship) is not a prerequisite for this phenomenon to occur.

Multilocus sequence typing has allowed the identification of at least four subpopulations of *S. agalactiae* to be present among aquatic isolates; they are the sequence types (ST) ST260, ST261, ST283 and ST491. Both the sequence type ST283, serotype III-4 and its novel single locus variant ST491, were detected in fish from Southeast Asia and shared a 3-set identical genotype to the emerging ST283 clone associated with invasive disease of adult humans in Asia. The ST283 serotype Ia, a subpopulation that is normally associated with human carriage, was found in gray seals, suggesting that human effluents may contribute to microbial pollution of surface waters and exposure of sea mammals to human pathogens. The subpopulations ST260 and ST261 serotype Ib consist of non-hemolytic isolates and belong to fish-associated clonal complexes that have never been reported in humans (Delannoy *et al.*, 2013). Finally, the human pathogen *S. agalactiae* strain ST7, serotype Ia was also detected in fish from Asia (Evans *et al.*, 2008). These findings indicate that some *S. agalactiae* strains may be an anthropozoonotic hazard.

A number of *S. agalactiae* isolates from tilapia farmed in Colombia were subjected to routine microbiological tests, molecular (16S RNA gene sequencing, amplification of surface protein-coding genes and mobile genetic elements) and phylogenetic (PFGE and MLST) analyses. From 25 evaluated isolates (period from 2003 to 2011), it was found that all strains corresponded to non-hemolytic mucoid colonies of *S. agalactiae* serotype Ib, which did not amplify for surface protein-coding genes (*bca*, *rib*, *alp*1 *epsilon*, *alp*2/3, *alp*4, and *bac*) nor to mobile genetic elements for 3 isolates (IS1381, IS861, IS1548, GBSi1, ISSa4, ISSag2, ISSag1). In addition, all 25 strains were ST260 and formed two pulsotypes by PFGE, one of them grouped 24 isolates and the other one slightly differed but has 95% similarity (Barato *et al.*, 2014, submitted). These results indicate that Colombian's *S. agalactiae* isolates have high similarity to strains that affect only fish and had been described in America, Europe and Australia (Delannoy *et al.*, 2013).

3   Pathology and Pathogenesis

The main clinical signs observed in tilapia with streptococcosis by *S. agalactiae* are loss of appetite, unilateral or bilateral exophthalmos, eye hemorrhages, corneal opacity, distended abdomen, curvature of the spinal cord, stiffness, erratic swimming, and bleeding at the base of the fins; some animals may have difficulty to breath, however, other may not show clinical signs before death (Yanong & Francis-Floyd, 2002; Pulido *et al.*, 2004).

Gross findings in tilapia with streptococcosis are the accumulation of bloody fluid in the abdominal cavity (hemorrhagic ascites), mucous content with reddish-brown color in the intestine, pale and sometimes enlarged liver, splenomegaly, deposition of a fibrinoid material on the epicardium, and a hemorrhagic brownish appearance of the retro-bulbar tissue and meninges (Pulido *et al.*, 2004; Zamri-Saad *et al.*, 2010).

Microscopically, most tilapias develop a primary inflammatory response of mononuclear cells with the subsequent formation of granulomatous nodules. Lesions include severe meningoencephalitis that can be hemorrhagic and/or granulomatous in nature with large areas of encephalomalacia (softening of the brain tissue); similar tissue lesions are found in the choroid, sclera and the eyeball. Inflammation may be present at different degrees on the epicardium, whereas other organs are less frequently involved (Pulido *et al.*, 2004).

Recognizing the entry route of a systemic pathogen such as *S. agalactiae* in tilapia, may provide a better understanding of the pathogenesis. In addition, this information is essential to develop novel prevention and control measures against the microorganism. To this end, we setup an experiment where juvenile tilapia (10g-body-weight) were infected with *S. agalactiae* by two different routes: first by dipping the fish in water with a high concentration of the microorganism (8.5 x 10^7 CFU/0.1ml), the fish in this group underwent mucus removal and skin (epidermis) scraping before infection. The second group of fish was subjected to an intragastric inoculation with bacteria (7 x 10^7 CFU/0.1ml) by gavages. The animals in both groups were euthanized periodically beginning at 30 min up to 96 hours post-infection (hpi) and the tissues were collected and processed for indirect immunoperoxidase technique (IIP) to monitor the pathogen under the microscope.

The result of those experiments showed that the main route of entry of *S. agalactiae* in tilapia was the gastrointestinal tract regardless of the route of exposure (oral vs. immersion). Of note, *S. agalactiae* was not consistently found on the skin of fish infected by the immersion route, and after 48hpi it was no more possible to detect *S. agalactiae* in this organ despite the fact that the fish developed systemic infection. Based on these findings, it was concluded that invasion of *S. agalactiae* in tilapia through skin or gills is of low frequency, in addition, in our experience with the natural disease by this microorganism, the skin, subcutaneous tissue and muscles are little affected. Interestingly, infection by both oral and immersion routes caused severe mucus secretion in the gastric and intestinal lumen of tilapia exposed to *S. agalactiae* when compared to non-infected control fish; the mucus secretion indicates that an immediate host defense response against the pathogen was stimulated, wherein the mucus substance forms a biological mesh which may trap large amounts of bacteria (Figure 1). Under the above experimental conditions some bacteria in the oral (0.5h) or immersion (1h) treated fish had reached the gastric and intestinal epithelium despite the abundant mucus secretion. This would indicate that although *S. agalactiae* can be found in large quantities in the water with easy access to the skin, the main route of entry is the gastrointestinal tissue of tilapia. Our findings also suggest that *S. agalactiae* is able to replicate in the lumen of the gastrointestinal tract and perhaps this replication process is a major pathogenic mechanism that may allow permanent colonization of the mucosal epithelium (Comas, 2005; Iregui *et al.*, 2014, Submitted).

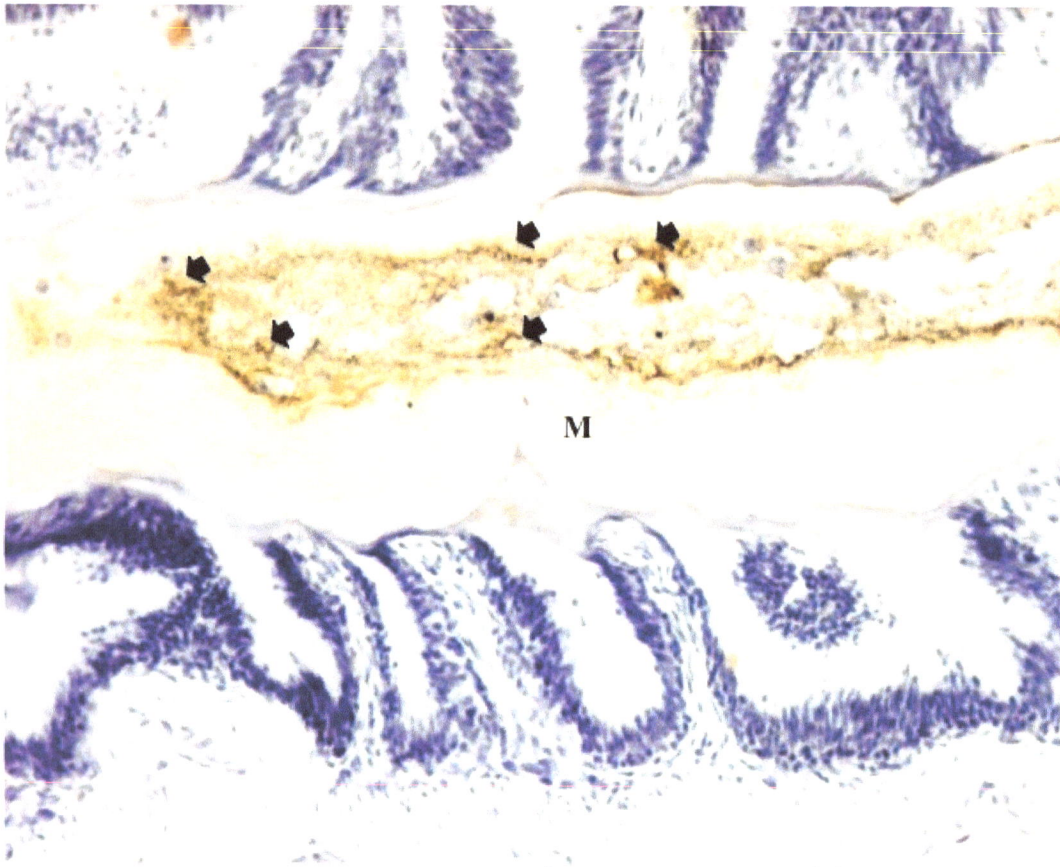

Figure 1: Immunohistochemical detection of *S. agalactiae* in the small intestine of tilapia hybrid experimentally infected by immersion route. Abundant mucus (**M**) and cell debris are present in the intestinal lumen where the mucus substance forms a biological mesh which appears to trap large amounts of bacteria (arrows).

4 Interaction of *S. agalactiae* with Host Tissues and Some Virulence Factors

In human infections by *S. agalactiae*, the amount of group B streptococci transmitted from mother to newborn is considered an important risk factor to infection and disease progression. Infants born from highly infected mothers are more likely to acquire the bacteria on their mucosal surfaces than newborn from mothers with low colony counts at the time of delivery (Ancona *et al.*, 1980; Jones *et al.*, 1984). Subsequently, the first step that any pathogen should meet during interaction with the host is the adhesion to the host cell surface where the entry process takes place, usually at a mucosal surface. In infections by GBS it is suggested that a microbial alpha C protein mediates the adhesion of the microorganism to epithelial cells of the cervix of the woman. In addition, it has been proposed that the bacterial cell wall-associated lipoteichoic acid, given their amphiphilic properties, could mediate low affinity interactions of GBS with host epithelial cells, whereas higher affinity interactions are mediated by hydrophobic surface proteins. Once the pathogen has invaded and traversed the epithelial cell layer, high affinity adhesions are largely mediated by extracellular matrix components such as fibronectin, fibrinogen and laminin; degradation of glycosaminoglycans like sulfated hyaluronan and chrondroitin sulfate by secreted hydrolytic enzymes from the pathogen may favor bacterial replication. The capsular polysaccharide has essential role in avoiding the immune system during invasion to different target tissues. It provides antiphagocytic protection by impairing surface deposition of opsonically active complement C3 on the bacterial surface (Maisey *et al.* 2008). Also, capsular sialic acid plays a role in molecular mimicry of GBS immune avoidance (Carlin *et al*, 2007). Finally, capsule permits resistance to lysis and the beginning of an intracellular stage that facilitates the progression from local to a systemic infection (Baron *et al.*, 2004; Baron *et al.*, 2007).

Growth of GBS in human tissues is attributed to multiple bacterial products that contribute to its virulence, perhaps among the most important are the β-hemolysins that produce lysis of epithelial cells and erythrocytes from different animal species (Weiser & Rubens, 1987). GBS also produces peptidases, enzymes that inactivate the complement component C5a by cleavage of a peptide at the carboxyl terminus (Bohnsack *et al.*, 1991). The hyaluronate lyase which cleaves sulfated hyaluronan and chondroitin sulfate is suggested to promote bacterial spread through host tissues, whereas the CAMP factor lyses host cells (co-hemolysin) and causes direct tissue injury. In bovine GBS isolates, a diverse and large number of proteins that are often encoded on pathogenicity islands, are coordinately expressed with capsule components on the surface of *S. agalactiae* and seem to have important roles in adhesion, invasion, iron binding, metabolism, transport, and inhibition of phagocytosis (Lindahl *et al.*, 2005).

The capsular polysaccharide (CPS) of many GBS is a virulence factor that seems to play a significant role after *S. agalactiae* has traversed the epithelial surfaces and begins its systemic dissemination into the host. Ten serotypes of GBS have been identified based on the CPS (serotypes Ia, Ib, and II-IX), which vary depending on the arrangement of four sugars into a unique repeated unit and are thought to play a key role in virulence (Cieslewicz *et al.*, 2005; Johri *et al.*, 2006). Horizontal transfer of genes coding for capsule biosynthesis accounts for diversity in capsule serotype (Martins *et al.*, 2010; Timoney, 2010), whereas conjugative transfer of large segments of chromosomal DNA among strains of *S. agalactiae* (Brochet *et al.*, 2008) accounts for both strain diversity and the emergence of clonal complexes with combinations of virulence factors and capsular types that are suited to a particular host niche (Timoney, 2010).

The properties of the GBS capsule have been investigated most intensively in members of the serotype III. A critical element in the epitope of this capsular type is the sialic acid, which appears to confer protection to the microorganism against host immune mechanisms. After treatment with sialidase, the CPS is unable to induce protective antibodies against GBS, however, serotype III GBS treated with sialidase are apparently more effectively opsonized by complement components (alternative pathway) and are more rapidly engulfed by human PMN in vitro (Edwards *et al.*, 1982; Shigeoka *et al.*, 1983). GBS possess a highly conserved $\alpha2 \rightarrow 3$ sialic acid terminal on the capsule that is identical to a sugar epitope widely distributed over the surface of all mammalian cells (Angata & Varki, 2002) and it is suggested that the presence of this sialylated capsule on GBS, resembling the host cell surface may prevents host immune recognition. In addition, it has been demonstrated that GBS uses molecular mimicry mechanisms that involve binding of a host cell surface receptor named Siglec 9. This molecule is expressed in human neutrophils and possesses an intracellular immunoreceptor tyrosine-based inhibitory motif (ITIM) which leads to negative signaling cascades that dampen the respiratory burst and bactericidal activities of the phagocytic cells (Edwards *et al.*, 1982; Carlin *et al*, 2007).

Transmission electron microscopy (TEM) has been used to analyze the features of *S. agalactiae* in tissues of tilapia suffering the natural disease (Pulido *et al.*, 2004). Those studies demonstrated the presence of a thick capsule around the bacteria attached to the outer wall (Figure 2), and the ability of the microorganisms to divide within macrophages (Figure 3), suggesting that this layer may provide protection to the pathogen against destructive substances from the host defense cells.

Initially, it was suggested that a thick layer of rigid peptidoglycan external to the cytoplasmic membrane was surrounded by concentric layers of cell wall antigens; it was also thought that carbohydrates (CHO) specific to groups of GBS were also covered by specific types of CPS. However, the evidence now suggests a model in which a B-type CHO and the CPS are independently attached to the cell wall peptidoglycan (Deng *et al.*, 2000). Based on those findings, it would be important to characterize the capsular components of *S. agalactiae* in an attempt to understand deeply their structural organization and composition and particularly their roles in host cell interaction and immune recognition.

By using immunoelectron microscopy, it has been shown an abundant CPS in strains with Lancefield serotype Ia, II and III, while members of serotype Ib possess less dense capsules, furthermore, ultrastructural studies have also shown that the protein C is located on the surface of the bacterium (Kasper & Baker, 1979). TEM has also shown that GBS produce long surface structures like pili, which extend from the bacterial surface to the capsule and beyond (Lauer *et al.*, 2005). These pili are composed of proteins with adhesive properties and are involved in colonization, adhesion and invasion (Maisey *et al.*, 2007). It is also known that these pili are abundantly expressed on the surface of the bacterium and perform functions during paracellular translocation and migration between epithelial cells. Their association with secretion systems apparatus and conjugative transfer systems are responsible for nucleic acid uptake and exchange and those mechanisms need to be explored in *S. agalactiae*.

5   Transmission of *S. agalactiae*

According to Nguyen *et al.*, (2002) the most important factor for introducing *S. iniae* and *S. agalactiae* into the fish farms is the movement of infected fish between farms. Bacteria are usually excreted in the feces of these fish and survive in the water and are infective to other individuals. The use of dead fish as food for other animals and the cannibalistic behavior are believed to be responsible for outbreaks of streptococcosis in Olive flounder (*Paralichthys olivaceus*) in Korea (Kim *et al.*, 2007). Based on their experimental results, the cohabitation of dead fish with healthy fish results in the infection of the healthy ones; it is believed that horizontal transmission of the pathogen is the most common mechanism of bacterial spread.

Several studies from our group on *S. agalactiae* have failed to demonstrate the infection or disease in tilapia fry less than 20 g of body-weight and this finding has allowed us to hypothesize that there would be no vertical transmission of the bacteria, thus strengthening previous observations (Hernández *et al.*, 2009; Jimenez *et al.*, 2011). In addition to the no apparent vertical transmission of this microorganism, it has also been proposed that in tilapia fry below the 20 g body-weight the absence of infection and

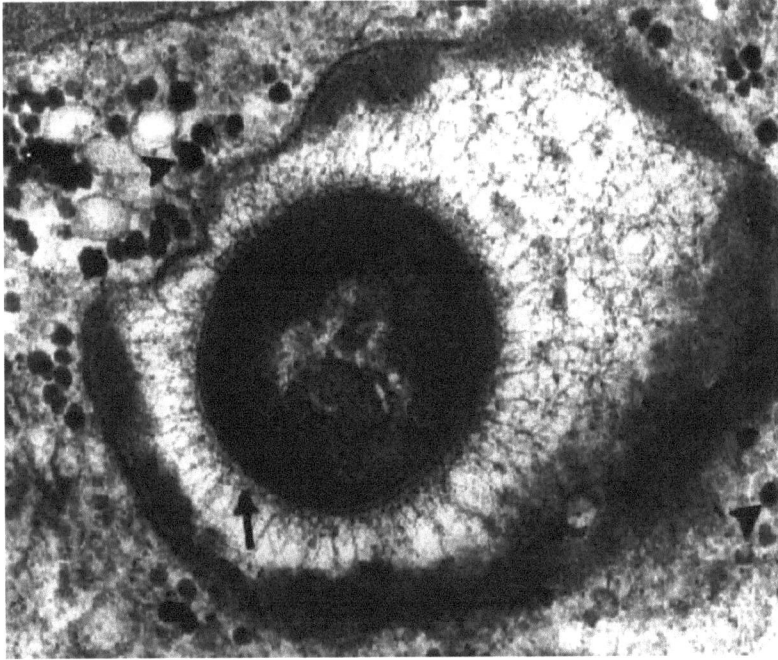

Figure 2: *S agalactiae*-containing phagosome from tilapia infected macrophages. Note the prominent filamentous capsule of a viable bacterium (→). There are also lysosomes close to the phagosome (▶). (Original magnification × 52000) (Used with permission of Revista AquaTic, Pulido et al., 2004).

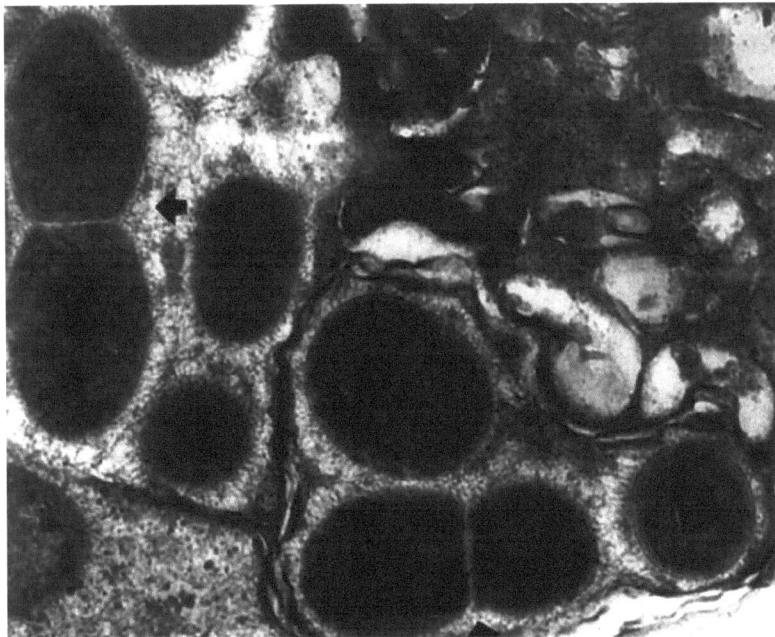

Figure 3: Close view of the phagosome where features of viable *S. agalactaie* are revealed, some of them in the process of cell division (→) (Original magnification × 28500) (Used with permission of Revista AquaTic, Pulido et al., 2004).

disease is due to reasons more relative than absolute in nature, this means that non-transmission of *S. agalactiae* from parents to offspring along with the absence of disease, should be more related to handling conditions of the fish in this age rather than an intrinsic resistance per se, and that infection and disease are more common in older animals due to intensive management practices applied to those individuals (Jimenez *et al.*, 2007; Hernández *et al.*, 2009).

Evans *et al.*, (2002) suggested that there may be *Streptococcus* transmission between farmed and wild animals that coexist in the same aquatic environment; a conclusion that apparently derives from the fact that *S. iniae* has been isolated from wild fish inhabiting the same aquatic environment of farmed fish in Israel (Colorni *et al.*, 2002). Perhaps this is the case of *S. iniae*, not that of *S. agalactiae*; in a study where it was demonstrated the infection and disease by this bacterium in cultivated tilapia, it was not possible to find *S. agalactiae* in white cachama (*Piaractus brachypomus*) that were cohabiting with tilapia and consumed those tilapia dying from the disease; *S. agalactiae* was not isolated in eighteen (18) wild fish species inhabiting the same aquatic environment including two kennels (*Hypostomus plecostomus*. L.), two black tilapia (*Oreochromis mossambicus*), three nicuros (*Pimelodus blochii*, Valenciennes), two bocachicos (*Prochilodus magdalenae*, Steindachner); however, two red tilapia that had escaped from the tilapia cage culture were positive to *S. agalactiae* isolation; in addition, seven individuals of different species of birds that were consuming diseased or dead tilapia, including two black Vulture (*Coragyps atratus*), two chanas (*Syrigma sibilatrix*) and two kingfishers (*Chlorceryle amazona*) were also processed and none of these individuals showed infection or disease by *S. agalactiae*. These findings led us to suggest that the transmission and maintenance of *S. agalactiae* infection in tilapia is only carried out by this fish species and not by any other assessed animal species (Hernández *et al.*, 2009).

5.1   Factors Contributing to the Development of Streptococcosis

As in many other infectious diseases of fish, in the case of streptococcosis, the single presence of the pathogen in the aquatic environment is not enough to induce the disease, and concomitant factors or risk factors that severely affect the physiology of tilapia appear to increase their susceptibility to the agent; within such risk factors the stress may play an important role (Yanong & Francis-Floyd, 2002). Some of the most common stressors related to outbreaks of streptococcosis include high temperatures or strong temperature fluctuations, high salinity and pH above 8, low concentration of dissolved O_2 (DO), poor water quality (with high concentrations of ammonium or nitrite), high stock density of individuals per unit-area of culture and the concomitant effects of routine handling and harvesting of animals (Chang & Plumb, 1996; Bunch and Bajerano, 1997; Bowser *et al.*, 1998; Yanong & Francis-Floyd, 2002; Mian *et al.*, 2009). Temperatures above 31°C are known to predispose to outbreaks *S. agalactiae* in tilapia (Evans *et al.*, 2006; Amal *et al.*, 2008; Mian *et al.*, 2009). Oxygen is the main limiting factor for fish health; it is claimed that the metabolism, growth and disease resistance are depressed when the DO falls below 1 mg/L for extended periods (Popma & Masser, 1999), which predispose tilapia to streptococcosis and other diseases. Furthermore, an increase in water temperature also reduces the rate of DO in the water. Currently, our research group is analyzing the data obtained from an observational study carried out from 2008 to 2010 that involved both cage (pens) and pond (earth) intensively cultivated tilapia. Among the results, a significant association ($p<0.05$) between fish diagnosed with streptococcosis (by H&E technique) and environmental factors such as daily temperature fluctuations (> 1 °C) and stocking density >25 kg/m^2 were found for fish cultivated in cages; while stocking densities higher than 0.5 kg/m^2 were found to be a risk factor to develop streptococcosis in pond-farmed tilapia. Additionally, the study also showed that tilapia with body-weight from 200 to 400 g cultivated in pens and tilapia from 100 to 200 g cultivated in ponds were more susceptible to the disease than fish with body-weight <20 g. Thus, those results also confirm our previous observations (Unpublished data) and suggest that the infection and the diseases might be slightly delayed in fish farmed in pens compared to those farmed in ponds, however, these observations need to be addressed experimentally.

6   Diagnosis

The diagnosis of *S. agalactiae* infection and of streptococcosis require several steps, initially it is recommended a formal visit to the fish farm where it is possible to observe the animals in their environment and to enable that those fish showing clinical signs listed above could be selected; the fish are then sacrificed and an immediate gross examination is performed followed by tissue sampling for bacterial isolation. Samples for histopathology are preferably taken from different specimens given the high lability of fish tissues. The fish tissues are fixed in 3.7% buffered formalin and processed by routine histotechnique (H&E technique). A presumptive diagnosis should be established if both clinical signs and gross findings coincide with those reported for the entity. Organs such as the brain, retro-orbital region, heart, kidney, spleen and liver usually give the best results by bacteriology technique (Sugiyama & Kusuda, 1981; Hernández *et al.*, 2009). The culture media of choice for *Streptococcus* is usually bovine blood tryptose agar, brain heart infusion (BHI) broth; nutrient agar supplemented with rabbit blood and Todd-Hewitt Agar (THA). Our experience indicates that temperature between 28°C to 30°C perform better than 37°C when the microorganism is cultured in BHI broth and THA agar plates (Delannoy *et al.*, 2013).

   To complement the basic H&E technique for diagnosis of *S. agalactiae*, an immunohistochemistry (IHC) assay was developed to detect *S. agalactiae* in fish tissues based on polyclonal antibodies generated in rabbits. The polyclonal antibodies were immunoadsorbed with gastrointestinal tissue of tilapia to eliminate cross-reactivity antibodies that could bind shared antigenic epitopes between the fish tissues and *S. agalactiae* capsule or other structural components such as the sialic acid. The results showed that the S. agalactiae-specific IHC was more sensitive and specific to detect the microorganism in several tissues of tilapia than the microbiology test (Hernández *et al.*, 2009, Iregui *et al.*, 2014, submitted).

   By using a set of primers described previously (Berridge *et al.*, 2001), PCR amplification of 16S-23S intergenic region of rRNA gene of *S. agalactiae*, followed by DNA sequencing allowed us to identify *S. agalactiae* at the species level. Subsequently, the VPG-UNC implemented for the first time the PCR technique in frozen and paraffin embedded tissues of tilapia and were able to detect *S. agalactiae* DNA on the order of fentograms and picograms, respectively, indicating this technique had high specificity and sensitivity (Jimenez *et al.*, 2011). However, it is important to note that a positive PCR result for *S. agalactiae* in fish tissues or a bacteriological isolation may indicate the presence of the microorganism or its DNA and not necessarily that *S. agalactiae* is the cause of disease and mortality, therefore it would be ideal to rely on the hematoxylin-eosin (H&E) technique to ensure that the disease in question truly is due to *S. agalactiae*. It is also important not to forget that this microorganism can be found in the water or even in tissues of apparently healthy tilapia (see infection above).

   The cited studies carried out by the VPG have shown that the H&E technique has a higher sensitivity and specificity to detect *S. agalactiae* than the microbiological culture or even the immunohistochemistry technique that use specific antibodies against *S. agalactiae* (Hernández *et al.*, 2009). The sensitivity of the histological technique to diagnose streptococcosis by *S. agalactiae* increases even more when the source of fish samples are highly infected farms, and the experience on this disease indicates that streptococcosis is the dominant bacterial pathology if not the exclusive one in some tilapia farms in Colombia. Bacteriological isolation provides high specificity, however, isolation is usually difficult and the reasons of why this is so are unknown. On the other hand, histological lesions such as epicarditis, meningoencephalitis and choroiditis, alone or in combination, when the agent is *S. agalactiae*, have high probability (90%) to be present, whereas the involvements of other tissues and organs have low frequency.

In conclusion, visit to the fish farm, histological evaluation of sick fish, and isolation of bacteria from tissues, immunohistochemistry and molecular identification from culture and tissues are the preferred tools to diagnose streptococcosis in farmed tilapia.

7   Prevention and Control

The aquatic environment where fish are grown is considered an important reservoir of microorganisms, however it is currently unclear to what extent *S. agalactiae* could be found in both the water and in the mud of the ponds of tilapia farms. In the case of tilapia farmed in Colombia, it has not been possible to reliably confirm or refute this hypothesis, despite of what is known from other members of the *Streptococcus* genus affecting fish, which are present in the mud and water of fish ponds (Al-Harbi & Uddin, 2005). Thus, preventing infection by those microorganisms is not an easy task and consequently it is always better to purchase specific pathogen free fish and quarantine new individuals entering the farm, in addition to maintain good routine production practices.

Based on our findings and those from other research groups, it is believed that a very important preventive measure is to reduce the stocking density of fish per-unit-area of culture, and although this management practice alone would not be the most effective to eliminate the infection or disease on a farm, it may significantly reduce morbidity and mortality. In addition, avoiding overfeeding, keeping separated the waters to use in various activities of the fish culture, reducing handling and transport of animals to a minimum, frequently removing sick and dead fish, feeding pathogen free rations and implementing excellent sanitary measures, are among the most important strategies to reduce pathogens spread within and between fish farms (Inglis *et al.*, 1993; Klesius *et al.*, 2008). Finally, cleaning and disinfecting the equipment, instruments and all facilities, as well as maintaining good water quality are common sense recommendations. Similar to biosecurity practices commonly used in other animal production systems, efforts must be directed to test the efficacy of "breaking the cycle" as a measure to reduce the spread of pathogens to susceptible fish (Amal *et al.*, 2008). This measure is directed to harvest adult fish of more than 200g before the coming critical period (with high water temperature) and to ensure that only fish of less than 100g are available in cages at critical months. Farmers who still keep fish of 150-300g during critical period are advised to reduce overcrowding by redistributing the fish in cages (Amal & Zamri-Saad, 2011).

To control streptococcosis some antibiotics have been used such as the oxytetracycline, which has been effective in controlling *S. iniae* in blue tilapia (Darwish & Griffin, 2002). Other reports have documented the effectiveness of antibiotics such as the erythromycin, doxycycline, kitasamycin and lincomycin. It should be noted that even in those studies where fish with *Streptococcus* infections appear to recover by antibiotic therapy, the disease cannot be controlled all the way to the slaughter of animals, since the time of antibiotic retirement is higher compared to the time taken by the infection to return. Furthermore, it is a matter of time for *Streptococcus* to develop antibiotic resistance; in fact, some *Streptococcus* strains are known to have developed resistance to some of these substances (Darwish & Hobbs, 2005).

Vaccination is another practice used to prevent streptococcosis and some reports have documented positive results using vaccines especially against *S. iniae* in rainbow trout (Eldar *et al.*, 1997). In that study, a formalin-killed *S. iniae* was used to immunize intraperitoneally rainbow trout and the recorded mortality was only 5% compared to 50% mortality in non-immunized fish in field trials. In experiments with *S. agalactiae*, Evans *et al.* (2004) showed relative percentage survival rates from 25 to 80 % in tilapias of 5-30g that were vaccinated via intraperitoneally (IP) and by immersion routes and subsequently challenged via IP. They suggested that the vaccine could be effective against *S. agalactiae* infection by a single IP injection in 30g tilapia. However, those vaccines although are widely used in the US, are not approved in Colombia. Nevertheless, the problem does not seems to lie in the vaccine but in the vaccination procedure that should be applied to immunize hundreds of thousands of small fish such as tilapia at the age they need to be vaccinated, sometimes with a booster dose. It is not an easy task when fish should be inoculated fish by fish, given that the oral route of immunization has not provided good results. Under these circumstances it seems to be appropriate to develop alternative strategies and tools in an attempt to address the problem of streptococcosis by *S. agalactiae* in tilapia.

8   Future Prospects

Although important developments have been made on fish vaccinology, the development of effective vaccines for fish pathogens is still in its infancy, particularly to control Gram-positive bacteria. This drawback, together with the steady increase in antibiotic resistance, precludes the control of *S. agalactiae* based on those strategies. In summary, we believe that our findings may contribute to the development of more ecologically feasible prevention and control measures to fish streptococcosis. Importantly, the entry route used by *S. agalactiae* into the fish appear to be dominated by the gastrointestinal tissue, thus efforts should be focused to stop the entry of the microorganism at this site before it gets distributed systemically. Further, it seems to be true that pathogens are more vulnerable as they are free and have not made contact with its host than after they have adhered to the host surfaces. Therefore, preventing pathogen adhesion without destroying them seems evolutionarily more strategic than applying biochemical pressure, which only appears to ensure their survival by developing new forms of virulence, as revealed by numerous failures on their control.

Within the mechanisms developed by nature to face pathogen encounter there is the production of abundant sticky substances such as sugars, polysaccharides and multiple forms of glycosidic conjugates that based on their physicochemical properties are able to trap and coat foreign material at any mucosal surface. These glycol-conjugates seem to be useful mechanisms to remove microorganisms, and potentially harmful substances such as microbial toxins. Consistent with this principle, the VPG-UNC is currently investigating the feasibility to prevent and control infection and disease by *S. agalactiae*, through the use of sugars that may inhibit specifically its adhesion to the gastrointestinal epithelium of tilapia.

References

Al-Harbi, A.H. (1994). First isolation of Streptococcus sp. from hybrid tilapia (Oreochromis niloticus x O. aureus) in Saudi Arabia. Aquaculture, 128, 195-201.

Al-Harbi, A.H. & Uddin, N. (2005). Bacterial diversity of tilapia (Oreochromis niloticus) cultured in brackish water in Saudi Arabia. Aquaculture, 250, 566–572.

Amal, A.M.N., Siti-Zahrah, A., Zulkafli, R., Misri, S., Ramley, A. & Zamri-Saad, M. (2008). *The effect of water temperature on the incidence of Streptococcus agalactiae infection in cage-cultured tilapia. International Seminar on Management Strategies on Animal Health and Production Control in Anticipation of Global Warming (pp. 48-51).*

Amal, M.N.A. & Zamri-Saad, M. (2011). *Streptococcosis in Tilapia (Oreochromis niloticus): A Review. Pertanika Journal of Tropical Agricultural Sciences, 34 (2), 195 – 206.*

Ancona, R.J., Ferrieri, P., & Williams, P.P. (1980). *Maternal factors that enhance the acquisition of Group B streptococci by newborn infants, Journal of Medical Microbiology, 13, 273–280.*

Angata, T. & Varki, A. (2002). *Chemical diversity in the sialic acids and related alphaketo acids: an evolutionary perspective, Chemical Reviews, 102, 439–469.*

Balarin, J.D. & Hatton, J.P. (1979). *Tilapia: A guide to their biology and culture in Africa. Stirling, UK.: University of Stirling.*

Barato P., Martins E.R., Melo-Cristino J., Iregui C., Ramirez M. (2014) *Persistence of a single clone of Streptococcus agalactiae causing disease in tilapia (Oreochromis sp) cultured in Colombia over 8 years. Journal of Fish Diseases. Submitted*

Baron, M., Bolduc, G., Goldberg, M., Auperin, T., & Madoff, L. (2004). *Alpha C protein of group B Streptococcus binds host cell surface glycosaminoglycan and enters cells by an actin-dependent mechanism. Journal of biological chemistry, 279, 24714-23.*

Baron, M., Filman, D., Prophete, G., Hogle, J., & Madoff, L. (2007). *Identification of a glycosaminoglycan binding region of the alpha C protein that mediates entry of group B Streptococci into host cells. Journal of biological chemistry, 282, 10526-36.*

Berridge, B.R., Fuller, J.D., de Azavedo, J., Low, D.E., Bercovier, H., & Frelier, F. (2001). *Development of a specific nested oligonucleotide PCR primer for S. iniae 16s-23s ribosomal DNA intergenic spacer. Journal of Clinical Microbiology, 36, 2778-2781.*

Berry, A.M., Yother, J., Briles, D.E., Hansman, D. & Paton, J.C. (1989) *Reduced virulence of a defined pneumolysin-negative mutant of Streptococcus pneumoniae. Infection and Immunity, 57, 2037-2042.*

Beveridge, M.C.M., & Baird, D.J. (1998). *Feeding mechanism and feeding ecology. In Beverigde M.C.M. & McAndrew, B.J. (Eds.), Tilapias: Their biology and exploitation. London: Chapman and Hall.*

Bohnsack, J.F., Mollison, K.W., Buko, A.M., Ashworth, J.C., & Hill, H.R. (1991). *Group B streptococci complement component C5a by enzymic cleavage at the C – terminus, Biochemical Journal, 273, 635-640.*

Bowser, P.R., Wooster, G.A., Getchell, R.G., & Timmons, M.B. (1998). *S. iniae infection of tilapia O. niloticus in a recirculation production facility. Journal of World Aquaculture Society, 29, 335-339.*

Brochet, M., Couvé, E., Glaser, P., Guédon, G., & Payot, S. (2008). *Integrative conjugative elements and related elements are major contributors to the genome diversity of Streptococcus agalactiae. Journal of Bacteriology, 190 (20), 6913.*

Bunch, E.C. & Bajerano, Y. (1997). *The effect of environmental factors on the susceptibility of hybrid tilapia Oreochromis niloticus x Oreochromis aureus to streptococcosis. Israeli Journal of Aquaculture, 49, 56-61.*

Carlin A.F., Lewis A.L., Varki A & Nizet V (2007) *Group B Streptococcal Capsular Sialic Acids Interacts with Siglecs (Immunoglobulin-Like Lectins) on Human Leukocytes. Journal of Bacteriology, 189, 1231-1237.*

Chang, P.H. & Plumb, J.A. (1996). *Histopathology of experimental Streptococcus sp. infection in tilapia, O. niloticus and channel catfish, Ictalarus punctatus. Journal of Fish Diseases, 19, 235-241.*

Cieslewicz, M.J., Chaffin, D., Glusman, G., Kasper, D., Madan, A., Rodrigues, S., Fahey, J., Wessels, J.R., & Rubens, C.E. (2005). *Structural and Genetic Diversity of Group B Streptococcus Capsular Polysaccharides. Infection and Immunity, 73(5), 3096–3103.*

Colorni, A., Diamant, A., Eldar, A., Kvitt, H., & Zlotkin, A. (2002). *S. iniae infections in Red Sea cage cultured and wild fish. Diseases of Aquatic Organisms, 49, 165-170.*

Comas, J. (2005). Replicación de la Estreptococosis en Tilapia roja e implementación de la inmunoperoxidasa como técnica diagnóstica de la enfermedad en Colombia, Tesis de pregrado, Facultad de Medicina Veterinaria, Universidad Nacional de Colombia.

CCI-MADR. Encuesta nacional piscícola 2012. Sistema de información de la oferta agropecuaria, Colombia.

Darwish, A.M. & Griffin, B.R. (2002). Study shows oxytetracycline controls Streptococcus in tilapia. Global Aquaculture Advocate, 5, 34-35.

Darwish, A.M. & Hobbs, M.S. (2005). Laboratory efficacy of amoxicillin for the control of S. iniae infection in blue tilapia. Journal of Aquatic Animal Health, 17, 197-202.

Delannoy, C.M.J., Crumlish, M. Fontaine, M.C., Pollock, J., Foster, G., Dagleish, M.P., Turnbull, J.F., & Zadoks, R.N. (2013). Human Streptococcus agalactiae strains in aquatic mammals and fish. BMC Microbiology, 13, 41.

Deng, L., Kasper, D.L., Krick, T.P., & Wessels, M.R. (2000). Characterization of the linkage between the type III capsular polysaccharide and the bacterial cell wall of group B Streptococcus, Journal of Biological Chemistry 275, 7497–7504.

Duremdez, R., Al-Marzouk, A., Qasem, J.A., Al-Harbi, A., & Gharaball. H. (2004). Isolation of S. agalactiae from cultured silver pomfret, Pampus argenteus, in Kuwait. Journal of Fish Diseases, 27, 307-310.

Edwards, M.S., Kasper, D.L., Jennings, H.J., Baker, C.J., & Nicholson-Weller, A. (1982). Capsular sialic acid prevents activation of the alternative complement pathway by type III, group B streptococci, Journal of Immunology, 128, 1278–1283.

Edwards, M. & Nizet, V. (2011). Group B Streptococcal Infections, chapter 12. In: Infectious Diseases of the Fetus and Newborn. Jack S. Remington et al., editors. 7th ed. Elsevier Inc (pp. 419-46).

Eldar, A., Bejerano, Y., Livoff, A., Horovitz, A., & Bercovier, H. (1995). Experimental streptococcal meningo-encephalitis in cultured fish. Veterinary Microbiology, 43, 33-40.

Eldar, A., Horovitz, A., & Bercovier, H. (1997). Development of a vaccine against S. iniae infection in farmed rainbow trout. Veterinary Immunology and Immunopathology, 56, 175-183.

El-Sayed, A.F.M. (2006). Tilapia culture. Oceanography Department, Faculty of Science, Alexandria University, Egypt. CABI Publishing.

Elliot, J.A., Facklam, R.R., & Ritchter, C.B. (1990). Whole-cell protein patterns of nonhemolytic group B, types 1b, streptococci isolated from humans, mice, cattle, frogs, and fish. Journal of Clinical Microbiology. 28, 628–630.

Evans, J.J., Klesius, P.H., Gilbert, P.M., Shoemaker, C.A., Al-Sarawi, M.A., Landsberg J., Durendez, R., Al-Marzouk, A., & Al-Zenki, S. (2002). Characterization of β-hemolytic group B Streptococcus agalactiae in cultured seabream, Sparus auratus and mullet, Liza klunzingeri, in Kuwait. Journal of Fish Diseases, 25, 505-513.

Evans, J.J., Klesius, P.H., & Shoemaker, C.A. (2004). Efficacy of Streptococcus agalactiae (group B) vaccine in tilapia (Oreochromis niloticus) by intraperitoneal and bath immersion administration. Vaccine, 22, 3769–3773.

Evans, J.J., Pasnik, D.J., Klesius, P.H., & Shoemaker, C.A. (2006). Identification and epidemiology of Streptococcus iniae and Streptococcus agalactiae in tilapia, Oreochromis spp. International Symposium on Tilapia in Aquaculture 7. Charles Town, WV, USA, American Tilapia Association (pp. 25-42).

Evans, J., Bohnsack, J.F., Klesius, P.H., Whiting, A.A., Garcia, J.C., Shoemaker, C.A., & Takahashi, Shinji. (2008). Phylogenetic relationships among Streptococcus agalactiae isolated from piscine, dolphin, bovine and human sources: a dolphin and piscine lineage associated with a fish epidemic in Kuwait is also associated with human neonatal infections in Japan. Journal of Medical Microbiology, 57, 1369 -1376.

FAO (Food and Agriculture Organization of the United Nations). (2004). Fishstat plus. FAO. Rome.

FAO (Food and Agriculture Organization of the United Nations). (2012). Yearbook 2010, Fishery and Aquaculture Statistics. Rome.

Finch, L.A. & Martin, D.R. (1984). Human and bovine group B streptococci: two distinct populations, Journal of Applied Bacteriology, 57, 273–278.

Garcia, J.C., Klesius, P.H., Evans, J.J., & Shoemaker, C.A. (2008). Non infectivity of cattle S. agalactiae in Nile tilapia (O. niloticus) and channel catfish (Ictalurus ounctatus). Aquaculture, 281, 151-154.

Hernández, E., Figueroa, J., & Iregui, C.A. (2009). Streptococcosis on a red tilapia, Oreochromis sp., farm: a case study Journal of Fish Diseases, 32, 247–252.

Hetzel, U., Ko¨nig, A., Yildirim, A.O¨., La¨mmler, C., & Kipar, A. (2003). Septicaemia in emerald monitors (Varanus prasinus Schlegel 1839) caused by Streptococcus agalactiae acquired from mice. Veterinary Microbiology 95, 283–293.

Hoshina, T., Sano, T., & Marimoto, Y. (1958). A Streptococcus pathogenic to fish. Journal of Tokyo University Fisheries, 44, 57-58.

Inglis, V., Robert, R.J., & Bromage, N.R. (1993). Bacterial disease of fish (pp. 196-207).

Iregui C.A. Comas J., Vasquez G., Verjan N. (2014) Experimental early pathogenesis of Streptococcus agalactiae infection in red tilapia (Oreochromis spp.). Journal of Fish Diseases, submitted.

Iregui, C.A., Hernández, E., Jiménez, A.P., Pulido, E.A., Rey, A.L., Comas, J., Peña, L.C., & Rodríguez, M. (2004). Primer Mapa Epidemiológico de las lesiones y enfermedades de los peces en Colombia [First epidemiological map of lesions and diseases of fish in Colombia]. Universidad Nacional de Colombia, MADR, Bogotá DC, Colombia.

Jimenez, A.P., Rey A.L., Penagos, L.G., Ariza, M.F., Figueroa, J., & Iregui, C.A. (2007). Streptococcus agalactiae: Hasta ahora el único Streptococcus patógeno de tilapias cultivadas en Colombia. Revista de Medicina Veterinaria y de Zootecnia, 54, 285-294.

Jimenez, A., Tibatá, V.M., Junca, H., Ariza, F., Verjan, N., & Iregui, C.A. (2011). Evaluating a nested-PCR assay for detecting Streptococcus agalactiae in red tilapia (Oreochromis sp.) tissue. Aquaculture, 321, 203–206.

Johri, A.K., Paoletti, L.C., Glaser, P., Dua, M., Sharma, P.K., Grandi, G., & Rappuolli, R. (2006). Group B Streptococcus: global incidence and vaccine development. Nature Reviews of Microbiology, 4, 932–942.

Jones, D., Kanarek, K., & Lim, D. (1984). Group B Streptococcal colonization patterns in mothers and their infants. Journal of clinical microbiology, 20, 438-440.

Kasper, D.L. & Baker, C.J. (1979). Electron microscopic definition of surface antigens of group B Streptococcus. Journal of Infection Diseases, 139, 147–151.

Kim, J.H., Gomez, D.K., Choresca, C.H., & Park, S.C. (2007). Detection of major bacterial and viral pathogens in trash fish used to feed cultured flounder in Korea. Aquaculture, 272, 105-110.

Klesius, P.H., Shoemaker, C.A., & Evans, J.J. (2008). Streptococcus: A worldwide fish health problem. 8th International Symposium on Tilapia in Aquaculture. Cairo, 83-107.

Lindahl, G., Stålhammar-Carlemalm, M., & Areschoug, T. (2005). Surface proteins of Streptococcus agalactiae and related proteins in other bacterial pathogens. Clinical Microbiology Rev., 18, 102-127.

Lauer, P., Rinaudo, C.D., Soriani, M., Margarit, I., Maione, D., Rosini, R., Taddei, A.R., Mora, M., Rappuoli, R., Grandi, G., & Telford, J.L. (2005). Genome analysis reveals pili in group B Streptococcus. Science, 309, 105.

Maisey, H.C., Hensler, M., Nizet, V., & Doran, K.S. (2007). Group B streptococcal pilus proteins contribute to adherence to and invasion of brain microvascular endothelial cells. Journal of Bacteriology, 189, 1464–1467.

Maisey H.C., Doran K.S. & Nizet V. (2008) Recent advances in understanding the molecular basis of group B Streptococcus virulence. Expert Reviews in Molecular Medicine, 10, e27.

Martins, E.R., Melo-Cristino, J., & Ramirez, M. (2010). Evidence for Rare Capsular Switching in Streptococcus agalactiae. Journal of Bacteriology, 192(5), 1361–1369.

Mian, G.F., Godoy, D.T., Leal, C.A.G., Yuhara, T.Y., Costa, G.M., & Figueiredo, H.C.P. (2009). Aspects of the natural history and virulence of S. agalactiae infection in Nile tilapia. Veterinary Microbiology, 136, 180–183.

Mitchell, T.J. (2003). The pathogenesis of streptococcal infections: from tooth decay to meningitis. Nature Reviews of Microbiology, 1, 219–230.

Nandlal, S. & Pickering, T. (2004). Tilapia fish farming in Pacific Island countries. Vol 1. Tilapia Hatchery Operation. Noumea, New Caledonia: Secretariat of the Pacific Community.

Netto, L.N., Leal, C.A., & Figueiredo, H.C. (2011). Streptococcus dysgalactiae as an agent of septicaemia in Nile tilapia, Oreochromis niloticus (L.), Journal of Fish Diseases, 34(3), 251-254.

Nguyen, H.T., Kanai, K., & Yoshikoshi, K. (2002). Ecological investigation of S. iniae isolated in cultured Japanese Flouder, Paralicthys olivaceus using selective isolation procedure. Aquaculture, 205, 7-17.

Oliveira, I.C.M., Mattos, M.C. de, Areal, M.F.T., Ferreira-Carvalho, B.T., Figueiredo, A.M.S., & Benchetrit, L.C. (2005). Pulsed-field gel electrophoresis of human group B streptococci isolated in Brazil. Journal Chemotherapy, 17, 258–263.

Pattison, I.H., Matthews, P.R.J., & Maxted, W.R. (1955). Type classification by Lancefields precipitin method of human and bovine group B streptococci isolated in Britain. Journal of Pathology and Bacteriology, 69, 43-50.

Pereira, U.P., Mian, G.F., Oliveira, I.C.M., Benchetrit, L.C., Costa, G.M., & Figueiredo H.C.P. (2010). Genotyping of Streptococcus agalactiae strains isolated from fish, human and cattle and their virulence potential in Nile tilapia. Veterinary Microbiology, 140, 186-192.

Pillay, T.V.R. (1990). Aquaculture principles and practices. Fishing News Books, Blackwell Science, Oxford, UK.

Plumb, J.A., Schachte, J.H., Gaines, J.L., Peltier, W., & Carrol, B. (1974). Streptococcus sp. from marine fishes along the Alabama and northwest Florida coast of the Gulf of Mexico. Transactions of the American Fisheries Society, 103, 358-361.

Popma, T. & Masser, M. (1999). Tilapia life story and biology. Southern Regional Aquaculture Center Publication No. 283.

Pulido, E.A., Iregui, C.A., Figueroa, J., & Klesius, P. (2004). Estreptococosis en tilapias (Oreochromis spp.) cultivadas en Colombia. Revista AquaTic, 20, 97-106.

Rasheed, V. & Plumb, J.A. (1984). Pathogenicity of non-hemolytic group B Streptococcus sp. in gulf killfish, Fundulus grandis. Aquaculture, 37, 97-105.

Robinson, J.A. & Meyer, F.P. (1966). Streptococcal fish pathogen. Journal of Bacteriology, 92, 512.

Salvador, R., Muller, E.E., Freitas, J.C., Leonhadt, J.H., Giordano, L.G.P., & Dias, J.A. (2005). Isolation and characterization of Streptococcus spp. group B in Nile Tilapia (Oreochromis niloticus) reared in hapas nets and earth nurseries in the northern region of Parana State, Brazil. Ciencia Rural. Santa Maria, 35, 1374-1378.

Sharon, N. (2006). Carbohydrates as future anti-adhesion drugs for infectious diseases. Biochimie, 1760(4), 527-37.

Shigeoka, A.O., Rote, N.S., Santos, J.I., & Hill, H.R. (1983). Assessment of the virulence factors of group B streptococci: correlation with sialic acid content, Journal of Infection Diseases, 147, 857–863.

Sorensen U.B, Poulsen K, Ghezoo C., Margarit I & Kilian M. (2010) Emergence and global dissemination of host-specific Streptococcus agalactiae clones. MBio, 1, e00178-10.

Suanyuk, N., Kanghear, H., Khongpradit, R., & Supamattaya, K. (2005). S. agalactiae infection in tilapia (O. niloticus) Songklanakarin. Journal of Science and Technology in Aquaculture Science, 27, 307-319.

Sugiyama, A. & Kusuda, R. (1981). Studies on the characters of Staphylococcus epidermidis isolated from diseased fishes. Fish Pathology, 16, 35-41.

Sukhanand, S., Dogam, B., Ayodele, M.O., Zadoks, R.N., Graver, M.P.J., Dumas, N.B., Schukken, Y.H., Boor, K.J., & Wiedmann, M. (2005). Molecular subtyping and characterization of bovine and human Streptococcus agalactiae isolates. Journal of Clinical Microbiology, 43, 1177–1186.

Timoney, J.F. (2010). Streptococcus. In: Gyles, C.L., Prescott, J.F., Songer, J.G., Thoen, C.O. Pathogenesis of Bacterial Infections in Animals, 4th Edition. Blackwell Publishing. (pp. 51-74)

Trewaves, E. (1983). Tilapia fishes of the Genera Sarotherodon, Oreochromis. Danakilia. British Museum (Natural History).

Vandamme, L., Devriese, L.A., Kersters, P.K., & Melin, P. (1997). S. difficile is a non-hemolytic group B, type Ib Streptococcus. International Journal of Systemic Bacteriology, 47, 81-85.

Weiser, J.N., & Rubens, C.E. (1987). Transposon mutagenesis of group B streptococcus beta-hemolysin biosynthesis. Infection and Immunity, 55, 2314-2316.

Wilkinson, H.W., Thacker, L.G., & Facklam, R.R. (1973). Nonhemolytic group B streptococci of human, bovine, and ichthyic origin. Infection and Immunity, 7, 496-498.

Yanong, R.P.E. & Francis-Floyd, R. (2002). Streptococcal infections of fish. Report from University of Florida. Series from the Department of Fisheries and Aquatic Sciences, Florida Cooperative Extension Service, Institute of Food and Agricultural Sciences, University of Florida.

Yildirim, A.O, La¨mmler, C., & Weiß, R. (2002a). Identification and characterization of Streptococcus agalactiae isolated from horses. Veterinary Microbiology, 85, 31–35.

Yildirim, A.O, La¨mmler, C., Weiß, R., & Kopp, P. (2002b). Pheno and genotypic properties of streptococci of serological group B of canine and feline origin. FEMS Microbiology, 212, 187–192.

Zamri-Saad. M., Amal, M.N., & Siti-Zahrah, A. (2010). Pathological changes in red tilapias (Oreochromis spp.) naturally infected by Streptococcus agalactiae. Journal of Comparative Pathology, 143(2-3), 227-229.

www.ingramcontent.com/pod-product-compliance
Lightning Source LLC
Chambersburg PA
CBHW050819220326

41598CB00006B/257